Congenital and Other Related Infectious Diseases of the Newborn

PERSPECTIVES IN MEDICAL VIROLOGY

Volume 13

Series Editors

A.J. Zuckerman

Royal Free and University College Medical School
University College London
London, UK

Isa K. Mushahwar

Abbott Laboratories (Retired)
Congenital Infectious Diseases
Abbott Park, IL 60064, USA

Congenital and Other Related Infectious Diseases of the Newborn

Editor

Isa K. Mushahwar

Abbott Laboratories (Retired)
Congenital Infectious Diseases
Abbott Park, IL 60064, USA

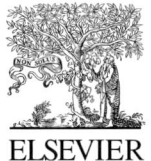

ELSEVIER

Amsterdam – Boston – Heidelberg – London – New York – Oxford – Paris
San Diego – San Francisco – Singapore – Sydney – Tokyo

Elsevier
Radarweg 29, PO Box 211, 1000 AE Amsterdam, The Netherlands
The Boulevard, Langford Lane, Kidlington, Oxford OX5 1GB, UK

First edition 2007

Notice
No responsibility is assumed by the publisher for any injury and/or damage to persons
or property as a matter of products liability, negligence or otherwise, or from any use
or operation of any methods, products, instructions or ideas contained in the material
herein. Because of rapid advances in the medical sciences, in particular, independent
verification of diagnoses and drug dosages should be made

Library of Congress Cataloguing-in-Publication Data
A catalog record for this book is available from the Library of Congress

British Library Cataloguing in Publication Data
A catalogue record for this book is available from the British Library

ISBN-13: 978-0-444-52073-9
ISBN-10: 0-444-52073-2
ISSN: 0168-7069

For information on all Elsevier publications
visit our website at books.elsevier.com

Printed and bound in The Netherlands

07 08 09 10 11 10 9 8 7 6 5 4 3 2 1

Working together to grow
libraries in developing countries

www.elsevier.com | www.bookaid.org | www.sabre.org

ELSEVIER   BOOK AID
            International   Sabre Foundation

I dedicate this book to my wife, Mary, my sons, Stephen and Mark, and my grandchildren, Stephen Isa II and Michael Taylor, whose patience and support sustain me through all my endeavors.

Contents

List of Contributors

Asad Ansari
School of Medicine
University of South Dakota
Sioux Falls, SD, USA

James F. Bale Jr.
Division of Pediatric Neurology
Departments of Pediatrics and Neurology
The University of Utah School of Medicine
    and Primary Children's Medical Center
Salt Lake City, UT, USA

Javier Bartolomé
Fundación para el Estudio de las Hepatitis Virales
Madrid, Spain

Vicente Carreño
Fundación para el Estudio de las Hepatitis Virales
Madrid, Spain

Inmaculada Castillo
Fundación para el Estudio de las Hepatitis Virales
Madrid, Spain

Amanda Corcoran
Biotrin International, The Rise
Mount Merrion Co. Dublin
Ireland

Sean Doyle
  National Institute for Cellular Biotechnology
  Department of Biology
  National University of Ireland Maynooth
  Maynooth, Co. Kildare, Ireland

Tomiko Koyama
  Health Service Association
  Iwate, Japan

Maria Paola Landini
  Department of Clinical and Experimental Medicine
  Clinical Unit of Microbiology and Virology
  St. Orsola Malpighi General Hospital
  University of Bologna, Bologna, Italy

Tiziana Lazzarotto
  Department of Clinical and Experimental Medicine
  Clinical Unit of Microbiology and Virology
  St. Orsola Malpighi General Hospital
  University of Bologna, Bologna, Italy

Lonnie Miner
  Department of Neonatal Medicine
  Dixie Regional Medical Center
  St. George, UT, USA

Hidetoshi Mito
  Health Service Association
  Shizuoka, Japan

Isa K. Mushahwar
  Abbott Laboratories (Retired)
  Congenital Infectious Diseases
  Abbott Park, IL 60064, USA

Andreas Sauerbrei
Institute of Virology and Antiviral Therapy
Friedrich-Schiller University
Jena, Germany

Gabriella Scarlatti
Unit of Viral Evolution and Transmission
DIBIT, Fondazione San Raffaele del Monte Tabor
Via Olgettina 58, 20132 Milano, Italy

Alejandro Gabriel Schijman
Laboratorio de Biología Molecular de la Enfermedad de Chagas
(LABMECH), Instituto de Investigaciones en Ingeniería
Genética y Biología Molecular (INGEBI)
Consejo Nacional de Ciencia y Tecnología (CONICET)
Vuelta de Obligado 2490, Buenos Aires, 1428, Argentina

Augusto E. Semprini
Department of Obstetrics and Gynaecology
University of Milan, Hospital L. Sacco
Via G.B. Grassi, 20157 Milan, Italy

Kazuaki Takahashi
Department of Medical Sciences
Toshiba General Hospital
Tokyo, Japan

Junko Tanaka
Department of Epidemiology
Infectious Disease Control and Prevention
Graduate School of Biomedical Sciences
Hiroshima University, Hiroshima, Japan

Elisabetta Tanzi
Department of Public Health-Microbiology-Virology
University of Milan, Via Pascal 36/38
20133 Milan, Italy

Adriana Weinberg
University of Colorado Health Sciences Center
Denver, CO, USA

Hiroshi Yoshizawa
Department of Epidemiology
Infectious Disease Control and Prevention
Graduate School of Biomedical Sciences
Hiroshima University, Hiroshima, Japan

Alessandro R. Zanetti
Department of Public
Health-Microbiology-Virology
University of Milan, Via Pascal 36/38
20133 Milan, Italy

Preface

Despite the introduction of efficacious vaccines against rubella, Varicella-zoster and hepatitis B viruses; the use of effective drugs for the treatment of herpes, toxoplasma and Chagas diseases; and the development of highly sensitive, specific and reproducible immunoassays and nucleic acid tests for the diagnosis of a variety of bacterial, viral and parasitic diseases, congenital infections continue to pose a substantial threat throughout the world. Congenital and other related diseases of the newborn remain important causes of malformation and death among infants worldwide. The incidence of intrauterine infections during pregnancy has been estimated to be about 14% when highly sensitive diagnostic procedures are used. Perinatal infections account for 2–3% of all congenital anomalies in western countries. A variety of etiologic agents are responsible for congenital infections. These agents can cause remarkably similar manifestations such as a rash, deafness, vision loss, growth retardation, stillbirth, ventriculitis, hepatomegaly, hepatitis, myocarditis and many other ailments involving the kidneys, liver and the digestive system.

Many congenital diseases are caused by bacterial, parasitic and viral agents. This book is directed mostly toward the molecular composition, pathogenesis, diagnosis, treatment and control of congenital and other related diseases of the newborn that are caused by a variety of viruses. These viruses comprise several families that include Herpesviridae (HSV-1, HSV-2, HSV-6, HSV-7, CMV and Varicella-zoster); Parvoviridae (parvovirus B19); Lentiviridae (HIV); Hepadnaviridae (HBV); Flaviviridae (HCV) and Togaviridae (RV). In addition, Chagas, a parasitic disease has been included in a series dedicated mainly to discussions on human viral disease. This was done intentionally because I do realize that a detailed volume on human congenital diseases will be incomplete without including this chapter, and because unlike toxoplasmosis, Chagas disease is neither fully understood nor frequently encountered by pediatricians outside South and Central America.

In this book, leading researchers in childhood diseases and virology from Brazil, Germany, Ireland, Italy, Japan, Spain and the United States of America report on the up-to-date advances in the molecular virology, immunology, biochemistry, pathology, diagnosis, prevalence and treatment of selected congenital and other related diseases of the newborn. It is hoped that the contents of this book will encourage new and innovative approaches to future congenital disease research and a better understanding of these diseases.

I have greatly enjoyed my interaction with the various authors whose love of medical sciences and commitment have led to the production of this book. Special thanks are due to Lisa Tickner, Joanna De Souza and Clare Rathbone of Elsevier for their excellent assistance, dedication and support, and also to Dr. Gregory Maine for introducing me to Dr. Tiziana Lazzarotto. Special thanks to Dr. Dominick Pucci for his encouragement and support.

Isa K. Mushahwar
Abbott Laboratories, Abbot Park, IL, USA

Congenital and Other Related Infectious
Diseases of the Newborn
Isa K. Mushahwar (Editor)
© 2007 Elsevier B.V. All rights reserved
DOI 10.1016/S0168-7069(06)13001-3

Diagnosis of Maternal and Congenital Cytomegalovirus Infection

Tiziana Lazzarotto, Maria Paola Landini

Department of Clinical and Experimental Medicine, Clinical Unit of Microbiology and Virology, St. Orsola Malpighi General Hospital, University of Bologna, Bologna, Italy

Introduction

Human cytomegalovirus (CMV) is one of the eight viruses belonging to the *Herpesviridae* family to infect humans. CMV belongs to the *Betaherpesvirinae* subfamily of viruses characterized by a restricted host spectrum, *in vitro* replication in fibroblasts of the natural host species *in vivo*, a slow replication cycle, the induction of intranuclear and intracytoplasmic inclusions and the ability to induce latency mainly in the myeloid cell linage.

Although rarely pathogenic in immunocompetent individuals, the virus poses a significant health threat to immunocompromised individuals. CMV is an important post-transplant pathogen as between 50% and 100% allograft recipients (depending on serological status of donor/recipient and type of immunosuppression) develop CMV infection.

Congenital CMV infection is the leading cause of congenital virus infection in developed countries, occurring in 0.3–2.4% (mean value 1%) of all live births depending on the seroprevalence of the population examined.

Intrauterine primary infections are second only to Down's syndrome as a known cause of mental retardation.

The virus

CMV virions are pleomorphic and measure between 150 and 300 nm in diameter. The CMV genome is made up of a double-stranded DNA and it is the largest of all known human viruses. It contains over 235 kilobase pairs, and has a potential protein encoding content of approximately 200 open reading frames (ORFs) (Chee et al., 1990).

Sequential genome expression is temporally regulated in productive infection. The first phase of transcription is commonly called the "immediate-early" phase, and immediately follows entry of the virus into the host cell. Immediate-early antigens accumulate in the nucleus. These antigens are non-structural viral proteins, i.e. not part of the virion itself, but instead exert important regulatory functions in the switch to the early phase of CMV infection by transactivating early gene promoters (Mocarski, 2001).

The early phase of CMV infection is defined as occurring before the onset of viral DNA synthesis. This phase starts about 2–4 h after infection, and proceeds until about 24–48 h after infection when viral DNA synthesis starts. About 75% of the viral genome is transcribed during the early phase of infection, and many structural and non-structural proteins are produced. Furthermore, cell rounding occurs during this phase. Finally, late genes are expressed at high levels after DNA replication. They mostly encode structural viral antigens such as the viral capsid proteins, the matrix or tegument proteins, and the envelope glycoproteins. During the late period of infection, more than 90% of the CMV genome is transcribed. This period extends from 24 to 48 h after infection until cell death occurs, and it is the phase in which cytopathology proceeds towards cell lysis, infectious virus is produced and mature virions appear in the culture supernatant (Stinksi, 1999; Mocarski, 2001; Murphy et al., 2003).

Epidemiology

CMV infection is endemic and ubiquitous and not subject to seasonal fluctuations. During their lives, from 40% to 80% of individuals in the industrialized countries and almost all those in the developing world will be infected by CMV. The seroprevalence of CMV infection increases with age in every group that has been studied (Ho, 1990; Britt et al., 1996).

Human beings are the only reservoir for human CMV. The virus is transmitted by direct contact and only indirectly in rare cases. Because of viral fragility towards environmental factors, close contact is required for horizontal propagation of infection.

Sources of infection include: oropharyngeal secretions, urine, cervical and vaginal secretions, sperm, breast milk, tears, faeces and blood. Propagation is fostered by prolonged elimination of the virus and the fact that most infections produce no symptoms.

The infection is generally acquired during childhood, with an incidence of 30–40% during the first year of life, mainly by breast milk, and subsequently by close personal contact in day-care centers and schools (Pass et al., 1984; Handsfield et al., 1985). Among the adult population, especially fertile women, sexual activity and close daily contact with children play a significant role in the spread of CMV infection (Taber et al., 1985; Pass et a., 1987). Blood products, solid organ and bone marrow transplant can also transmit active as well as latent CMV (Barbara et al., 1987).

In most cases, CMV infection in normal hosts leads to a clinically inapparent infection (primary and non-primary infection). Although rarely pathogenic in immunocompetent individuals, the virus poses a significant health threat to immunocompromised individuals. Infection can occur by reactivation of latent virus, by reinfection in patients who are already infected (non-primary infection) or by primary infection (Pass, 2001). CMV infection in immunocompromised individuals causes different clinical syndromes in different groups of patients and the severity of the infection parallels the degree of the immunosuppression.

The infants may acquire infection from the mother as a result of intrauterine infection (congenital infection), or through contact with infected genital secretions during passage through the birth canal (perinatal infection) or postpartum through breast feeding (postnatal infection).

The congenital CMV infection in the developed countries occurs with an incidence between 0.3% and 2.4% of all live births (Alford et al., 1990; Peckham, 1991). Only 10–15% of congenitally infected babies present symptoms of infection at birth and these infants have a perinatal mortality rate of around 30% with 70–80% of surviving babies presenting major neurological sequelae (Boppana et al., 1992). Despite infection, 85–90% of babies have no symptoms at birth, but 8–15% of them will suffer delayed injury (Boppana et al., 1992; Fowler et al., 1992).

Mother-to-child transmission is mainly the result of primary maternal CMV infection which carries a risk of transmission varying from 24% to 75% (mean value 40%) (Alford et al., 1990; Fowler et al., 1992). Cases of CMV transmission due to non-primary infection have been reported in 1–2.2% of cases, i.e. at a much lower rate than those resulting from primary infection (Fowler et al., 1992). Nevertheless, increasing evidence shows that the outcome of non-primary maternal infection may be symptomatic and severe (Boppana et al., 1999; Gaytant et al., 2003). Recently, the possibility that recurrences and unfavourable outcome might be related to reinfection by a new viral strain has been suggested (Boppana et al., 2001). Congenital CMV infection is strongly dependent on maternal serological status.

Fowler et al. (2003) reported that the older maternal age ($\geqslant 25$ years) and gravidity (> 2) were associated with decreased risk of congenital CMV infection. The presence of maternal antibody at the previous delivery was highly protective against delivering a future newborn with congenital CMV infection (RR, 0.32; 95% CI, 0.17–0.62).

Since the prevalence of maternal antibody increases rapidly with age in young women, it is likely that a greater proportion of younger women would have been seronegative near the time of their first pregnancy. It has been gauged that about 30–40% of the young population (< 25 years) in northern Italy is seronegative for CMV making the same proportion of fertile women at risk of contracting CMV infection during pregnancy (unpublished data).

Clinical manifestations in symptomatic newborns range from severe multiorgan involvement with jaundice (with high direct bilirubin levels), thrombocytopenic purpura, hepatomegaly, splenomegaly, pneumonia and encephalitis. Mild clinical manifestations usually include liver problems with hepatosplenomegaly (60% of cases) and thrombocytopenia (53–77% of cases), and around half the babies present delayed intrauterine growth with low birth weight (Ramsay et al., 1991; Boppana et al., 1992). Structural abnormalities mainly affect the central nervous system (ventriculomegaly, intracranial calcifications and cerebral atrophy), whereas other organs are seldom involved. Associated visual impairment and hearing loss have also been reported and CMV has been implicated in non-immunological hydrops (Inoue et al., 2001).

In addition 8–15% of asymptomatic newborns develop long-term sequelae, namely psychomotor delay and hearing loss (Fowler et al., 1997). CMV is the leading non-genetic cause of deafness in children: more than half the babies born with symptomatic infection and 10% of asymptomatic newborns will develop mild-to-severe neurosensory hearing loss which is progressive in 50% of cases (Stagno et al., 1986; Dahle et al., 2000). Hearing loss is bilateral in 50% of cases leading to language impairment and learning delay whose severity is directly proportional to the delay in diagnosis precluding prompt rehabilitation (Kimberlin et al., 2003).

In summary, around 30–40% of congenitally CMV infected newborns will present problems varying in severity at birth and/or throughout life.

Transmission of CMV from mother to foetus occurs with the same frequency throughout all three trimesters of pregnancy (Stagno et al., 1986). More recently, Bodeus reported an overall rate of transmission of 57.5% with maternal seroconversion during pregnancy; however, the transmission rate was lower, 36% with first-trimester infection than with third-trimester infection, 77.6% (Bodeus et al., 1999).

CMV can also be transmitted to the foetus when primary maternal infection occurs before conception. Revello et al. (2002b) showed that preconception primary CMV infection (3 months before the last menstrual period) carries a low risk of intrauterine transmission, one (9.1%) infected newborn out of 12 examined. In the periconceptional CMV infection (4 weeks after the last menstrual period) the virus was transmitted to 4 newborns (30.8%) of 13 pregnancies. The authors conclude that periconceptional primary CMV infection seems to bear a higher risk of unfavourable outcome than preconceptional infection, and counselling should be adjusted accordingly.

The extent of foetal–newborn injury, namely severe brain damage, is correlated to the gestational epoch in which vertical transmission occurs: the most severe is correlated to primary maternal infected contracted in the first 2 months of pregnancy (Stagno et al., 1986). A report by Pass et al. (2006) demonstrated that children with congenital CMV infection following first-trimester maternal infection are more likely to have CNS sequelae, especially sensorineural hearing loss, than are those whose mothers were infected later in pregnancy. However, some degree of CNS impairment can follow even late gestational infection .

Most CMV infections encountered in pregnant women are asymptomatic even during the acute stage. Less than 5% of pregnant women with primary infection are reported to be symptomatic, and an even smaller percentage suffer from a mononucleosis syndrome (Pass et al., 1999). Even in rare cases with symptoms, the manifestations are non-specific and mild such as persistent low fever, muscle ache and gland enlargement. Laboratory tests may sometimes disclose atypical lymphocytosis and slightly raised transaminase levels.

Pathogenesis of congenital infection

Congenital infection is transmitted through the placenta. The virus in maternal leucocytes infects the placenta and replicates until it comes into contact with the foetal circulation (Fisher et al., 2000). *In vitro* studies have clearly demonstrated how CMV productively infects the placental trophoblasts (Halwachs-Baumann et al., 1998; Hemmings et al., 1998). It has also been shown how inflammation triggers the expression of adhesion molecules (namely ICAM-1) on the trophoblast membranes, thereby enhancing the adhesion of maternal blood cells (Xiao et al., 1997).

The placenta acts as a portal of entry for the virus, but it also acts as a barrier because even during maternal primary infection, transmission occurs in only 40% of cases. Twin pregnancies represent an interesting model because different foetuses are simultaneously exposed to the same maternal influences and had a completely different outcome. In our recent studies, we described three cases of CMV-infected twin pregnancies. Only six of seven newborns were infected and three of whom were symptomatic (Lazzarotto et al., 2003; Gabrielli et al., 2003).

During primary infection of the mother, leucocytes carrying infectious virus may transmit CMV infection to trophoblasts and from these cells the virus seems to spread cell-to-cell into the stroma replicating in fibroblasts and then reaching foetal endothelial cells. Recent studies indicate a complete but limited CMV replication in trophoblast cells and a subsequent high virus replication within the stromal cells (Fig. 1). Therefore, even if a low viraemia phase occurs in the mother a congenital infection might occur as a result of virus amplification at placental level (Gabrielli et al., 2001).

After an initial foetal viraemic stage (dissemination stage), the virus can invade and productively replicate in target organs like the central nervous system, liver, inner ear, spinal cord, kidney, duct epithelium and vascular epithelium, etc. In particular, the tubular epithelium within the kidney appears to be a major site of viral replication. Cleared by foetal diuresis into the amniotic fluid (AF), the virus can be newly ingested by the foetus and replicate in the oropharyngeal epithelium giving rise to more extensive dissemination via the blood (Fig. 2).

Diagnosis of maternal infection

Since pregnancy generally does not affect the clinical course of infection, usually symptom-free in immmunocompetent subjects, laboratory tests (virology and serology) are the best means of establishing diagnosis. It is up to the physician to decide on the basis of maternal status prior to conception whether to test for CMV

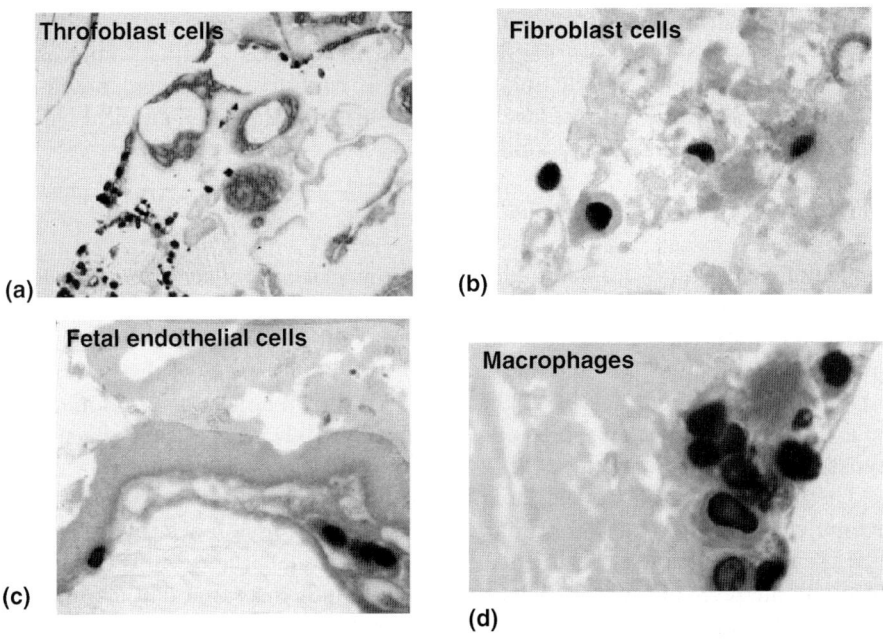

Fig. 1 Immunohistochemical double detection of viral and cellular in CMV-infected placenta explants. (A) In blue, the cytokeratin marker showing the trophoblast layer and in brown CMV-early antigen ($\times$ 200); (B) In blue, the vimentin-positive cells showing fibroblast cells and in brown CMV-immediate early antigen ($\times$ 400); (C) In blue, the endothelial cell marker and in brown CMV-early antigen ($\times$ 400); (D) In blue, the CD68 marker showing macrophages and in brown CMV-early antigen ($\times$ 500). From Gabrielli et al. (2001) (for color version: see color section on page 261).

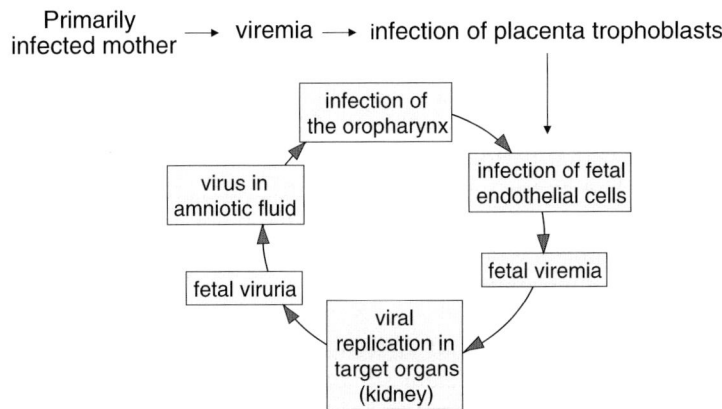

Fig. 2 Transmission of CMV through the placenta barrier and infection of the foetus.

in pregnancy and which tests to prescribe and then to interpret the results accurately.

Women seropositive for CMV before conception

IgG-specific antibodies in serum disclosed at the first test in pregnancy (8–10th week) is indicative of past infection and no further investigations are required. There is tacit agreement among the international community that no laboratory testing for CMV needs to be carried out, unless indicated by particular clinical conditions such as abnormal ultrasonographic findings. Even though it does not offer full protection, acquired immunity will defend the mother from primary infection in pregnancy which carries a much greater risk of foetal damage. Any reinfection or reactivation of infection carries the same risk as pregnancy itself.

For these reasons, the information on maternal status prior to conception precludes the need for screening during pregnancy.

Women seronegative for CMV within the 6 months before conception

Non-immune pregnant women are therefore at risk of acquiring primary infection. First and foremost they must be informed of hygiene and behaviour measures (avoiding direct contact with organic materials, close contact with pre-school children and frequent thorough hand-washing) to reduce the chance of infection (Cannon et al., 2005). A recent study reported that pregnant women who received an intervention involving hygienic practices were significantly less likely to acquire CMV infection than were non-pregnant women (Adler et al., 2004).

Seronegative pregnant women must also undergo periodic serological testing. Although there are no universally accepted guidelines, monthly testing until the 18–20th week of pregnancy is reasonable to implement foetal investigations in case of seroconversion. If the mother continues to be seronegative, serological follow-up testing can be limited or confined to one more test at 35–37 weeks to select newborns at risk of congenital infection in the case of late seroconversion (Guerra et al., 2000).

Women whose pre-pregnancy serological status is unknown

Diagnosis of CMV infection is more complex in women unaware of their serological status before pregnancy. As most infections are asymptomatic, the only way to disclose primary infection is to implement specific testing as early in pregnancy as possible.

Serological findings

Testing for anti-CMV IgM antibodies is the most widely used procedure for screening pregnant women. However, there is currently some concern over the fact that different commercially available kits frequently yield discordant results, limiting their diagnostic value. Agreement between kits varies from 56% to 75% with a sensitivity between 30% and 88% (Lazzarotto et al., 1997a).

When anti-CMV IgM antibodies are detected in a pregnant woman the diagnosis remains open.

Anti-CMV IgM antibodies are a good indicator of acute or recent infection, but cannot always be correlated to primary infection. Findings indicate that fewer than 10% of IgM-positive women congenitally infect their foetus/newborn (Lazzarotto et al., 2004). This is because pregnant women can produce IgM during reactivations or reinfections (Lazzarotto et al., 1997b). In addition, anti-CMV IgM antibodies have been detected in some pregnant women 6–9 months after the end of the acute phase of primary infection (Stagno et al., 1986) and false-positive results are common (Lazzarotto et al., 1997a, 2004).

Hence, the detection of IgM in the serum of pregnant women may simply be a starting point for further diagnostic investigation.

The anti-CMV IgG avidity test is currently the most reliable procedure to identify primary infection in pregnant women (Grangeot-Keros et al., 1997; Lazzarotto et al., 1997b; Eggers et al., 2000; Mace et al., 2004). Antibody avidity indicates the strength with which a multivalent antibody binds to a multivalent antigen. The antibodies produced during the primary response have a much lower antigen avidity than the antibodies produced during the non-primary response. For this reason, low-avidity antibodies are found after primary antigenic stimulation. The degree of antibody avidity increases progressively and slowly reflecting the maturation of the immune response.

Low-avidity indices indicate low-avidity IgG antibodies in serum caused by acute or recent primary CMV infection, whereas high-avidity indices (high-avidity serum IgG) indicate no current or recent primary infection (Lazzarotto et al., 1997b). Low-avidity anti-CMV IgG are found in more than 90% of primary infections in both immunocompetent and immunocompromised subjects, whereas they are never detected in non-primary infection (Lazzarotto et al., 1997b).

Low-avidity indices are encountered 18–20 weeks after the onset of symptoms in immunocompetent subjects. The test is reliable and 100% sensitive before the 16–18th week of pregnancy after which sensitivity is drastically reduced (62.5%) (Lazzarotto et al., 2000b).

Immunoblot is the gold standard test to confirm the presence of IgM antibodies in serum (Lazzarotto et al., 1998). In addition, analysis of the virus-specific IgM response to individual structural and non-structural CMV proteins will disclose fairly typical reactive profiles to distinguish primary from non-primary infection. Moreover, counting the number of bands recognized by IgM present in sera from CMV-infected women, we observed that serum IgM from women who transmit CMV infection reacts with a higher number of bands than does serum IgM from those who do not transmit the infection ($P < 0.0001$) (Lazzarotto et al., 1998).

Figure 3 shows some examples of IgM-reactive profiles against viral and recombinant CMV proteins in serum samples from pregnant women IgM-positive and IgM-negative for CMV.

A management scheme for CMV serology in pregnant women is proposed in Fig. 4.

Virological findings

Virological tests play a secondary role in the diagnosis of primary CMV infection in pregnant women. During and after pregnancy CMV is commonly cleared in

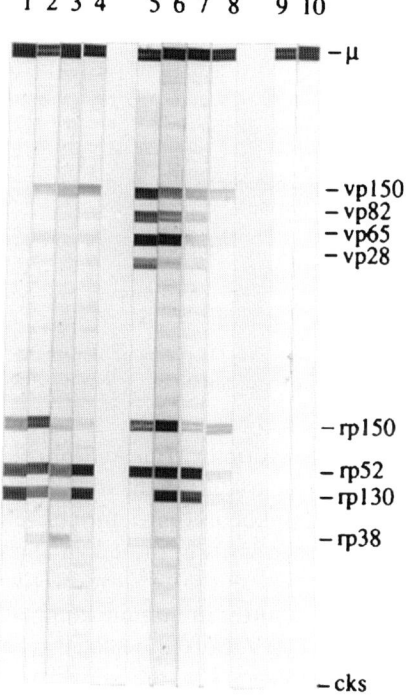

Fig. 3 The new immunoblot. Individual suspensions of each of the four purified viral proteins (vp150, vp82, vp65 and vp28) and the four purified recombinant proteins (rp150, rp52, rp130 and rp38) were deposited onto the nitrocellulose strip. Furthermore, two additional control proteins were added: the CKS protein (negative control) and human μ chain (IgM) (positive control). Representative examples of serum reactivity with the immunoblot. Viral and recombinant proteins are identified on the right. CKS is the negative control, and μ is the IgM heavy chain and represents the positive control. Lanes: 1–8, IgM-positive sera from pregnant women; 9 and 10, IgM-negative sera from pregnant women. Sera 1–4 preferentially reacted with recombinant proteins, while sera 5–8 reacted with both viral and recombinant proteins. Sera 5 and 6 were from pregnant women who transmitted the infection. From Lazzarotto et al. (1998).

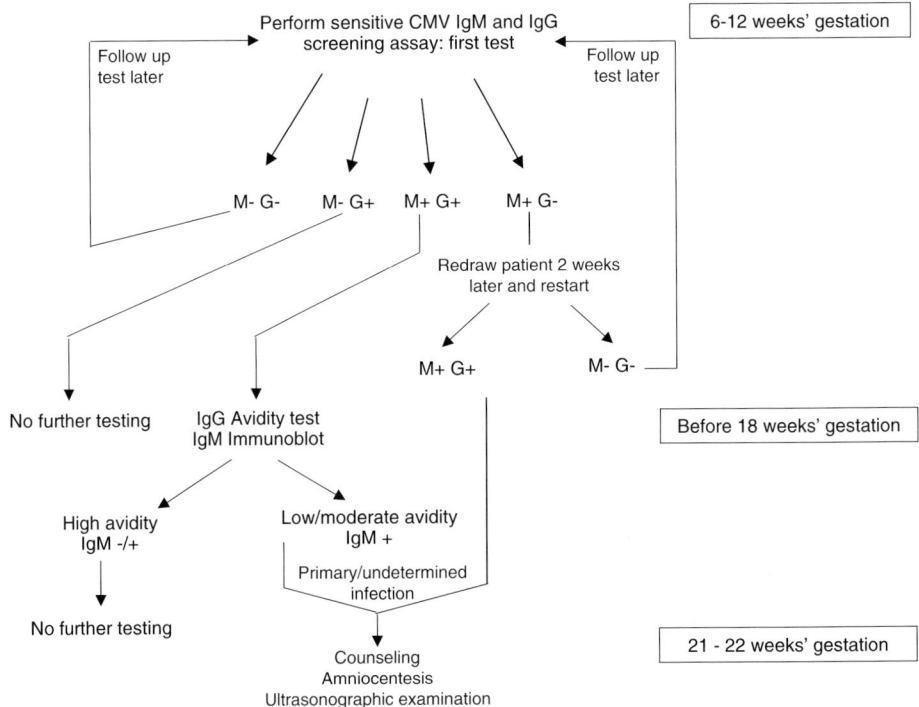

Fig. 4 A management scheme for CMV serology in pregnant women. M, CMV-specific IgM; G, CMV-
specific IgG; – negative for antibody; + positive for antibody.

organic secretion so that virus isolation in urine and/or cervical secretions is a poor
indicator of the risk of intrauterine transmission and the severity of foetal/neonatal
damage. We found low positive prediction rates for congenital CMV infection and
foetal injury when the mother shed virus in the saliva and/or urine during the first
two trimesters of pregnancy (29.2% and 57.1%, respectively) (Table 1).

The viraemic phase is much shorter in immunocompetent subjects with respect
to immunodepressed patients. CMV can be detected in blood by virus isolation
and/or the search for viral components by the antigenaemia tests and qualitative
and quantitative polymerase chain reaction (PCR). Findings demonstrated that
CMV may be found in the blood of pregnant women during acute or recent primary infection (Revello et al., 1998b).

Nevertheless, the results of these diagnostic tests also fail to correlate with either
the clinical course of infection and/or the risk of intrauterine transmission and the
severity of foetal/neonatal injury (Lazzarotto et al., 2004), confirming literature
reports (Revello et al., 1998b). Both antigenaemia and qualitative PCR tests
undertaken in a group of pregnant women infected between 4 and 30 weeks' gestation with primary CMV had a low sensitivity (equal to 14.3% and 47.6%, respectively) with respect to the number of cases of mother–foetus viral transmission.

Table 1

CMV detection in the urine and/or saliva of primarily infected women in relation to congenital CMV infection. Urine samples were obtained from pregnant women during the first and second trimester (range 7–24 weeks' gestation) at the time of diagnosis of primary infection with serologic methods

		CI yes	CI no	Total	Sens (%)	Spec (%)	PPV (%)	NPV (%)
Urine and/or saliva[a]	pos	7	17	24	36.8	75	29.2	80.9
	neg	12	51	63				
Total		19	68	87				

Abbreviations: CI, congenital infection; pos, positive; neg, negative; SENS, sensitivity; SPEC, specificity; PPV and NPV, positive and negative predictive value.
[a]Virus isolation (shell vial).

Specificity and positive and negative prediction rates were also poor (Lazzarotto et al., 2004).

The outcome of studies designed to identify and quantify the viral genome and/ or viral components in maternal blood in relation to symptomatic infection in the foetus/newborn also yielded disappointing results from a diagnostic standpoint.

These findings suggest that CMV may or may not be detected in maternal blood in pregnant women undergoing primary infection at the time of diagnosis. Positive viral detection is not associated with a greater risk of infection and/or foetal/neonatal injury (Lazzarotto et al., 2004).

Immunological findings

Revello et al. (2006) investigated the CMV-specific T cell response in pregnant women and, for comparison, in immunocompetent non-pregnant individuals experiencing primary CMV infection. The authors reported that the cellular immune response to CMV did not differ significantly between pregnant and non-pregnant patients with symptomatic primary CMV infection. In addition, the study indicate that a sustained deficit in the cellular immune response, as evaluated by the lymphoproliferative response analysis, appears to be significantly associated with intrauterine transmission of the virus, confirming literature reports. This work is still at the investigational stage and because exceptions were observed in the study, as well as in previous studies, the authors indicate that, at the moment, the lymphoproliferative response analysis cannot be used to reliably predict intrauterine transmission in individual cases (Revello et al., 2006).

Diagnosis of foetal infection

The foetal compartment can be studied by invasive prenatal diagnostic investigation and ultrasound. The risks linked to invasive testing are counterbalanced by certain diagnosis of foetal infection. Ultrasound has the advantage of not being invasive and will disclose any structural and/or growth abnormalities caused by CMV infection, but its sensitivity is poor and it correctly identifies not more than 5% of infected babies (Ville, 1998). In addition, a structural abnormality may be disclosed, a long time, after with initial negative tests and borderline structural changes detected early in pregnancy could be temporary.

In other words, normal ultrasound findings are reassuring for the pregnant woman, but poorly predictive of a normal newborn. Frankly pathological findings (e.g. multiple cerebral calcifications, severe ventriculomegaly, hydrocephalus, hydrothorax, ascites, etc.) carry a definitely unfavourable prognosis. On the other hand, borderline ultrasound findings (e.g. mild ventriculomegaly) can sometimes regress spontaneously and should not have a major effect on counselling.

Invasive prenatal diagnosis is currently established by amniocentesis. Recent studies have demonstrated that the AF is the most appropriate material (Donner et al., 1994; Lipitz et al., 1997; Revello et al., 1998a; Enders et al., 2001; Grangeot-Keros and Cointe, 2001), obviating the need for cordocentesis, an invasive technique with a two-fold higher risk to the foetus (1–2% vs. 0.5–1%) (Weiner, 1988).

Studies of prenatal diagnosis of foetal CMV infection such as detection of virus or virus components in foetal blood were found to be of poor sensitivity to significantly improve prenatal diagnosis of intrauterine transmission of the virus. The statistical analysis of the data of different test for diagnosis of congenital infection on foetal blood showed that the sensitivity of antigenaemia was 57.9%; of viraemia, 55.5%; and of leukoDNAemia, 82.3% (Revello et al., 1999b).

Tests performed on foetal blood may provide prognostic information, in particularly when performed quantitatively. In retrospective studies (Revello et al., 1999b; Enders et al., 2001), it was observed that the presence and the level of CMV-specific IgM in foetal blood identified foetuses with abnormal findings with high probability. Moreover, low CMV load in foetal blood at 20–24 weeks of gestation may have a more favourable outcome (Revello and Gerna, 2002a).

Given the high risk of mother–foetus transmission and foetal damage, prenatal diagnosis is recommended to women with primary and undetermined CMV infection contracted in the first half of pregnancy (documented by antibody seroconversion or advanced serological tests) and in case of foetal abnormalities suggestive of infection (Guerra et al., 2000; Lazzarotto et al., 2000a).

Invasive prenatal diagnosis

Amniocentesis entails sampling the AF under ultrasound control and is undertaken exclusively between the 21st and 22nd weeks of gestation. This period has been chosen for the following reasons: (1) CMV is a slow replication virus and 6–9 weeks are required after maternal infection for the virus to be eliminated in the foetus's urine in amounts large enough to be detected in the AF (Ruellan-Eugene et al., 1996) and (2) foetal disease is more severe if the infection is contracted in the first 12–16 weeks of gestation (Pass et al., 2006). In addition, false-negative results are common when amniocentesis is carried out earlier in pregnancy and some viruses are shed by the foetal kidney, the elective site of replication, due to limited diuresis early on.

The AF is subject to direct search for CMV virus in culture and for the viral genome by qualitative PCR. Viral isolation from the AF is an indicative of congenital infection, but the procedure is not sensitive (70–80%). False-negative results are partly due to transporting and maintaining the AF in optimal conditions as the viral particles must be infective to be detected in culture.

The qualitative search for CMV DNA in AF has a good sensitivity and specificity (90–98% and 92–98%, respectively) with respect to viral transmission from mother to foetus (Ruellan-Eugene et al., 1996; Lipitz et al., 1997; Revello et al., 1998a; Guerra et al., 2000; Enders et al., 2001).

If both techniques are negative, foetal infection can be ruled out with a high degree of certainty. If results are positive, investigation is completed by DNA quantification by quantitative PCR (Guerra et al., 2000; Lazzarotto et al., 2000a; Gouarin et al., 2002). There is a low risk of symptomatic infection in the presence of viral loads $< 10^3$ copies/ml (Guerra et al., 2000; Lazzarotto et al., 2000a). We recently observed that among 81 positive samples of AF from mothers who transmitted the virus to their babies, 18 had a result below 1000 copies. These 18 congenitally infected babies were asymptomatic at birth and subsequent monitoring in 16 of them confirmed normal development and the absence of late-onset sequelae. Twelve of 16 infected infants were followed up for at least 12 months and the remaining four infants for at least 6 months.

In agreement with other literature reports (Gouarin et al., 2002; Revello and Gerna, 2002a), these findings suggest that low viral loads in the AF, sampled at the appropriate times (at 20–22 weeks gestation and the time interval between onset of maternal infection is $\geqslant$6–8 weeks) may be a good indicator ruling out foetal damage at birth and/or subsequent exacerbation of infection with the onset of sequelae like hearing loss and/or delayed psychomotor development.

In conclusion, negative results of invasive prenatal diagnosis can rule out CMV infection in almost 100% of cases. This discourages parents from seeking pregnancy termination on the grounds of primary infection at high risk of mother–foetus transmission and reassures the mother in continuing her pregnancy. Reassuring results are also obtained when minimal amounts or traces of the virus are found in the AF since the newborns are infected but asymptomatic at birth and subsequent follow-up checks.

Diagnosis of infection in newborns

At birth, it is essential to use appropriate tests for the diagnosis of CMV congenital infection. The gold standard for the diagnosis of congenital CMV infection in newborns remains viral isolation in the urine and/or saliva within the first 2 weeks of life. Detection of specific IgM in neonatal serum also discloses congenital infection, but IgM antibodies are only present in 70% of infected babies (Revello et al., 1999a).

After 2 weeks of life, virological and serological tests will no longer distinguish pre from perinatal CMV infection and the diagnosis of congenital infection can only be suspected on clinical grounds.

The determination of DNA in blood by PCR at birth seems to be as sensitive and specific as recovery from urine for diagnosis of congenital CMV infection (Revello and Gerna, 2002a; Ross et al., 2005; Lanari et al., 2006).

Interesting findings recently emerged from viral genome research using PCR on blood adsorbed on Guthrie cards, collected at birth for neonatal screening (Barbi et al., 2000). However, these virological tests are made highly delicate by the complexity of the extraction and purification phase of viral DNA. This test only sometimes offers retrospective confirmation of congenital infection in selected cases with a strong clinical suspicion, and cannot be utilized as a diagnostic test for congenital CMV infection (Barbi et al., 2006).

If urine is positive for viral isolation, various clinical, laboratory and instrumental findings are monitored in the infected babies for subsequent weeks and the newborns classified as symptomatic or asymptomatic (Boppana et al., 1992). If viral isolation is negative, the baby is considered uninfected and no further tests are warranted (Fig. 5).

The mortality rate among symptomatic newborns is high and 70–80% of surviving babies are at high risk of developing major neurological sequelae (Boppana et al., 1992). Most infected babies (85–90%) are asymptomatic at birth. The

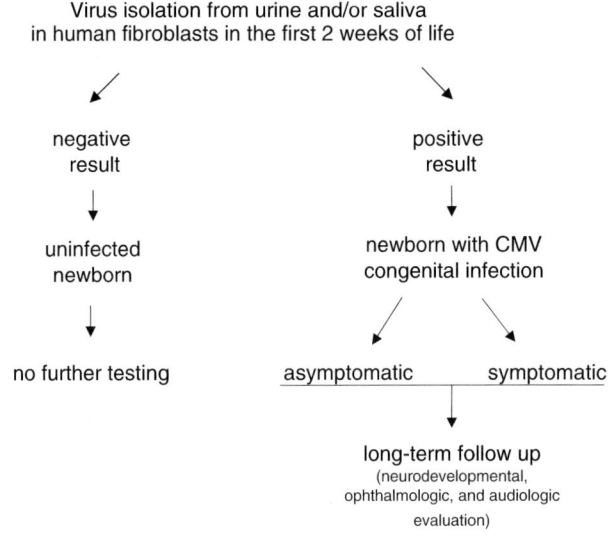

Fig. 5 A management scheme for diagnosis of congenital CMV infection in the newborn.

majority of them will develop normally, but 8% will develop progressive hearing loss (Fowler et al., 1997).

For these reasons, all infected babies undergo follow-up monitoring at 1, 3, 6 and 12 months of life and annually thereafter until school age. Monitoring includes physical, neurological and anthropometric evaluation; neurodevelopmental evaluation; auditory brainstem responses; *fundus oculi*; blood sampling for laboratory tests (complete blood count, platelet count, transaminase level, bilirubin levels— direct and indirect); and urine sampling for virus isolation.

In recent years, one of the most widely discussed topics in the management of congenital CMV infection has been the possibility to predict the long-term outcome of infection more accurately in the neonatal period. This would offer a series of advantages including appropriate parent counselling and the implementation of prompt interventions for babies at high risk of handicap. Pinpointing reliable prognostic markers of favourable outcome would attenuate parental anxiety. Patients could also be stratified in terms of varying risk of neurological sequelae to devise more accurate treatments such as antiviral therapies to improve the prognosis.

A report by Rivera et al. (2002) demonstrated that a high viral load in early infancy, expressed by a high amount of virus in urine, is highly predictive of audiological impairment.

Bradford et al. (2005) observed that viraemic infants (presence of CMV DNA in baseline serum sample) were more likely to have (1) hearing loss both at enrollment ($P = 0.045$) and at 6-month follow-up testing ($P = 0.035$) and (2) other indicators of active CMV disease, including elevated levels of alanine aminotransferase, petechial rash and organomegaly.

Finally, we recently obtained encouraging results in this direction studying the role of CMV DNA load in infant blood measured on polymorphonuclear leucocyte (PMNLs) samples taken in the first month of life as a possible prognostic indicator of sequelae. Low neonatal viral load detected by pp65 antigaenemia test and quantitative PCR (qPCR) was highly predictive or absence of sequelae: DNAemia <1000 copies per 10^5 PMNLs has a negative predictive factor of 95%. Different viraemia value ranges are correlated to a different risk of sequelae: $\sim$70% sequelae were found in newborns with a qPCR higher than 10,000 copies per 10^5 PMNLs (Lanari et al., 2006).

Conclusions

Although the diagnosis of congenital CMV infection is still complex, important goals have been achieved in recent years, among which are: the availability of more reliable IgM tests for screening pregnant women whose pre-pregnancy serological status for CMV is unknown (Maine et al., 2001); tests to determine the avidity index of anti-CMV IgG, allowing the diagnosis of a primary CMV infection; and, innovative and traditional, virological tests to detect the virus in AF. We are confident that the risk of terminating potentially normal babies would be largely contained by a comprehensive diagnostic approach to CMV infection in pregnancy. Furthermore, a fully standardized diagnostic algorithm should lessen the anxiety felt by pregnant women, which is mainly due to concerns about mismanagement. We believe that it is time to rethink current strategies, recommendations and attitudes among health authorities, clinicians and pregnant women in order to control congenital CMV infection. Possible future advances in our understanding of the natural history of intrauterine CMV infection and antiviral chemotherapy may allow the prenatal identification of affected foetus to lead to the treatment of the mother with an anti-CMV agent that crosses the placenta and thus provides pre-emptive foetal therapy.

References

Adler SP, Finney JW, Manganello AM, Best AM. Prevention of child-to-mother transmission of cytomegalovirus among pregnant women. J Pediatr 2004; 145: 485–491.

Alford CA, Stagno S, Pass RF, Britt WJ. Congenital and perinatal cytomegalovirus infections. Rev Infect Dis 1990; 12: S745–S753.

Barbara JA, Tegtmeier GE. Cytomegalovirus and blood transfusion. Blood Rev 1987; 1: 207–211.

Barbi B, Binda S, Primache V, Caroppo S, Dido P, Guidotti P, Corbetta C, Melotti D. Cytomegalovirus DNA detection in Guthrie cards: a powerful tool for diagnosing congenital infection. J Clin Virol 2000; 17: 159–165.

Barbi M, Binda S, Caroppo S, Primache V. Neonatal screening for congenital cytomegalovirus infection and hearing loss. J Clin Virol 2006; 35: 206–209.

Bodeus M, Hubinont C, Goubau P. Increased risk of cytomegalovirus transmission in utero during late gestation. Obstet Gynecol 1999; 93: 658–660.

Boppana S, Pass RF, Britt WS, Stagno S, Alford CA. Symptomatic congenital cytomegalovirus infection: neonatal and mortality. Pediatr Infect Dis 1992; 11: 93–99.

Boppana SB, Fowler KB, Britt WJ, Stagno S, Pass RF. Symptomatic congenital cytomegalovirus infection infants born to mothers with preexisting immunity to cytomegalovirus. Pediatrics 1999; 104: 55–60.

Boppana SB, Rivera LB, Fowler KB, Mach M, Britt WJ. Intrauterine transmission of cytomegalovirus to infants of women with preconceptional immunity. N Engl J Med 2001; 344: 1366–1371.

Bradford RD, Cloud G, Lakeman AD, Boppana S, Kimberlin DW, Jacobs R, Demmler G, Sanchez P, Britt W, Soong SJ, Whitley RJ, National Institute of Allergy and Infectious Diseases Collaborative Antiviral Study Group. Detection of cytomegalovirus (CMV) DNA by polymerase chain reaction is associated with hearing loss in newborns with symptomatic congenital CMV infection involving the central nervous system. J Infect Dis 2005; 191: 227–233.

Britt WJ, Alford CA. Cytomegalovirus. In: Fields Virology (Fields BN, Knipe D, Howley P, editors). Vol. 2. Philadelphia: Lippincott Williams and Wilkins; 1996; p. 2493.

Cannon MJ, Davis KF. Washing our hands of the congenital cytomegalovirus disease epidemic. BMC Public Health 2005; 5: 70.

Chee MS, Bankier AT, Beck S, Bohni R, Brown CM, Cerny R, Horsnell T, Hutchison III CA, Kouzarides T, Martignetti JA. Analysis of the protein-coding content of the sequence of human cytomegalovirus strain AD169. Curr Top Microbiol Immunol 1990; 154: 125–169.

Dahle AJ, Fowler KB, Wright JD, Boppana SB, Britt WJ, Pass RF. Longitudinal investigation of hearing disorders in children with congenital cytomegalovirus. J Am Acad Audiol 2000; 11: 283–290.

Donner C, Liesnard C, Brancart F, Rodesch F. Accuracy of amniotic fluid testing before 21 weeks' gestation in prenatal diagnosis of congenital cytomegalovirus infection. Prenat Diagn 1994; 14: 1055–1059.

Eggers M, Bader U, Enders G. Combination of microneutralization and avidity assays: improved diagnosis of recent primary human cytomegalovirus infection in single serum sample of second trimester pregnancy. J Med Virol 2000; 60: 324–330.

Enders G, Bader U, Lindemann L, Schalasta G, Daiminger A. Prenatal diagnosis of congenital cytomegalovirus infection in 189 pregnancies with known outcome. Prenat Diagn 2001; 21: 362–377.

Fisher S, Genbacev O, Maidji E, Pereira L. Human cytomegalovirus infection of placental cytotrophoblasts *in vitro* and *in utero*: implications for transmission and pathogenesis. J Virol 2000; 74: 6808–6820.

Fowler KB, McCollister FP, Dahle AJ, Boppana S, Britt WJ, Pass RF. Progressive and fluctuating sensorineural hearing loss in children with asymptomatic congenital cytomegalovirus infection. J Pediatr 1997; 130: 624–630.

Fowler KB, Stagno S, Pass RF. Maternal immunity and prevention of congenital cytomegalovirus infection. JAMA 2003; 289: 1008–1011.

Fowler KB, Stagno S, Pass RF, Britt WJ, Boll TJ, Alford CA. The outcome of congenital cytomegalovirus in relation to maternal antibody status. N Engl J Med 1992; 326: 663–667.

Gabrielli L, Lazzarotto T, Foschini MP, Lanari M, Guerra B, Eusebi V, Landini MP. Horizontal in utero acquisition of cytomegalovirus infection in a twin pregnancy. J Clin Microbiol 2003; 41: 1329–1331.

Gabrielli L, Losi L, Varani S, Lazzarotto T, Eusebi V, Landini MP. Complete replication of human cytomegalovirus in explants of first trimester human placenta. J Med Virol 2001; 64: 499–504.

Gaytant MA, Rours GI, Steegers EA, Galama JM, Semmekrot BA. Congenital cytomegalovirus infection after recurrent infection: case reports and review of the literature. Eur J Pediatr 2003; 162: 248–253.

Gouarin S, Gault E, Vabret A, Cointe D, Rozenberg F, Grangeot-Keros L, Barjot P, Garbarg-Chenon A, Lebon P, Freymuth F. Real-time PCR quantification of human cytomegalovirus DNA in amniotic fluid samples from mothers with primary infection. J Clin Microbiol 2002; 40: 1767–1772.

Grangeot-Keros L, Cointe D. Diagnosis and prognostic markers of HCMV infection. J Clin Virol 2001; 21: 213–221.

Grangeot-Keros L, Mayaux MJ, Lebon P, Freymuth F, Eugene G, Stricker R, Dussaix E. Value of cytomegalovirus (CMV) IgG avidity index for the diagnosis of primary infection in pregnant women. J Infect Dis 1997; 175: 944–946.

Guerra B, Lazzarotto T, Quarta S, Lanari M, Bovicelli L, Nicolosi A, Landini MP. Prenatal diagnosis of symptomatic congenital cytomegalovirus infection. Am J Obstet Gynecol 2000; 183: 476–482.

Halwachs-Baumann G, Wilders-Truschnig M, Desoye G, Hahn T, Kiesel L, Klingel K, Rieger P, Jahn G, Sinzger C. Human trophoblast cells are permissive to the complete replicative cycle of human cytomegalovirus. J Virol 1998; 72: 7598–7602.

Handsfield HH, Chandler SH, Caine VA, Meyers JD, Corey L, Medeiros E, McDougall JK. Cytomegalovirus infection in sex partners: evidence for sexual transmission. J Infect Dis 1985; 151: 344–348.

Hemmings DG, Kilani R, Nykiforuk C, Guilbert LJ. Permissive cytomegalovirus infection of primary villous term and first trimester trophoblasts. J Virol 1998; 72: 4970–4979.

Ho, M. Epidemiology of CMV infection. Rev Infect Dis 1990; 12: S701–S710.

Inoue T, Matsumura N, Fukuoka M, Sagawa N, Fujii S. Severe congenital cytomegalovirus infection with fetal hydrops in a cytomegalovirus-seropositive healthy woman. Eur J Obstet Gynecol 2001; 95: 184–186.

Kimberlin DW, Lin CY, Sanchez PJ, Demmler GJ, Dankner W, Shelton M, Jacobs RF, Vaudry W, Pass RF, Kiell, JM, Soong, SJ, Whitley, RJ, National Institute of Allergy and Infectious Diseases Collaborative Antiviral Study Group. Effect of ganciclovir therapy on hearing in symptomatic congenital cytomegalovirus disease involving the central nervous system: a randomized, controlled trial. J Pediatr 2003; 143: 16–25.

Lanari M, Lazzarotto T, Venturi V, Papa I, Gabrielli L, Guerra B, Landini MP, Faldella G. Neonatal cytomegalovirus blood load and risk of sequele in symptomatic and asymptomatic congenitally infected newborns. Pediatrics 2006; 117: e76–e83.

Lazzarotto T, Brojanac S, Maine GT, Landini MP. Search for cytomegalovirus-specific immunoglobulin M: comparison between a new Western blot, conventional western blot, and nine commercially available assays. Clin Diagn Lab Immunol 1997a; 4: 483–486.

Lazzarotto T, Gabrielli L, Foschini MP, Lanari M, Guerra B, Eusebi V, Landini MP. Congenital cytomegalovirus infection in twin pregnancies: viral load in the amniotic fluid and pregnancy outcome. Pediatrics 2003; 112: e153–e157.

Lazzarotto T, Gabrielli L, Lanari M, Guerra B, Bellucci T, Sassi M, Landini MP. Congenital cytomegalovirus infection: recent advances in the diagnosis of maternal infection. Hum Immunol 2004; 65: 410–415.

Lazzarotto T, Ripalti A, Bergamini G, Battista MC, Spezzacatena P, Campanini F, Pradelli P, Varani S, Gabrielli L, Maine GT, Landini MP. Development of a new cytomegalovirus (CMV) immunoglobulin M (IgM) immunoblot for detection of CMV-specific IgM. J Clin Microbiol 1998; 36: 3337–3341.

Lazzarotto T, Spezzacatena P, Pradelli P, Abate DA, Varani S, Landini MP. Avidity of immunoglobulin G directed against human cytomegalovirus during primary and secondary infections in immunocompetent and immunocompromised subjects. Clin Diagn Lab Immunol 1997b; 4: 469–473.

Lazzarotto T, Varani S, Guerra B, Nicolosi A, Lanari M, Landini MP. Prenatal indicators of congenital cytomegalovirus infection. J Pediatr 2000a; 137: 90–95.

Lazzarotto T, Varani S, Spezzacatena P, Gabrielli L, Pradelli P, Guerra B, Landini MP. Maternal IgG avidity and IgM detected by blot as diagnostic tools to identify pregnant women at risk of transmitting cytomegalovirus. Viral Immunol 2000b; 13: 137–141.

Lipitz S, Yagel S, Shalev E, Achiron R, Mashiach S, Schiff E. Prenatal diagnosis of fetal primary cytomegalovirus infection. Obstet Gynecol 1997; 89: 763–767.

Mace M, Sissoeff L, Rudent A, Grangeot-Keros L. A serological testing algorithm for the diagnosis of primary CMV infection in pregnant women. Prenat Diagn 2004; 24: 861–863.

Maine GT, Lazzarotto T, Landini MP. New developments in the diagnosis of maternal and congenital CMV infection. Exp Rev Mol Diagn 2001; 1: 89–99.

Mocarski ES. Cytomegalovirus and their replication. In: Fields Virology (Fields BN, Knipe D, Howley P, editors). Vol. 2. Philadelphia: Lippincott Williams and Wilkins; 2001; p. 2629.

Murphy R, Yu D, Grimwood J, Schmutz J, Dickson M, Jarvis MA, Hahn G, Nelson JA, Myers RM, Shenk TE. Coding potential of laboratory and clinical strains of human cytomegalovirus. Proc Natl Acad Sci USA 2003; 100: 14976.

Pass RF. Cytomegalovirus and their replication. In: Fields Virology (Knipe D, Howley P, editors). Vol. 2. Philadelphia: Lippincott Williams and Wilkins; 2001; p. 2675.

Pass RF, Boppana S. Cytomegalovirus. In: Viral Infection in Obstetrics and Gynaecology (Jeffries DJ, Hudson CN, editors). New York, NY: ARNOLD; 1999; pp. 35–36.

Pass RF, Fowler KB, Boppana SB, Britt WJ, Stagno S. Congenital cytomegalovirus infection following first trimester maternal infection: symptoms at birth and outcome. J Clin Virol 2006; 35: 216–220.

Pass RF, Hutto SC, Reynolds DW, Polhill RB. Increased frequency of cytomegalovirus infection in children in group day care. Pediatrics 1984; 74: 121–126.

Pass RF, Little EA, Stagno S, Britt WJ, Alford CA. Young children as a probable source of maternal and congenital cytomegalovirus infection. N Engl J Med 1987; 316: 1366–1370.

Peckham CS. Cytomegalovirus infection: congenital and neonatal disease. Scand J Infect Suppl 1991; 78: 82–87.

Ramsay ME, Miller E, Peckham CS. Outcome of confirmed symptomatic congenital cytomegalovirus infection. Arch Dis Child 1991; 66: 1068–1069.

Revello MG, Gerna G. Diagnosis and management of human cytomegalovirus infection in the mother, fetus, and newborn infant. Clin Microbiol Rev 2002; 15: 680–715.

Revello MG, Lilleri D, Zavattoni M, Furione M, Genini E, Comolli G, Gerna G. Lympho-proliferative response in primary human cytomegalovirus (HCMV) infection is delayed in HCMV transmitter mothers. J Infect Dis 2006; 193: 269–276.

Revello MG, Sarasini A, Zavattoni M, Baldanti F, Gerna G. Improved prenatal diagnosis of congenital human cytomegalovirus infection by modified nested polymerase chain reaction. J Med Virol 1998a; 56: 99–103.

Revello MG, Zavattoni M, Sarasini A, Baldanti F, De Julio C, De-Giuli L, Nicolini U, Gerna G. Prenatal diagnostic and prognostic value of human cytomegalovirus load and IgM antibody response in blood of congenitally infected fetuses. J Infect Dis 1999b; 180: 1320–1323.

Revello MG, Zavattoni M, Baldanti F, Sarasini A, Paolucci S, Gerna G. Diagnostic and prognostic value of human cytomegalovirus load and IgM antibody in blood of congenitally infected newborns. J Clin Virol 1999a; 14: 57–66.

Revello MG, Zavattoni M, Furione M, Lilleri D, Gorini G, Gerna G. Diagnosis and outcome of preconceptional and periconceptional primary human cytomegalovirus infections. J Infect Dis 2002; 186: 553–557.

Revello MG, Zavattoni M, Sarasini A, Percivalle E, Simoncini L, Gerna G. Human cytomegalovirus in blood of immunocompetent persons during primary infection: prognostic implications for pregnancy. J Infect Dis 1998b; 177: 1170–1175.

Rivera LB, Boppana SB, Fowler KB, Britt WJ, Stagno S, Pass RF. Predictors of hearing loss in children with symptomatic congenital cytomegalovirus infection. Pediatrics 2002; 110: 762–767.

Ross SA, Boppana SB. Congenital cytomegalovirus infection: outcome and diagnosis. Semin Pediatr Infect Dis 2005; 16: 44–49.

Ruellan-Eugene G, Barjot P, Campet M, Vabret A, Herlicoviez M, Muller G, Levy G, Guillois B, Freymuth F. Evaluation of virological procedures to detect fetal human

cytomegalovirus infection: avidity of IgG antibodies, virus detection in amniotic fluid and
    maternal serum. J Med Virol 1996; 50: 9–15.
Stagno S, Pass RF, Cloud G, Britt WJ, Henderson RE, Walton PD, Veren DA, Page F,
    Alford CA. Primary cytomegalovirus infection in pregnancy. Incidence, transmission to
    fetus, and clinical outcome. JAMA 1986; 256: 1904–1908.
Stinksi MF. Cytomegalovirus promoter for expression in mammalian cells. In: Gene Ex-
    pression System: Using Nature for the Art of Expression (Fernandez JM, Hoeffler JP,
    editors). San Diego, CA: Academic Press; 1999; pp. 211–233.
Taber LH, Frank AL, Yow MD, Bagley A. Acquisition of cytomegaloviral infections in
    families with young children: a serological study. J Infect Dis 1985; 151: 948–952.
Ville Y. The megalovirus [editorial]. Ultrasound Obstet Gynecol 1998; 12: 151–153.
Weiner CP. Cordocentesis. Obstet Gynecol Clin North Am 1988; 15: 283–301.
Xiao Y, Garcia-Lloret M, Winkler-Lowen B, Miller R, Simpson K, Guilbert LJ. ICAM-1
    mediated adhesion of peripheral blood monocytes to the maternal surface of placental
    syncytiotrophoblasts: implications for placental villitis. Am J Pathol 1997; 150:
    1845–1860.

Congenital and Other Related Infectious
Diseases of the Newborn
Isa K. Mushahwar (Editor)
DOI 10.1016/S0168-7069(06)13002-5

Herpes Simplex Virus Infections of the Newborn

Lonnie Miner[a], James F. Bale Jr.[b]

[a]*Department of Neonatal Medicine, Dixie Regional Medical Center, St. George, UT, USA*
[b]*Division of Pediatric Neurology, Departments of Pediatrics and Neurology, The University of Utah School of Medicine and Primary Children's Medical Center, Salt Lake City, UT, USA*

Introduction

Herpes simplex virus (HSV) infection of the newborn is an important, potential source of morbidity and mortality among young children. Neonatal HSV infections can be categorized as (1) mucocutaneous (infection localized to the skin, eye, and/or mouth); (2) disseminated (infection involving multiple organs or tissues, including the central nervous system (CNS)); or (3) encephalitic (infection of the CNS with or without skin lesions). In addition, 5–10% of HSV infections in the neonatal period result from intrauterine (also called, congenital) infection. The polymerase chain reaction (PCR) has greatly improved the detection of HSV infection at all ages, including the neonate. However, as many as 25% of the infants with proven CNS HSV infections have negative PCR studies of the cerebrospinal fluid. Despite impressive advances in the development of antiviral therapies and in the medical management of infants with perinatal HSV infections, many infants die or have permanent neurodevelopmental disabilities. Early recognition of HSV infection remains a major barrier in improving the outcome of this potentially devastating infection. This chapter describes the virology, epidemiology, clinical features, diagnosis, management and prognosis for infants with HSV infections (Table 1).

Virology

Though certain clinical manifestations of human herpes have been recognized since the Greco-Roman era, the precise nature of the infectious agents and the spectrum

Table 1

Morbidity and mortality in neonatal HSV infections[a]

Disease category	Mortality[b] (%)	Morbidity[c] (%)
SEM	0	<5
Disseminated infection	50	25
CNS infection (encephalitis)	~15	70
Congenital infection	~30	>90

[a]Adapted from Kimberlin et al., 2001a; Whitley et al., 1980b; Hutto et al., 1987.
[b]Percent of HSV-infected infants who died by 1 year of age.
[c]Percent of the surviving infants with mild, moderate or severe ophthalmologic or neurodevelopmental sequelae at 1 year of age (mild = ocular sequelae, speech or mild motor delay; moderate = hemiparesis, epilepsy, <3-month developmental delay; severe—microcephaly, spastic quadriplegia, blindness/chorioretinitis, >3-month developmental delay (see Kimberlin, 2001 for additional details)]

of disease caused by these viruses were not fully established until the 20th century. In the 1930s neonatal HSV infections were initially described (Batignani, 1934; Haas, 1935). With the advent of electron microscopy and techniques of modern molecular biology, HSV types 1 and 2 were identified as enveloped, icosahedral, double-stranded DNA viruses with linear genomes of approximately 150,000 base pairs. HSV-1 and HSV-2 display approximately 50% nucleotide homology, and each encodes for approximately 70 proteins (Taylor et al., 2002; Kimberlin, 2004a). Of the eight human herpesviruses identified to date (HSV-1, HSV-2, cytomegalovirus, Epstein–Barr virus, varicella-zoster virus, and human herpesviruses 6, 7, and 8), HSV-1 and HSV-2 serve as the prototypes for the herpesviridae.

HSV-1 and HSV-2 can infect numerous cell types of both humans and animals. Virus glycoproteins (g), especially gB and gD, interact with heparin sulfate molecules on the host cell surface to initiate adherence to host cells and virus entry (Taylor et al., 2002; Kimberlin 2004a). Upon infection of human cells HSV-1 and HSV-2 replicate via a highly regulated molecular cascade involving host cell elements and immediate-early (alpha), early (beta), and late (gamma) genes encoded by the viruses (Taylor et al., 2002). DNA replication and initial virus assembly occur in the cell nucleus; the herpesviruses become enveloped as the virus particles emerge through the nuclear membrane. The viral DNA encodes for several glycoproteins, as well as other polypeptides, that contribute to virus infectivity and participate in host immune responses to the virus.

Acute primary maternal infection with HSV-1 or HSV-2 occurs without symptoms or causes localized disease of the oropharyngeal or genital areas. Either virus can be detected at either site. When mucocutaneous replication continues unabated in neonates, viremia ensues, leading to dissemination of HSV to numerous target organs, including the brain, liver, or lung. Virus replication in host tissues produces lytic infection and hemorrhagic necrosis. As with other members of the herpesvirus family, HSV-1 and HSV-2 establish latent infections of host cells, typically sensory neurons, and periodically reactivate, producing mucocutaneous lesions or systemic disease (Taylor et al., 2002).

Epidemiology

The incidence of neonatal HSV infections ranges from 1 per 3000 to 1 per 40,000 live-born infants per year (Stone et al., 1989; Brown, 2004; Kimberlin, 2004a). This corresponds to approximately 500–2000 HSV-infected infants annually in the United States. In certain regions, such as Australia or the United Kingdom, the incidence of neonatal HSV is lower, apparently because of a lower seroprevalence of HSV-2 among women of child-bearing age (Brown, 2004; Freedman et al., 2004). Approximately two-thirds of neonatal cases result from infections with HSV-2, with the remainder due to HSV-1. During the past two decades the number of neonatal infections due to HSV-1 has increased considerably (Roberts, 2005), reflecting changing sexual behaviors and increasing numbers of women with genital HSV-1 infections (Lafferty et al., 2000).

The seroprevalence of HSV-2, the more common cause of neonatal infection, among women in the United States has risen steadily during the past three decades (Fleming et al., 1997; Buchacz et al., 2000; Armstrong et al., 2001). Nearly 30% of 30-year-old men and women have serologic evidence of prior HSV-2 infection (Fleming et al., 1997). Most seropositive persons have no history of genital herpes. HSV-2 seropositivity among women in the United States is associated with African-American race, Mexican-American ethnicity, poverty, greater lifetime number of sexual partners, earlier age of sexual intercourse, and drug use (Fleming et al., 1997; Sucato et al., 2001). Risk factors for HSV-2 acquisition by men include not using condoms and having sex when the female partner has active genital herpes (Rana et al., 2005).

Approximately 2% of adult women acquire HSV-2 annually (Fleming et al., 1997; Buchacz et al., 2000; Lafferty et al., 2000; Armstrong et al., 2001). Primary HSV-2 infection usually occurs without recognizable symptoms; up to 80% of women with HSV-infected infants lack histories of genital herpes (Brown et al., 1997; Kimberlin, 2004a). When primary HSV-2 infection occurs during pregnancy, women have increased risks of spontaneous abortion, still birth, or premature labor (Brown et al., 1997). Women can shed HSV-2 in the cervix asymptomatically after primary or recurrent (reactivated) infections, exposing infants to HSV-2 during passage through infected birth canals. Neonates can acquire HSV-1 during delivery by contact with infected cervical secretions or less often, by postnatal contact with persons with active oral HSV-1 infections. The majority of infants (> 80%) acquire HSV-1 or HSV-2 during the birth process (Brown, 2004; Kimberlin, 2004a); postnatal infection causes approximately 10% of neonatal HSV infections. As many as 40% of infants with neonatal HSV infections have had fetal scalp monitors placed during labor and delivery (Sucato et al., 2001; Brown, 2004), suggesting that this procedure facilitates virus entry and neonatal infection.

Clinical features

Neonatal HSV infections are categorized into three clinical syndromes (Whitley et al., 1980b; Koskiniemi et al., 1989; Kimberlin et al., 2001a; Kimberlin, 2004a,b): (1) mucocutaneous infection (skin, eye and/or mouth (SEM) involvement without obvious signs of disseminated or CNS disease), usually labeled SEM infection; (2) disseminated infections, during which the virus affects numerous tissues or organs; and (3) encephalitis with or without recognized skin lesions. Approximately 5–10% of HSV-infected neonates have congenital infections (Montgomery et al., 1973; Chalhub et al., 1977; Hutto et al., 1987; Grose 1994). Infants with either SEM or disseminated infections usually become symptomatic at an average age of 10–12 days, whereas infants with encephalitis are an average age of ~17 days at presentation (Whitley et al., 1980b; Kimberlin et al., 2001a). However, signs or symptoms of HSV infections, especially those acquired *in utero*, can be evident on the first day of life (Koskiniemi et al., 1989).

Skin, eye, and/or mouth infections

Mucocutanous infections currently account for approximately 45% of all neonatal HSV disease (Kimberlin, 2004a). This proportion has risen coincident with improved recognition and management of neonatal herpes (Whitley et al., 1988; Kimberlin et al., 2001a). Infants with SEM infections can have conjunctivitis, keratitis, or vesicular rash. The cutaneous rash consists of single lesions or clusters of vesicles (Fig. 1), often appearing first on the presenting part of the infant (i.e. face or head in vertex deliveries; buttocks in breech deliveries). Rarely, HSV infection localizes to the laryngeal mucosa and produces stridor (Sharp et al., 1998). Infants with pure SEM infections lack signs of systemic or neurologic infections, such as hepatitis, pneumonitis, coagulopathy, seizures, or CSF abnormalities (Kimberlin, 2004a,b).

Disseminated disease

Disseminated HSV infections currently account for approximately 25% of neonatal HSV infections and begin with poor feeding, temperature instability, irritability, or lethargy (Whitley et al., 1980b, 1988; Kimberlin et al., 2001a; Kimberlin, 2004a). These signs and symptoms may be subtle during the early stages of infection and mimic enteroviral or bacterial disease. Later signs of disseminated neonatal HSV infection include fever, jaundice, tachypnea, petechiae, or vesicular rash, although the absence of rash or fever does not eliminate HSV from consideration. As many as 40% of infants with disseminated HSV infections do not have vesicular rashes that might suggest HSV (Arvin et al., 1982; Kimberlin et al., 2001a). With disease progression, hypotension, acidosis, cardio-respiratory failure, and organ dysfunction, such as liver or renal insufficiency, adrenalitis, pneumonitis, seizures, and disseminated intravascular coagulopathy (DIC), may develop (Whitley et al., 1980b;

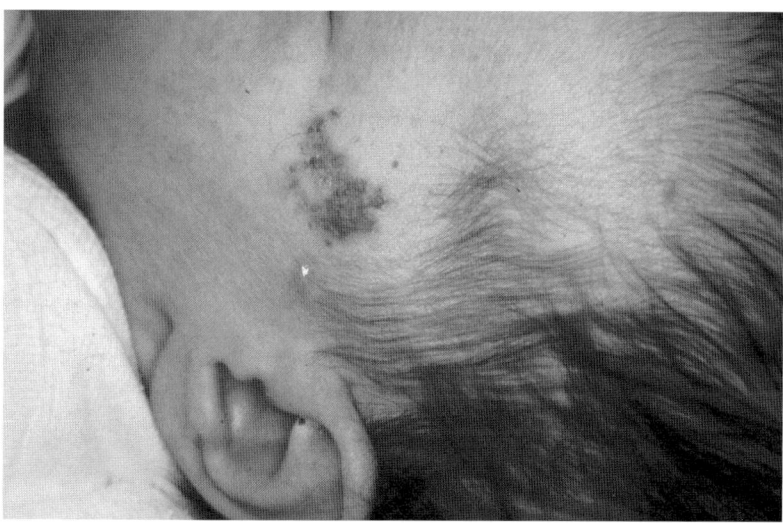

Fig. 1 Facial vesicular rash indicative of neonatal HSV infection (for color version: see color section on page 262). (Photograph courtesy of Andrew Pavia, Division of Infectious Diseases, Department of Pediatrics, University of Utah School of Medicine.)

Anderson, 1987; Kimberlin et al., 2001a). The presence of pneumonia is particularly concerning as these neonates can experience early respiratory failure and have a more severe course (Meyer et al., 1997).

Encephalitis

Approximately 30% of neonates with HSV infections have encephalitis with or without skin lesions (Whitley et al., 1980b; Arvin et al., 1982; Kimberlin, 2004a). CNS manifestations, such as seizures, lethargy, or coma, can also be part of disseminated neonatal HSV infections. The early signs of HSV encephalitis, like those of disseminated infections, can be non-specific, consisting only of poor oral intake, temperature instability, fussiness, or inactivity. As the disease progresses, neurologic features, such as apnea, lethargy, coma, seizures, or hypotonia appear. More than half of the infants with encephalitis have seizures, either partial (focal) or generalized, and approximately 50% are lethargic (Kimberlin et al., 2001a). Approximately two-thirds of infants with HSV encephalitis have skin vesicles (Arvin et al., 1982; Kimberlin et al., 2001a); a small number have pneumonia or conjunctivitis (Kimberlin et al., 2001a).

Congenital infection

Approximately 5% of HSV-infected neonates acquire the virus, typically HSV-2, *in utero* (Hutto et al., 1987); roughly 1 of every 300,000 live born infants has congenital HSV disease (Baldwin and Whitley, 1989). Infants with congenital HSV infections closely resemble neonates with other intrauterine infections, especially the fetal varicella syndrome (Grose, 1994; Cliff et al., 1997). HSV-infected infants have a relatively characteristic disorder with vesicular skin lesions or scarring at birth, chorioretinitis, cataracts, optic atrophy or microphthalmia, and microcephaly, hydranencephaly, cystic encephalomalacia, or intracranial calcifications. Approximately 60% of the infants have ophthalmologic abnormalities; 25% have intrauterine growth retardation (Hutto et al., 1987). In rare instances, segmental cutaneous scarring may be the only sign of intrauterine HSV infection (Cliff et al., 1997), further underscoring the potential similarities between congenital HSV infection and varicella embryopathy (Grose, 1994).

Laboratory studies and diagnosis

Routine laboratory studies

Infants with disseminated or CNS HSV infections can have thrombocytopenia, hemolytic anemia, elevated serum transaminases, metabolic acidosis, or CSF abnormalities consisting of a mixed pleocytosis, xanthochromia, modest hypoglycorrachia, and an elevated protein content (Whitley et al., 1980b; Koskiniemi et al., 1989; Kimberlin et al., 2001a). Infants with severe disseminated HSV infections may have laboratory evidence of DIC, and chest radiographs may reveal pneumonitis (Anderson, 1987). Infants with encephalitis have CSF abnormalities, as above, and may have elevated serum transaminases, reflecting seeding of the liver during hematogenous dissemination of the virus. By contrast, infants with SEM infections, by definition, have normal laboratory studies.

Microbiologic studies

Infants with suspected HSV infection should undergo virus cultures at multiple sites, including the conjunctiva, oropharynx, rectum, circulating leukocytes, CSF, and skin. Neonatal infection can be confirmed by isolating HSV-1 or 2 from any of these sites. Conjunctiva cultures have the highest yield (>90%) in neonatal HSV infections; the yield of oropharyngeal cultures is less (~40%) (Kimberlin et al., 2001a). Herpes simplex virus can be detected in CSF samples in 40–50% of infants with CNS involvement (Koskiniemi et al., 1989; Kimberlin, 2001). HSV types 1 and 2 grow rapidly, usually enabling a specific diagnosis within 72–96 h. For maximum sensitivity, cultures should be obtained prior to acyclovir treatment (however, CSF PCR can remain positive for HSV DNA for 24–48 h or longer after initiation of acyclovir therapy).

The diagnosis of HSV infection can be established specifically by studying cerebrospinal, serum, or vesicle fluid using the PCR (Kimberlin et al., 1996a; Diamond et al., 1999; Romero and Kimberlin, 2003). Emerging PCR methods can also be used to distinguish HSV-1 and HSV-2 (Corey et al., 2005; Issa et al., 2005). The likelihood of detecting HSV in CSF depends greatly upon the category of infection. In one study, positive CSF results were observed in 93% and 76% of the infants with disseminated and CNS disease, respectively (Kimberlin et al., 1996a). Remarkably, HSV DNA can also be detected in the CSF of approximately one-quarter of the infants categorized as SEM infections. The latter data may explain why occasional infants with SEM infections have neurodevelopmental sequelae, as discussed further below. HSV DNA can be detected in the serum of approximately two-thirds of neonates with proven HSV infections (Diamond et al., 1999; Malm et al., 1999). Such data clearly indicate that negative PCR results must be interpreted cautiously.

Neurodiagnostic studies

Because neonatal herpes encephalitis results from hematogenous dissemination of the virus to the brain, neurodiagnostic studies (electroencephalography (EEG), computed-tomography (CT), or magnetic resonance imaging (MRI)) usually reveal diffuse or multifocal abnormalities (Mizrahi and Tharp, 1982; Chang et al., 1990; Bale, 1999). In the natural history study performed by the National Institutes of Health-sponsored Collaborative Antiviral Study Group (CASG) 82% (36 of 44) of the infants with neonatal HSV encephalitis had abnormal EEGs, and 65% (31 of 48 infants) had abnormal imaging studies compatible with HSV infection (Kimberlin et al., 2001a). Early features of CNS involvement consist of brain edema (Fig. 2), and infants who survive disseminated infection or HSV encephalitis may later show cystic encephalomalacia, intracranial calcifications, or diffuse brain atrophy (Chang et al., 1990). Infants with congenital HSV infections have intracranial calcifications of the deep nuclei, cortical dysplasia, and cystic encephalomalacia (Hutto et al., 1987; Bale, 1999).

Treatment

Prevention

In neonatal herpes simplex virus infections the majority of mothers (up to 80%) do not recall having herpes infections, making prevention by obstetrical measures complex (Leung and Sacks, 2003; Brown, 2004; Kimberlin, 2004a). Serologic studies employing type-specific assays can identify sexually active women at high risk (i.e., HSV seronegative) as well as HSV-2 seropositive women who may benefit from close monitoring for active genital herpes (Brown, 2004). However, serial viral cultures in women with histories of genital herpes are not cost effective (Brown, 2004). Behavioral strategies, such as abstinence or condom use, that might reduce acquisition of HSV by women during pregnancy have considerable appeal, but such measures are difficult to implement (Brown, 2004).

Cesarean section can reduce the risk of HSV infection among infants born to mothers with active HSV lesions or prodromal symptoms suggesting genital HSV

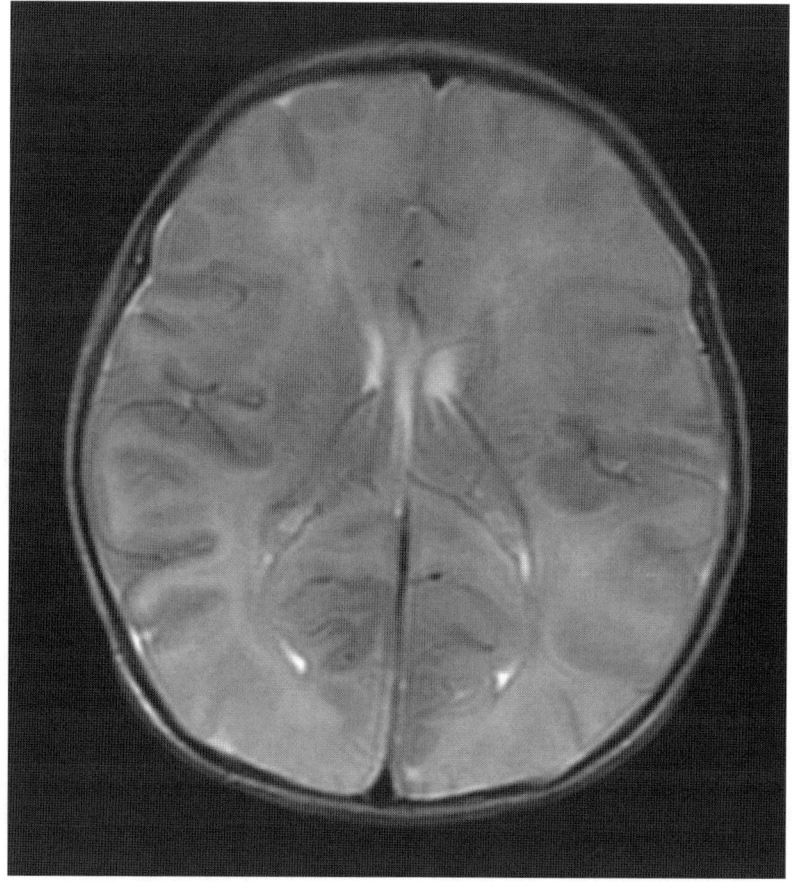

Fig. 2 Axial T2-weighted MRI shows diffuse loss of the cortical ribbon, especially posteriorly, indicating cerebral edema secondary to neonatal HSV encephalitis.

infection (Brown, 2004; Kimberlin, 2004a). In a prospective study of >40,000 women Brown and colleagues reported that Cesarean section significantly reduced the risk of neonate HSV infections among women from whom HSV was isolated during labor (Brown et al., 2003). However, some infants acquire HSV despite Cesarean section (Brown et al., 2003; Brown, 2004; Gallardo et al., 2005). Brown and colleagues conclude that neonatal infections could also be reduced by limiting the use of invasive fetal monitors in HSV-2 seropositive women and in women shedding HSV at the time of delivery (Brown, 2004). Limited data regarding the use of acyclovir during maternal HSV infections indicate that the drug modifies the clinical course of maternal genital herpes (Greenspoon et al., 1994; Scott, 1999; Scott et al., 2001, 2002; Brown, 2004); data are insufficient regarding an effect on HSV transmission to the neonate (Brown, 2004). No vaccine is available to prevent

HSV infections, although modest efficacy has been observed with subunit vaccines based on HSV-2 gD (Stanberry, 2004).

Pharmacologic treatment of neonates

In 1980, vidarabine (adenine arabinoside) was found to be beneficial in neonatal herpes simplex virus infections in a randomized controlled trial (Whitley et al., 1980a; Whitley, 1993). Approximately 10 years later, acyclovir (9-[(2-hydro-xyethoxy)methyl]guanine) was shown to be equally effective when compared with vidarabine in a multicenter, controlled trial of the CASG (Whitley et al., 1991a) Acyclovir, a well-tolerated antiviral drug, relies upon an HSV-encoded thymidine kinase to phosphorylate the drug to the active triphosphate form which inhibits viral DNA replication in infected cells. Acyclovir, using 30 mg/kg/day for 10–14 days, became the accepted approach in the early 1990s.

Because mortality and morbidity remained unacceptably high in severe disseminated and CNS HSV infections in neonates despite treatment with acyclovir, the CASG subsequently investigated the benefits of higher dose (60 mg/kg/day versus the previous standard of 30 mg/kg/day) and longer duration (21 days in CNS and disseminated infections versus 10–14 days) of acyclovir. An open labeled study determined that infants with disseminated HSV infections had improved survival when treated with high dose acyclovir (Kimberlin et al., 2001b), although morbidity remained problematic. Currently, high-dose acyclovir is the standard for treating infants with neonatal HSV infections (Kimberlin, 2001, 2004a; Kimberlin et al., 2001a,b).

Infants with suspected or proven HSV infections should receive acyclovir 60 mg/kg/day in divided doses every 8 h for 14 days if infections are SEM only and for a minimum of 21 days if the infection is disseminated or involves the CNS (Whitley, 1993; Kimberlin, 2004a). If the CSF has not been studied by culture or PCR, infants require 21 days of treatment (Kimberlin, 2004a). Because high-dose acyclovir therapy can cause marrow suppression and neutropenia, complete blood cell counts should be monitored twice weekly during acyclovir therapy (Kimberlin, 2004a). Significant neutropenia (absolute neutrophil counts $< 500/\mu l$) may require reductions in the acyclovir dose or therapy with granulocyte colony-stimulating factor.

Because improved outcome of neonatal HSV infections correlates with the early initiation of acyclovir therapy, parenteral treatment should begin as soon as the diagnosis of neonatal HSV infection is considered (Fig. 3) (Kimberlin, 2001; Sucato et al., 2001). However, given the subtlety of the early features of neonatal HSV infection, timely recognition of HSV infection remains a serious barrier for improving outcome (Fidler et al., 2004; Handsfield et al., 2005; Kimberlin and Whitley, 2005).

Infants who recover from neonatal HSV infections often have mucocutaneous reactivations (Fig. 4). Infants who initially have skin–eye–mucous membrane infections only and later experience three or more cutaneous reactivations have an

L. Miner, J.F. Bale Jr.

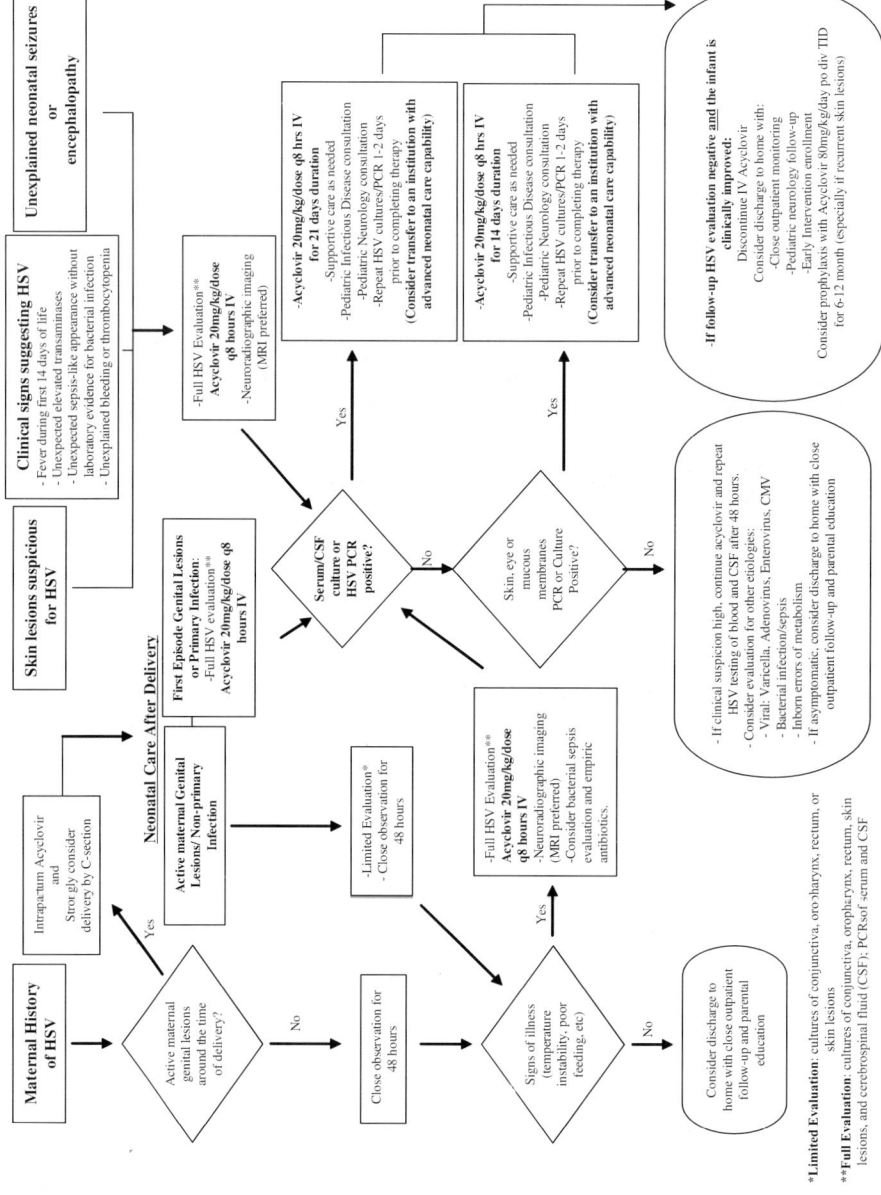

Fig. 3 Algorithmic approach to the diagnosis and management of suspected neonatal HSV infections.

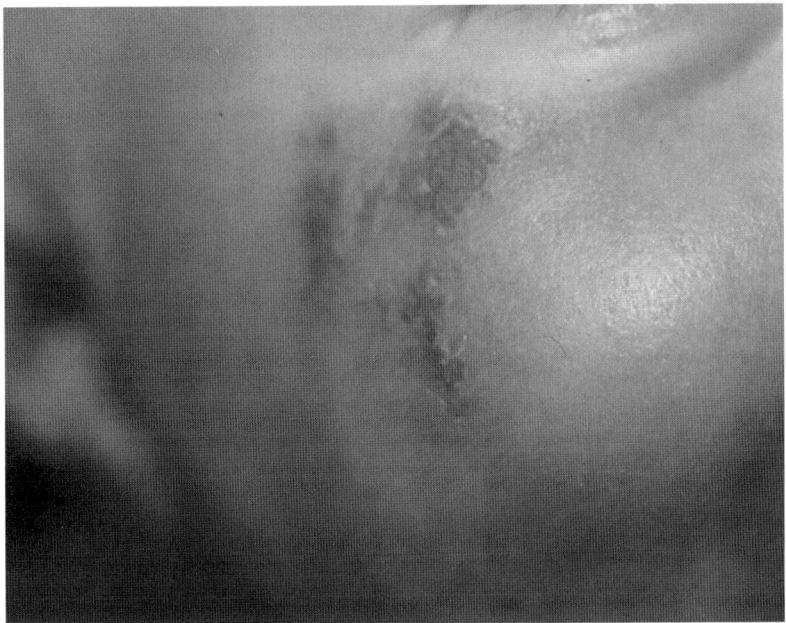

Fig. 4 Recurrent HSV rash in a young infant with a history of neonatal HSV infection (for color version: see color section on page 262). (Photograph courtesy of Andrew Pavia, Division of Infectious Diseases, Department of Pediatrics, University of Utah School of Medicine.)

increased risk of long-term neurodevelopmental sequelae (Kimberlin et al., 2001a). This presumably occurs because viremia develops during reactivations, and the virus invades the CNS. To address this problem, the role of suppressive antiviral therapy after treatment of neonatal HSV infections is being investigated. In placebo-controlled trials, oral acyclovir is administered to HSV-infected infants for six months (Kimberlin et al., 1996b). Information regarding this and other trials of HSV therapy can be obtained from the National Institutes of Health Collaborative Antiviral Study Group, Birmingham, AL [(205) 934-5316]. Because myelosuppression and nephrotoxicity are potential side effects of prolonged acyclovir therapy, laboratory studies should be obtained periodically.

Prognosis

The prognosis of neonatal HSV infection depends on the severity of the organ involvement and the response to acyclovir therapy (Kimberlin, 2004a). Infants who are detected early and treated aggressively with acyclovir generally fare better. Adverse neurologic sequelae occur rarely in infants with disease restricted to the skin, eyes, and mucous membranes (Whitley et al., 1980a; Whitley et al., 1991b; Kimberlin et al., 2001a); none of the infants with SEM infections treated in the acyclovir era have died. In nearly two decades of study by the CASG, 98% of the infants ($N = 48$) with SEM infections had normal development at 12 months of age.

By contrast, infants with encephalitis or disseminated disease have high rates of mortality and morbidity even with appropriate antiviral therapy (Whitley, 1991b). In the CASG studies, spanning nearly two decades 53% of the infants with disseminated infections and nearly 13% of the infants with CNS infections (encephalitis) died despite acyclovir therapy (Kimberlin, 2001). Prematurity, seizures, and lethargy are clinical factors associated with higher mortality rates. Only 30% of the infants who survived HSV encephalitis (13 of 43) and 75% of infants who survived disseminated infections (18 of 24) were normal at 1 year of age (Kimberlin, 2001). Among infants who survive CNS or disseminated HSV infections, seizures are associated with a higher likelihood of adverse outcomes.

Infants with congenital HSV infection have high rates of death and permanent neurodevelopmental sequelae (Hutto et al., 1987; Grose, 1994). In the study of Hutto and colleagues, ~30% of the infants with intrauterine HSV infections died, and none were developing normally at 2 years of age (Hutto et al., 1987). Sequelae include cerebral palsy, epilepsy, developmental delay and blindness.

References

Anderson RD. Herpes simplex virus infection of the neonatal respiratory tract. Am J Dis Child 1987; 141: 274–276.

Armstrong GL, Schillinger J, Markowitz L, et al. Incidence of herpes simplex virus type 2 infection in the United States. Am J Epidemiol 2001; 153: 912–920.

Arvin A, Yeager AS, Bruhn FW, Grossman M. Neonatal herpes simplex infection in the absence of mucocutaneous lesions.. J Pediatr 1982; 100: 715–721.

Baldwin S, Whitley RJ. Teratogen update: intrauterine herpes simplex virus infection. Teratology 1989; 39: 1–10.

Bale Jr. JF. Human herpesviruses and neurological disorders of childhood. Semin Pediatr Neurol 1999; 6: 278–287.

Batignani A. Congiuntivite da virus erpectico in neonato. Boll Ocul 1934; 1217–1220.

Brown ZA. Preventing herpes simplex virus transmission to the neonate. Herpes 2004; 11: 175A–185A.

Brown ZA, Selke S, Zeh J, et al. The acquisition of herpes simplex virus during pregnancy. N Engl J Med 1997; 337: 509–515.

Brown ZA, Wald A, Morrow RA, et al. Effect of serologic status and cesarean delivery on transmission rates of herpes simplex virus from mother to infant. JAMA 2003; 289: 203–209.

Buchacz K, McFarland W, Hernandez M, et al. Prevalence and correlates of herpes simplex virus type 2 infection in a population-based survey of young women in low-income neighborhoods of Northern California. The Young Women's Survey Team. Sex Transm Dis 2000; 27: 393–400.

Chalhub EG, Baenziger J, Feigen RD, et al. Congenital herpes simplex type II infection with extensive hepatic calcification, bone lesions, and cataracts: complete post-mortem examination. Develop Med Child Neurol 1977; 19: 527–534.

Chang Y, Soffer D, Horoupina DS, Weiss JM. Evolution of post-natal herpes simplex virus encephalitis to multicystic encephalomalacia. Acta Neuropathol 1990; 80: 666–670.

Cliff S, Osterle LS, Haque KS, et al. Segmental scarring following intrauterine herpes simplex virus infection. Clin Exp Dermatol 1997; 22: 96–98.

Corey L, Huang ML, Selke S, Wald A. Differentiation of herpes simplex virus types 1 and 2 in clinical samples by a real-time taqman PCR assay. J Med Virol 2005; 76: 350–355.

Diamond C, Mohan K, Hobson A, et al. Viremia in neonatal herpes simplex virus infection. Pediatr Infect Dis J 1999; 18: 487–489.

Fidler KJ, Pierce CM, Cubitt WD, et al. Could neonatal disseminated herpes simplex virus infections be treated earlier? J Infect 2004; 49: 141–146.

Fleming AL, McQuillan GM, Johnson RE, et al. Herpes simplex virus type 2 in the United States, 1976 to 1994. N Engl J Med 1997; 337: 1105–11011.

Freedman E, Mindel A, Jones CA. Epidemiological, clinical and laboratory aids for the diagnosis of neonatal herpes—an Australian perspective. Herpes 2004; 11: 38–44.

Gallardo MJ, Johnson DA, Gaviria J, et al. Isolated herpes simplex keratoconjunctivitis in a neonate born by cesarean delivery. JAAPOS 2005; 9: 285–287.

Greenspoon JS, Wilcox JC, Hutchinson LB, et al. Acyclovir for disseminated herpes simplex virus in pregnancy A case report. J Reprod Med 1994; 39: 311–317.

Grose C. Congenital infections caused by varicella zoster virus and herpes simplex virus. Sem Pediatr Neurol 1994; 1: 43–49.

Haas GM. Hepato-renal necrosis with intranuclear inclusion bodies: a case report. Am J Pathol 1935; 11: 127–142.

Handsfield HH, Waldo AB, Brown ZA, et al. Neonatal herpes should be a reportable disease. Sex Transm Dis 2005; 32: 521–525.

Hutto C, Arvin A, Jacobs R, et al. Intrauterine herpes simplex virus infections. J Pediatr 1987; 110: 97–101.

Issa NC, Espy MJ, Uhl JR, Smith TF. Sequencing and resolution of amplified herpes simplex virus DNA with intermediate melting curves as genotype 1 or 2 by LightCycler PCR assay. J Clin Microbiol 2005; 43: 1843–1845.

Kimberlin D, Whitley R. Neonatal herpes: what have we learned. Semin Pediatr Infect Dis 2005; 16: 7–16.

Kimberlin DW. Advances in the treatment of neonatal herpes simplex virus infections. Rev Med Virol 2001; 11: 157–163.

Kimberlin DW. Neonatal herpes simplex infection. Microbiol Rev 2004a; 17: 1–13.

Kimberlin DW. Herpes simplex virus, meningitis and encephalitis in the neonate. Herpes 2004b; 11(Suppl 2): 65A–76A.

Kimberlin DW, Lakeman FD, Arvin AM, et al. Application of the polymerase chain reaction to the diagnosis and management of neonatal herpes simplex virus disease. J Infect Dis 1996a; 174: 1162–1167.

Kimberlin DW, Lin C-Y, Jacobs RF, et al. Natural history of neonatal herpes simplex virus infections in the acyclovir era. Pediatrics 2001a; 108: 223–229.

Kimberlin DW, Lin C-Y, Jacobs RF, et al. Safety and efficacy of high-dose intravenous acyclovir in the management of neonatal herpes simplex virus infections. Pediatrics 2001b; 108: 230–238.

Kimberlin DW, Powell D, Gruber W, et al. Administration of oral acyclovir suppressive therapy after neonatal herpes simplex disease limited to skin, eyes, and mouth: results of a phase I/II trial. Pediatr Infect Dis J 1996b; 15: 247–254.

Koskiniemi M, Happonen JM, Jarvenpaa AL, et al. Neonatal herpes simplex virus infection: a report of 43 patients. Pediatr Infect Dis J 1989; 8: 30–35.

Lafferty WEL, Downey C, Celum C, Wald A. Herpes simplex virus type 1 as a cause of genital herpes: impact on surveillance and prevention. J Infect Dis 2000; 181: 1454–1457.

Leung DT, Sacks SL. Current treatment options to prevent perinatal transmission of herpes simplex virus. Expert Opin Pharmacother 2003; 10: 1809–1819.

Malm G, Forsgren M. Neonatal herpes simplex virus infections: HSV DNA in cerebrospinal fluid and serum. Arch Dis Child Fetal Neonatal Ed 1999; 81: F24–F29.

Meyer TA, Warner BW. Extracorporeal life support for the treatment of viral pneumonia: collective experience from the ELSO registry. Extracorporeal Life Support Organization. J Pediatr Surg 1997; 32: 232–236.

Mizrahi EM, Tharp BR. A characteristic EEG pattern in neonatal herpes simplex encephalitis. Neurology 1982; 32: 1215–1220.

Montgomery JR, Flanders RW, Yow MD. Congenital anomalies and herpesvirus infection. Am J Dis Child 1973; 126: 364–366.

Rana RK, Pimenta JM, Rosenberg DM, et al. Demographic, behavioral and knowledge factors associated with herpes simplex virus type 2 infection among men whose current female partner has genital herpes. Sex Transm Dis 2005; 32: 308–313.

Roberts C. Genital herpes in young adults: changing sexual behaviors, epidemiology and management. Herpes 2005; 12: 10–14.

Romero JR, Kimberlin DW. Molecular diagnosis of viral infections of the central nervous system. Clin Lab Med 2003; 23: 843–865.

Scott LL. Prevention of perinatal herpes: prophylactic antiviral therapy? Clin Obstet Gynecol 1999; 42: 134–148.

Scott LL, Hollier LM, McIntire D, et al. Acyclovir suppression to prevent clinical recurrences at delivery after first episode genital herpes in pregnancy: an open-label trial. Infect Dis Obstet Gynecol 2001; 9: 75–80.

Scott LL, Hollier LM, McIntire D, et al. Acyclovir suppression to prevent recurrent genital herpes at delivery. Infect Dis Obstet Gynecol 2002; 10: 71–77.

Sharp HR, Blaney SP, Morrison GA. Neonatal stridor in association with herpes simplex infection of the larynx. J Laryngol Otol 1998; 112: 1192–1193.

Stanberry LR. Clinical trials of prophylactic and therapeutic herpes simplex virus vaccines. Herpes 2004; 11(Suppl 3): 161A–169A.

Stone K, Brooks C, Guinan M, et al. National surveillance for neonatal herpes simplex virus infections. Sex Transm Dis 1989; 16: 152–156.

Sucato G, Celum C, Dithmer D, et al. Demographic rather than behavioral risk factors predict herpes simplex virus type 2 infection in sexually active adolescents. Pediatr Infect Dis J 2001; 20: 422–426.

Taylor TJ, Brockman MA, McNamee EE, Knipe DM. Herpes simplex virus. Front Biosci 2002; 7: d752–d764.

Whitley RJ. Neonatal herpes simplex virus infections. J Med Virol 1993; Suppl; 1: 13–21.

Whitley R, Arvin A, Prober C, et al. A controlled trial comparing vidarabine with acyclovir in neonatal herpes simplex virus infection. N Engl J Med 1991a; 324: 444–449.

Whitley R, Arvin A, Prober C, et al. Predictors of morbidity and mortality in neonates with herpes simplex virus infections. The National Institute of Allergy and Infectious Diseases Collaborative Antiviral Study Group. N Engl J Med 1991b; 324: 450–454.

Whitley RJ, Corey L, Arvin A, et al. Changing presentation of herpes simplex virus infection in neonates. J Infect Dis 1988; 158: 109–116.

Whitley RJ, Nahmias AJ, Soong SJ, et al. Vidarabine therapy of neonatal herpes simplex virus infection. Pediatrics 1980a; 66: 495–501.

Whitley RJ, Nahmias AJ, Visintine AM, et al. The natural history of herpes simplex virus infection of mother and newborn. Pediatrics 1980b; 66: 489–494.

Congenital and Other Related Infectious
Diseases of the Newborn
Isa K. Mushahwar (Editor)
© 2007 Elsevier B.V. All rights reserved
DOI 10.1016/S0168-7069(06)13003-7

Epidemiology of Herpes Viruses 6 and 7 in Children

Asad Ansari[a], Adriana Weinberg[b]

[a]*Avera Children's Hospital and Department of Pediatrics, University of South Dakota, Sioux Falls, SD, USA*
[b]*University of Colorado Health Sciences Center, Denver, CO, USA*

Abstract

Human herpes viruses (HHV) 6 and 7 are two of three recently identified members of the human herpes virus family. They infect most of the human population by early childhood and exhibit properties similar to other herpes viruses including life-long infection, asymptomatic shedding and periodic reactivations during periods of immune suppression, which may or may not be clinically relevant. The asymptomatic shedding, mainly in the saliva, is the major source of transmission, and hence a formidable barrier to disruption of transmission. These viruses cause self-limited infections in immunocompetent individuals, but have been associated with serious morbidity and mortality in immunocompromised hosts, especially HHV-6B. Patients with immunosuppression may be treated with manipulation of the immune system and use of antiviral medications. No vaccine candidate is being currently studied for either of the two viruses.

The viruses

Salahuddin et al. (1986) first isolated the human herpes virus (HHV) 6 from peripheral blood leukocytes of patients with lymphoproliferative diseases. In 1988, HHV-6 was linked to the childhood illness, roseola or exanthem subitum aka the sixth disease (Yamanishi et al., 1988). The virus measures 160–200 nm in diameter with a capsid of 90–110 nm and a genome of 162–162 kb (Braun et al., 1997; Campadelli-Fiume et al., 1999; Abdel-Haq and Asmar, 2004; Grose, 2004; De Bolle et al., 2005) (Image 1). A major research focus has been the five identified

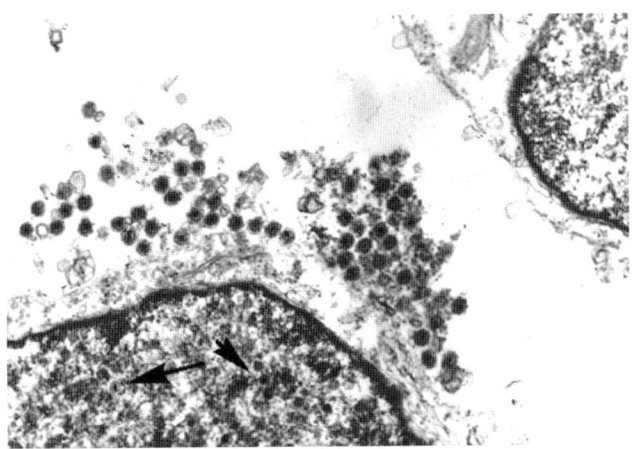

Image 1 HSB-2 cell lines are infected with HHV-6 (GS strain) and processed for electron microscopy at day 6. Arrows show HHV-6 capsids in the nucleus. Partially enveloped virus can be seen in the remains of the cytoplasm. With permission from Dr. Janos Luka, Ph.D, associate professor, Department of Pathology, Eastern Virginia Medical School (1993 to present). http://herpesvirus.tripod.com/gallery/pictures/electro/0001.jpg

glycoproteins of which glycoprotein H (gH) is thought to mediate viral entry and virus-induced cell fusion. HHV-6 utilizes gH to bind to a wide variety of cells through the widely distributed cell surface CD46 receptor but preferentially CD4 + T lymphocytes (Mori et al., 2002, 2003; Santoro et al., 2003). Molecular, biological and immunological differences between various isolates have resulted in two distinct variants: A (prototype strains are U1102 and GS) and B (prototype strains are Z29 and HST). Further comparison of the genome of HHV-6A and 6B sequences indicates between 95% and 98% homology in the middle portion of the genome with subsequent sequential decrease in the region of termini and immediate-early-1 region where divergence reaches 31% at the nucleotide level (Dominguez et al., 1999; Isegawa et al., 1999). Because of considerable differences, some researchers feel that they should be classified as two separate viruses (Ablashi et al., 1991; Aubin et al., 1993). Persistent infection with HHV-6 may involve true latent state (monocytes and early bone marrow progenitor cells) and a low-level chronic replication (salivary glands and brain tissue). HHV-6B has also been found in kidneys and genital secretions (Braun et al., 1997; Campadelli-Fiume et al., 1999; Ohashi et al., 2002; Abdel-Haq and Asmar, 2004; De Bolle et al., 2005).

Analysis of different genes and regions of HHV-6 variants show that intra-strain variation exists in DR regions (Thompson et al., 1994; De Bolle et al., 2005). This may account for reinfection with the same variant.

Frenkel et al. (1990) isolated HHV-7 after observing a cytopathic effect in culture of activated CD4 + T lymphocytes from healthy individuals. HHV-7 is 170 nm in diameter with a viral genome of 145 kb, which encodes for 84 different proteins including two major capsid proteins (Image 2). It shows homologies to

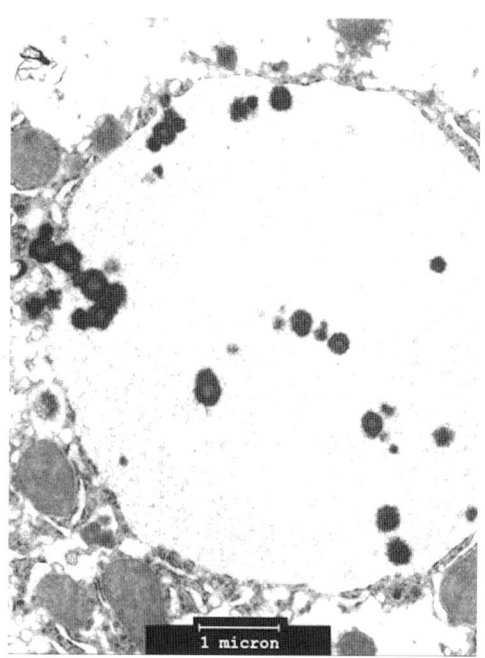

Image 2 Electron microscopic picture of a patient's liver biopsy showing HHV-7 engulfed by a large lysosome. With permission from Dr. Janos Luka, Ph.D, associate professor, Department of Pathology, Eastern Virginia Medical School (1993 to present). http://herpesvirus.tripod.com/gallery/pictures/electro/hhv-7liver2.JPG

HHV-6 and cytomegalovirus (CMV). Cell-surface receptor, CD4+ is necessary but not sufficient for infection and the virus persistently infects CD4+ T lymphocytes and salivary glands, and in HIV-infected individuals, macrophages (Lusso et al., 1994). However, the persistent, productive state of HHV-7 infection in the salivary glands contrasts with the latent infection that occurs in mononuclear cells. Asymptomatic shedding of HHV-7 DNA occurs in saliva, cervical secretions, mononuclear cells and breast milk (Fujisaki et al., 1998).

Both of these viruses belong to the beta subgroup of the human *herpesviridae* family along with human CMV, and share the common characteristics of containing double-stranded linear DNA, causing frequent human infections (except for HSV-2 and HHV-8) (De Bolle et al., 2005), and subsequently establishing the latency. This is followed by asymptomatic shedding and frequent reactivations when immune systems are stressed.

Epidemiology and pathogenesis

Humans are the only known hosts for HHV-6 and -7, although macaques and other monkey species have been successfully infected under experimental conditions

(Yalcin et al., 1992). A minority of HHV-6 infections, 1–2%, are deemed to be acquired *in utero* based on the encounter of viral DNA in the cord blood and other studies (Adams et al., 1998; Hall et al., 2004; Weinberg et al., 2005). However, transmission occurs primarily after birth via infected oral secretions with variant B causes the majority of early childhood infections, which are symptomatic. During the first few months of life, actively transported maternal antibodies may play a role in protecting most newborns against HHV-6 and -7 infections, along with other currently unknown factors (Ohashi et al., 2001; Sugimoto et al., 2002). Maternal antibodies against HHV-6 decline by 5–7 months of life, after which the infants start acquiring HHV-6B infection rapidly. Half of them acquire the infection in the second 6 months of life with the peak occurring between 9 and 21 months of life. It is unclear when infection with HHV-6A occurs, as it is typically asymptomatic. Maternal antibodies against HHV-7 decline slightly later and most of the children acquire HHV-7 by 3 years of age. Epidemiological serological surveys reveal that more than 95% of the adults in developed countries have been infected with HHV-6A and B and HHV-7, though antibody titers decline with age (De Bolle et al., 2005). Reinfections with similar variants of HHV-6 have been documented by genotypic analyses and may be related to intra-strain variation as reported earlier. The incubation period for HHV-6 is postulated to be between 7 and 14 days during which the child has asymptomatic viremia, followed by clinical illness in more than 90% of the children (Braun et al., 1997; Campadelli-Fiume et al., 1999; Abdel-Haq and Asmar, 2004; De Bolle et al., 2005). The major route of transmission for HHV-7, is oral secretions, and probably but less common, breast milk. Its incubation period is currently unknown (Pickering, 2003; Hall et al., 2004).

The role of these viruses in causing immunosuppression via downregulation of CD4+ T lymphocytes warrants more research, as secondary complications are still rare considering the widespread infections.

Clinical presentation

Congenital infection with HHV-6 differ from post-natal infections in terms of being mainly asymptomatic, demonstrating viral reactivation in 10% at birth, and frequent persistence of HHV-6 DNA in follow-up blood samples. One-third of congenital infections are HHV-6A (Hall et al., 2004). Sporadic cases of exanthema subitum, fulminant hepatitis, fatal pneumonitis with immunodeficiency and seizures with adverse outcome have been reported in the neonatal period, albeit rare (Knox et al., 1995; Mendel et al., 1995; Lanari et al., 2003; Yoshikawa et al., 2004). HHV-7 has not been associated with congenital and neonatal infections (Hall et al., 2004; Weinberg et al., 2005).

The majority of HHV-6B infections occur between the ages of 6 and 24 months, and are symptomatic. They includes an undifferentiated febrile or an afebrile illness, exanthem subitum or an afebrile exanthema subitum (Braun et al., 1997; Campadelli-Fiume et al., 1999; Abdel-Haq and Asmar, 2004; De Bolle et al., 2005; Ward, 2005). This has been recently reconfirmed by Zerr et al. (2005) who prospectively followed a cohort of 277 children from birth through 2 years with weekly testing of saliva for HHV-6. HHV-6 has also been associated with myelodysplastic syndrome, hemophagocytic syndrome, infectious mononucleosis, thrombocytopenia with and without purpura and in more rare instances, dilated cardiomyopathy and acute lymphadenitis including Rosai–Dorfman diseases (a rare, benign, pediatric lymphadenopathy) (Levine et al., 1992; Saijo et al, 1995; Syruckova et al., 1996; Yoshikawa et al., 2001; Hashimoto et al., 2002; Maric et al., 2004; Kagialis-Girard et al., 2005). Recently, a case of acute respiratory distress syndrome secondary to HHV-6 pneumonia has been described in an immunocompetent young female (Merk et al., 2005). HHV-6 has also been implicated in chronic fatigue syndrome without clear proof.

Roseola, which was first described by Zahorsky in 1913, typically involves fever up to 39–40°C for 2–4 days (may last up to 7 days), followed by a rash lasting from few hours to 4 days (Zahorsky, 1954). The rash may be papular, macular or maculopapular. Other associated findings may include diarrhea, Nagayama spots (papules on soft palate and uvula), otitis media, cough, cervical adenopathy, edematous eyelids, bulging fontanelle and seizures (Braun et al., 1997; Campadelli-Fiume et al., 1999; Abdel-Haq and Asmar, 2004; Grose, 2004; De Bolle et al., 2005).

HHV-6 has also been implicated in many different manifestations of central nervous system (CNS) illnesses including afebrile and febrile seizures, encephalitis, temporal-lobe epilepsy and infantile bilateral striatal necrosis, among others (Wilborn et al., 1994; Boutolleau et al., 2005; Murakami et al., 2005; Ward et al., 2005). However, considerable differences exist in the estimates of CNS disease attributed to HHV-6 especially in healthy children with primary HHV-6 infection, with recent studies pointing to a much lower prevalence rate (Ansari et al., 2004). Although variant A is thought to be more neurotropic, HHV-6B-associated acute encephalitis have been recently reported in immunocompetent adults (Birnbaum et al., 2005; Boutolleau et al., 2005; Isaacson et al., 2005). Active HHV-6 infection has also been found in patients with progressive multifocal leukoencephalopathy (PML) along with JC polyoma virus. It is suggested that HHV-6 may be a cofactor in causing PML in patients with impaired cell-mediated immunity (Daibata et al., 2001; De Bolle et al., 2005). The role of HHV-6 in multiple sclerosis, Guillain –Barre syndrome and acute disseminated encephalomyelitis remains controversial and is being studied further (Kamei et al., 1997; Fotheringham and Jacobson, 2005; Opsahl and Kennedy, 2005).

In immunosuppressed patients, especially transplant recipients, HHV-6 infection has associated with a wide variety of clinical manifestations. They include fever, rash, pneumonitis, encephalitis, bone marrow suppression, delayed platelets engraftment, hemophagocytic syndrome, cardiomyopathy, thrombotic microangiopathy and bronchiolotis obliterans (Carrigan et al., 1991; Drobyski et al., 1993; Chan et al., 1997; De Almeida Rodrigues et al., 1999; Karras et al., 2004; Boeckh et al., 2005; Neurohr et al., 2005; Savolainen et al., 2005). The incidence of such manifestations varies between 32% (range, 0–82%) for solid organ transplant

(SOT) recipients and 48% (range, 28–75%) for bone marrow transplant patients. The majority of such HHV-6 infections, mostly due to reactivation of HHV-6B, occur between 2 and 4 weeks post-transplantation. Less frequently, primary HHV-6 infection occurs in the setting of transmission of the virus in donor tissue or infection by a different HHV-6 strain (Chan et al., 1997; Boeckh et al., 2005; Savolainen et al., 2005). Another postulated role for HHV-6 is the increased CMV reactivation in SOT, either alone or in conjunction with HHV-7 (DesJardin et al., 2001; Humar et al., 2002; De Bolle et al., 2005).

Drug-induced hypersensitivity syndrome (DIHS) is a severe multi-organ system reaction caused by specific drugs. Many reports have revealed reactivation of HHV-6, HHV-7, Ebstein–Barr virus and CMV in DIHS. Several patients with DIHS have been treated with intra-venous immunoglobulin (IVIG) and systemic corticosteroids with encouraging clinical results. However, virus reactivation was not suppressed and hence causal relationship is not clearly established (Kano et al., 2005; Mitani et al., 2005).

The pathogenesis and disease association of HHV-7 have, to date, been poorly described, except for exanthem subitum, especially the second episode, a non-specific illness, encephalitis and postinfectious myeloradiculoneuropathy in normal hosts (Ueda et al., 1994; Chan et al., 1997; Pickering, 2003; Mihara et al., 2005; Ward, 2005).

Diagnosis

Multiple testing methods are available to detect the presence of HHV-6 and 7 in humans and include immunoglobulin M (IgM) and IgG, mainly by EIA, polymerase chain reaction (PCR) including real-time analysis, detection of viral antigens and viral culture (Images 3 and 4). Positive testing includes the presence of IgM and/or four-fold rise in IgG and positive antigenemia, PCR or shell–vial culture (Braun et al., 1997; Campadelli-Fiume et al., 1999; Pickering, 2003; Abdel-Haq and Asmar, 2004; Grose, 2004; Ward, 2005). Antibody testing for HHV-6 does not differentiate between the two variants. Virus isolation from blood is not practical, though it may be attempted by cultivating the patient's peripheral blood mononuclear cells in the presence of phytohemagglutinin for 3–6 days and then co-cultivated with similarly stimulated cord blood lymphocytes. Saliva has been used as a preferred specimen both for viral isolation and PCR. PCR for HHV-6 commonly use the following sequence for primers and probes: 5′ AAG CTT GCA CAA TGC CAA AAA ACA G (17627–17603), 5′ AAC TGT CTG ACT GGC AAA AAC TTT T (17405–17429), and 5′ AAC TGT CTG GCA AAA ACT6 TTT (17516–17492), and for HHV-7: 5′ TAT CCC AGC TGT TTT CAT ATA GTA AC, 5′ GCC TTG CGG TAG CAC TAG ATT TTT TG and 5′ AGA ATT CTG TAC CCA TGG GCA CAT TTG TAC (Gopal et al., 1990; Berneman et al., 1992).

Given the fact that HHV-6 and 7 reactivate under many conditions of biological stresses along with reactivation of other herpes viruses and cause elevations in IgM and IgG antibodies, the interpretation of such testing should be done

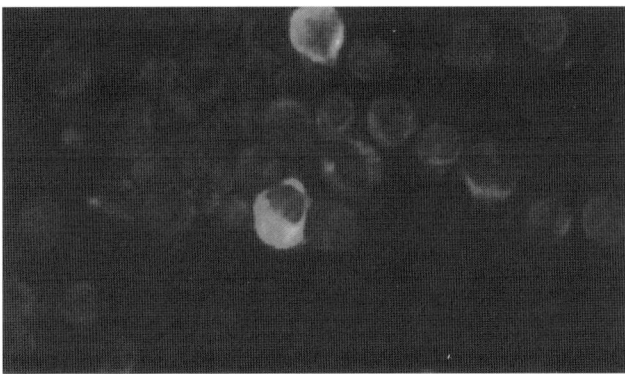

Image 3 Peripheral blood lymphocytes isolated on Ficoll from a patient with roseola infantum (caused by HHV-6) and stained with monoclonal antibody to gp 60/110. Approximately 2–3% of the cells are positive for HHV-6 antigens. With permission from Dr. Janos Luka, Ph.D, associate professor, Department of Pathology, Eastern Virginia Medical School (1993 to present) (for color version: see color section on page 263). http://herpesvirus.tripod.com/gallery/pictures/imfluo/ar202.JPG

cautiously when attempting to establish the etiologic diagnosis of clinical manifestations. Serial quantitative PCR, performed on serum or cerebrospinal fluid, has been increasingly used in immunocompromised hosts, in whom a primary infection or reactivation may be associated with disease (Boutolleau et al., 2005; Pradeau et al., 2005).

Treatment

Infections with HHV-6 and 7 are self-limited in healthy individuals, and require only supportive treatment as indicated. However, treatment should be considered in immunocompromised individuals, and possibly DIHS and hemophagocytic syndrome. This may include manipulating the immune system, and use of antiviral drugs and possibly IVIG (Chen et al., 1995; Pickering, 2003; Abdel-Haq and Asmar, 2004; Grose, 2004; Kano et al., 2005). Steriods have also been used in DIHS (Kano et al., 2005). However, none of these interventions have been studied in a randomized-controlled manner.

For HHV-6, a treatment pattern similar to CMV exists in that HHV-6 is inhibited by acyclovir at considerably higher levels than those required for the treatment of HSV-1, -2 and VZV. Ganciclovir is active in inhibiting DNA synthesis by inhibiting the binding of deoxyganosine triphosphate to DNA polymerase, due to the homologue of CMV pUL97, U69 found in HHV-6, which monophosphorylates the drug. Also active are foscarnet, an inorganic phosphatase which inhibits viral DNA polymerase and cidofovir (CDV), a cytosine analog, which targets viral DNA polymerase and prevents transcription (Ansari and Emery, 1999). *In vitro* data suggest that lipid ester analogs of CDV are more potent inhibitors of HHV-6 than CDV alone (Williams-Aziz et al., 2005). Ganciclovir seems an appropriate

A. Ansari, A. Weinberg

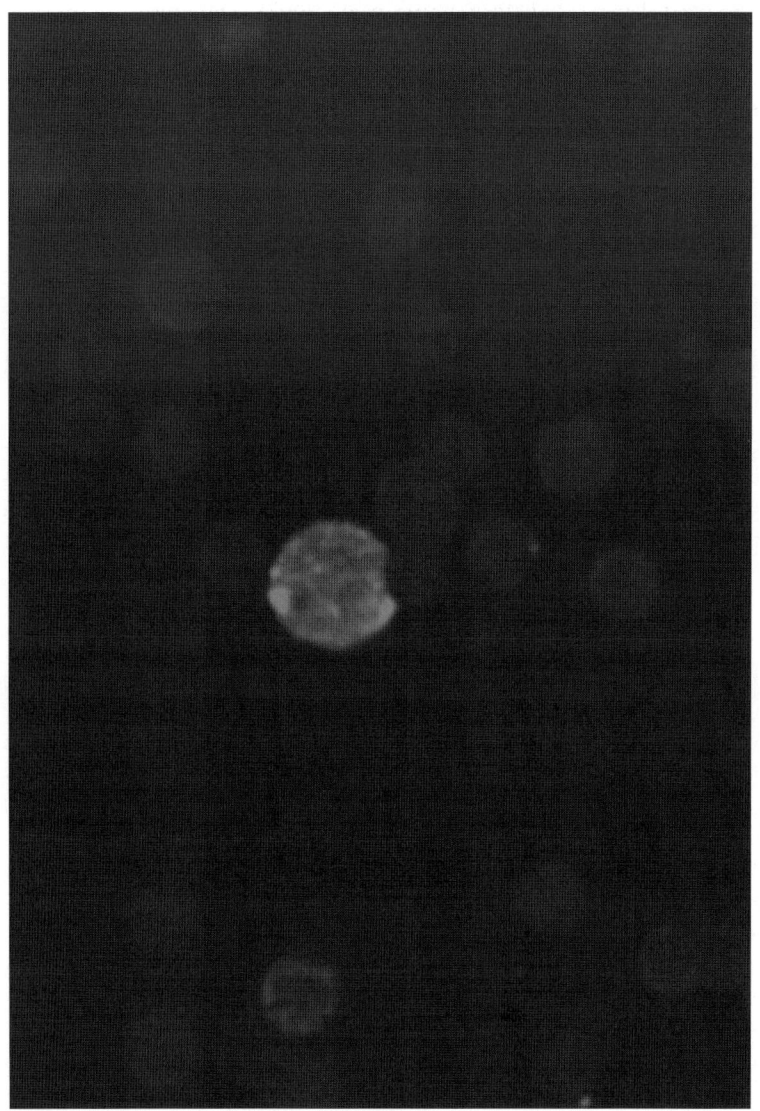

Image 4 SUP-T1 cell line infected with HHV-7 and stained at day 7 with monoclonal antibodies to gp 110 envelop antigen. With permission from Dr. Janos Luka, Ph.D, associate professor, Department of Pathology, Eastern Virginia Medical School (1993 to present) (for color version: see color section on page 264). http://herpesvirus.tripod.com/gallery/pictures/imfluo/7ve701.JPG

first-line antiviral for now. The use of these antivirals may be limited by their adverse effects including dose-dependent neutropenia and thrombocytopenia with ganciclovir, and nephrotoxicity with foscarnet and CDV.

Evidence indicates that HHV-7 is not inhibited by ganciclovir, though foscarnet and CDV may be used if indicated (Razonable et al., 2005). The literature on their uses in such instances is scarce.

Newer antivirals including maribavir, BDCRB and the 4-oxo-dihydroxyquinol-ones, effective against CMV, are not active against HHV-6 and 7 (Townsend et al., 1995; Thomsen et al., 2003; Wang et al., 2003).

Prevention

Infections with these viruses are currently not preventable. Though standard precautions have not been studied in the prevention of these infections, they should be practiced at all health care encounters. Antiviral prophylaxis for CMV in solid organ transplant recipients, with oral ganciclovir and valganciclovir, has been shown to reduce HHV-6B, but not HHV-7 DNAemia, though its implications are not clear (Razonable et al., 2005). Also, the lower dose of ganciclovir, used in prevention of CMV infection may facilitate development of resistance in these viruses. Ganciclovir resistance has been experimentally facilitated in HHV-6 (Manichanh et al., 2001). Currently, there are no vaccines in development.

References

Abdel-Haq NM, Asmar BI. Human herpesvirus 6 (HHV6) infection. Indian J Pediatr 2004; 71: 89–96.

Ablashi DV, Balachandran N, Josephs SF, Hung CL, Krueger GR, Kramarsky B, Salahuddin SZ, Gallo RC. Genomic polymorphism, growth properties, and immunologic variations in human herpesvirus-6 isolates. Virology 1991; 184: 545–552.

Adams O, Krempe C, Kogler G, Wernet P, Scheid A. Congenital infections with human herpesvirus 6. J Infect Dis 1998; 178: 544–546.

Ansari A, Emery VC. The U69 gene of human herpesvirus 6 encodes a protein kinase which can confer ganciclovir sensitivity to baculoviruses. J Virol 1999; 73: 3284–3291.

Ansari A, Li S, Abzug MJ, Weinberg A. Human herpesviruses 6 and 7 and central nervous system infection in children. Emerg Infect Dis 2004; 10: 1450–1454.

Aubin J, Agut H, Collandre H, Yamanishi K, Chandran B, Montagnier L, Huraux JM. Antigenic and genetic differentiation of the two putative types of human herpes virus 6. J Virol Methods 1993; 41: 223–234.

Berneman ZN, Ablashi DV, Li G, Eger-Fletcher M, Reitz Jr. MS, Hung CL, Brus I, Komaroff AL, Gallo RC. Human herpesvirus 7 is a T-lymphotropic virus and is related to, but significantly different from, human herpesvirus 6 and human cytomegalovirus. Proc Natl Acad Sci USA 1992; 89: 10552–10556.

Birnbaum T, Padovan CS, Sporer B, Rupprecht TA, Ausserer H, Jaeger G, Pfister HW. Severe meningoencephalitis caused by human herpesvirus 6 type B in an immunocompetent woman treated with ganciclovir. Clin Infect Dis 2005; 40: 887–889.

Boeckh M, Erard V, Zerr D, Englund J. Emerging viral infections after hematopoietic cell transplantation. Pediatr Transplant 2005; 7: 48–54.

Boutolleau D, Duros C, Bonnafous P, Caiola D, Karras A, Castro ND, Ouachee M, Narcy P, Gueudin M, Agut H, Gautheret-Dejean A. Identification of human herpesvirus 6 variants A and B by primer-specific real-time PCR may help to revisit their respective role in pathology. J Clin Virol 2006; 35(3): 257–263.

Braun DK, Dominguez G, Pellett PE. Human herpesvirus 6. Clin Microbiol Rev 1997; 10: 521–567.

Campadelli-Fiume G, Mirandola P, Menotti L. Human herpesvirus 6: an emerging pathogen. Emerg Infect Dis 1999; 5: 353–366.

Carrigan DR, Drobyski WR, Russler SK, Tapper MA, Knox KK, Ash RC. Interstitial pneumonitis associated with human herpesvirus-6 infection after marrow transplantation. Lancet 1991; 338: 147–149.

Chan PK, Peiris JS, Yuen KY, Liang RH, Lau YL, Chen FE, Lo SK, Cheung CY, Chan TK, Ng MH. Human herpesvirus-6 and human herpesvirus-7 infections in bone marrow transplant recipients. J Med Virol 1997; 53: 295–305.

Chen RL, Lin KH, Lin DT, Su IJ, Huang LM, Lee PI, Hseih KH, Lin KS, Lee CY. Immunomodulation treatment for childhood virus-associated haemophagocytic lymphohistiocytosis. Br J Haematol 1995; 89: 282–290.

De Almeida Rodrigues G, Nagendra S, Lee CK, De Magalhaes-Silverman M. Human herpes virus 6 fatal encephalitis in a bone marrow recipient. Scand J Infect Dis 1999; 31: 313–315.

De Bolle L, Naesens L, De Clercq E. Update on human herpesvirus 6 biology, clinical features, and therapy. Clin Microbiol Rev 2005; 18: 217–245.

DesJardin JA, Cho E, Supran S, Gibbons L, Werner BG, Snydman DR. Association of human herpesvirus 6 reactivation is associated with cytomegalovirus infection and syndromes in kidney transplant recipients. Clin Infect Dis 2001; 33: 1358–1362.

Diabata M, Taguchi T, Kamioka M, Nemoto Y, Hiroi M, Miyoshi I, Taguchi H. Detection of human herpesvirus 6 and JC virus in progressive multifocal leukoencephalopathy complicating follicular lymphoma. Am J Hematol 2001; 67: 200–205.

Dominguez G, Dambaugh TR, Stanley FR, Dewhurst S, Inoue N, Pellett PE. Human herpesvirus 6B genome sequence: coding content and comparison with human herpes virus 6A. J Virol 1999; 73: 8040–8052.

Drobyski WR, Dunne WM, Burd EM, Knox KK, Ash RC, Horowitz MM, Flomenberg N, Carrigan DR. Human herpesvirus-6 (HHV-6) infection in allogeneic bone marrow transplant recipients: evidence of a marrow-suppressive role for HHV-6 *in vivo*. J Infect Dis 1993; 167: 735–739.

Fotheringham J, Jacobson S. Human herpesvirus 6 and multiple sclerosis: potential mechanisms for virus-induced disease. Herpes 2005; 12: 4–9.

Frenkel N, Schirmer EC, Wyatt L, Katsafanas G, Roffman E, Danovich RM, June CH. Isolation of a new herpesvirus from human CD4+ T cells. Proc Natl Acad Sci USA 1990; 87: 748–752.

Fujisaki H, Tanka-Taya K, Tanabe H, Hara T, Miyoshi H, Okada S, Yamanishi K. Detection of human herpesvirus 7 (HHV-7) DNA in breast milk by polymerase chain reaction and prevalence of HHV-7 antibody in breast-fed and bottle-fed children. J Med Virol 1998; 56: 275–279.

Gopal MR, Thomson BJ, Fox J, Tedder RS, Honess RW. Detection by PCR of HHV-6 and EBV DNA in blood and oropharynx of healthy adults and HIV-seropositives. Lancet 1990; 335: 1598–1599.

Grose C. Human herpes viruses 6, 7 & 8. In: Textbook of Pediatric Infectious Diseases. 1957–62 (Feigin RD, Cherry JD, Demmler GJ, Kaplan SL, editors). 5th ed. USA: Saunders; 2004.

Hall CB, Caserta MT, Schnabel KC, Boettrich C, McDermott MP, Lofthus. GK, Carnahan JA, Dewhurst S. Congenital infections with human herpesvirus 6 (HHV6) and human herpesvirus 7 (HHV7). J Pediatr 2004; 145: 472–477.

Hashimoto H, Maruyama H, Fujimoto K, Sakakura T, Seishu S, Okuda N. J Pediatr Hematol Oncol 2002; 24: 211–214.

Humar A, Kumar D, Caliendo AM, Moussa A, Ashi-Sulaiman A, Levy G, Mazzulli T. Clinical impact of human herpesvirus 6 infection after liver transplantation. Transplantation 2002; 73: 599–604.

Isaacson E, Glaser CA, Forghani B, Amad Z, Wallace M, Armstrong RW, Exner MM, Schmid S. Evidence of human herpesvirus 6 infection in 4 immunocompetent patients with encephalitis. Clin Infect Dis 2005; 40: 890–893.

Isegawa Y, Mukai T, Nakano K, Kagawa M, Chen J, Mori Y, Sunagawa T, Kawanishi K, Sashihara J, Hata A, Zou P, Kosuge H, Yamanishi K. Comparison of the complete DNA sequences of human herpesviruses 6 variants A and B. Br J Virol 1999; 73: 8053–8063.

Kagialis-Girard S, Durand B, Mialou V, Pages MP, Galambrun C, Bertrand Y, Negrier C. Human herpesvirus 6 infection and transient acquired myelodysplasia in children. Pediatr Blood Cancer 2005; Dec 6: (Epub).

Kamei A, Ichinohe S, Onuma R, Hiraga S, Fujiwara T. Acute disseminated demyelination due to primary human herpesvirus-6 infection. Eur J Pediatr 1997; 156: 709–712.

Kano Y, Inaoka M, Sakuma K, Shiohara T. Virus reactivation and intravenous immunoglobulin (IVIG) therapy of drug-induced hypersensitivity syndrome. Toxicology 2005; 209: 165–167.

Karras A, Thervet E, Legendre C. Groupe Cooperatif de transplantation d'Ile de France. Hemophagocytic syndrome in renal transplant recipients: report of 17 cases and review of literature. Transplantation 2004; 77: 238–243.

Knox KK, Pietryga D, Harrington DJ, Franciosi R, Carigan DR. Progressive immunodeficiency and fatal pneumonitis associated with human herpesvirus 6 infection in an infant. Clin Infect Dis 1995; 20: 406–413.

Lanari M, Papa I, Venturi V, Lazarotto T, Faldella G, Gabrielli L, Guerra B, Landini MP, Salviolo GP. Congenital infection with human herpesvirus 6 variant B associated with neonatal seizures and poor neurological outcome. J Med Virol 2003; 70: 628–632.

Levine PH, Jahan N, Murari P, Manak M, Jaffe ES. Detection of human herpesvirus 6 in tissues involved by sinus histiocytosis with massive lymphadenopathy (Rosai-Dorfman disease). J Infect Dis 1992; 166: 291–295.

Lusso P, Secchiero P, Crowley RW, Garzino-Demo A, Berneman ZN, Gallo RC. CD4 is a critical component of the receptor for human herpesvirus 7: interference with human immunodeficiency virus. Proc Natl Acad Sci USA 1994; 91: 3872–3876.

Manichanh C, Olivier-Aubron C, Lagarde JP, Aubin JT, Bossi P, Gautheret-Dejean A, Huraux JM, Agut H. Selection of the same mutation in the U69 protein kinase gene of human herpesvirus-6 after prolonged exposure to ganciclovir *in vitro* and *in vivo*. J Gen Virol 2001; 82: 2767–2776.

Maric I, Bryant R, Abu-Asab M, Cohen JI, Vivero A, Jaffe ES, Raffeld M, Tsokos M, Banks PM, Pittaluga S. Human herpesvirus-6-associated acute lymphadenitis in immuno-competent adults. Mod Pathol 2004; 17: 1427–1433.

Mendel I, Matteis M, Bertin C, Delaporte B, Maguer D, Collandre H, Buffet-Janvresse C. Fulminant hepatitis in neonates with human herpesvirus 6 infection. Pediatr Infect Dis J 1995; 14: 993–997.

Merk J, Schmid FX, Fleck M, Schwarz S, Lehance C, Boehm S, Salzberger B, Birnbaum DE. Fatal pulmonary failure attributable to viral pneumonia with human herpes virus 6 (HHV6) in a young immunocompetent woman. J Intensive Care Med 2005; 20: 302–306.

Mihara T, Mutoh T, Yoshikawa T, Yano S, Asano Y, Yamamoto H. Postinfectious my-eloradiculoneuropathy with cranial nerve involvements associated with human herpesvi-rus 7 infection. Arch Neurol 2005; 62: 1755–1757.

Mitani N, Aihara M, Yamakawa Y, Yamada M, Itoh N, Mizuki N, Ikezawa Z. Drug-induced hypersensitivity syndrome due to cyanamide associated with multiple reactivation of human herpesviruses. J Med Virol 2005; 75: 430–434.

Mori Y, Seya T, Huang HL, Akkapaiboon P, Dhepakson P, Yamanishi K. Human herpesvirus 6 variant A but not variant B induces fusion from without in a variety of human cells through a human herpesvirus 6 entry receptor, CD46. J Virol 2002; 76: 6750–6761.

Mori Y, Yang X, Akkapaiboon P, Okuno T, Yamanishi K. Human herpesvirus 6 variant A glycoprotein H-glycoprotein L-glycoprotein Q complex associates with human CD46. J Virol 2003; 77: 4992–4999.

Murakami A, Morimoto M, Adachi S, Ishimaru Y, Sugimoto T. Infantile bilateral striatal necrosis associated with human herpes virus-6 (HHV-6) infection. Brian Dev 2005; 27: 527–530.

Neurohr C, Huppmann P, Leuchte H, Schwaiblmair M, Bittmann I, Jaeger G, Hatz R, Frey L, Uberfuhr P, Reichart B, Behr J, Munich Lung Transplant Group. Human herpesvirus 6 in bronchalveolar lavage fluid after lung transplantation: a risk factor for bronchiolitis obliterans syndrome? Am J Transplant 2005; 5: 2982–2991.

Ohashi M, Ihira M, Suzuki K, Suga S, Asano Y, Yoshikawa T, Saitto Y, Sakui H. Transfer of human herpesvirus 6 and 7 antibodies from mothers to their offspring. Pediatr Infect Dis J 2001; 20: 449–450.

Ohashi M, Yoshikawa T, Ihira M, Suzuki K, Suga S, Tada S, Udagawa Y, Saku H, Idia K, Saito Y, Nisiyama Y, Asano Y. Reactivation of human herpesvirus 6 and 7 in pregnant women. J Med Virol 2002; 67: 354–358.

Opsahl ML, Kennedy PG. Investigating the presence of human herpesvirus 7 and 8 in multiple sclerosis and normal control brain tissue. J Neurol Sci 2006; 240(1-2): 37–44.

Pickering LK (Ed.). American Academy of Pediatrics: Human herpesvirus 6 (Including Roseola) and 7. Red Book: Report of the Committee on Infectious Diseases. 2003; 357–359.

Pradeau K, Couty L, Szelag JC, Turlure P, Rolle F, Ferrat P, Bordessoule D, Le Meur Y, Denis F, Ranger-Rogez S. Multiplex real-time PCR assay for simultaneous quantitation of human cytomegalovirus and herpesvirus-6 in polymorphonuclear and mononuclear cells of transplant recipients. J Virol Methods 2005 (Epub ahead of print).

Razonable RR, Brown RA, Humar A, Covington E, Alecock E, Paya CV. PV16000 Study Group. Herpesvirus infections in solid organ transplant patients at high risk of primary cytomegalovirus disease. J Infect Dis 2005; 192: 1331–1339.

Saijo M, Saijo H, Yamamoto M, Takimoto M, Fujiyasu H, Murano K, Fujita K. Thrombocytopenic purpura associated with primary human herpesvirus 6 infcetion. Pediatr Infect Dis J 1995; 14: 405.

Salahuddin SZ, Ablashi DV, Markham PD, Josephs SF, Sturzenegger S, Kaplan M, Halligan G, Biberfeld P, Wong-Staal F, Kramarsky B, et al. Isolation of a new virus, HBLV, in patients with lymphoproliferatie disorders. Science 1986; 234: 596–601.

Santoro F, Greenstone HL, Insinga A, Liszewski MK, Atkinson JP, Lusso P, Berger A. Interaction of glycoprotein H of human herpesvirus 6 with the cellular receptor CD46. J Biol Chem 2003; 278: 25964–25969.

Savolainen H, Lautenschlager I, Piiparinen H, Saarinen-Pihkala U, Hovi L, Vettenranta K. Human herpesvirus-6 and -7 in pediatric stem cell transplantation. Pediatr Blood Cancer 2005; 45: 820–825.

Sugimoto T, Tanaka-Taya K, Ono J, Miyoshi H, Okada S, Yamanishi K. Human herpesvirus-6 infection in neonates: not protected by only humoral immunity. Pediatr Int 2002; 44: 281–285.

Syruckova Z, Stary J, Sedlacek P, Smisek P, Vavrinec J, Komrska V, Roubalova K, Vandasova J, Sintakova B, Houskova J, Hassan M. Infection-associated hemophagocytic syndrome complicated by infectious lymphoproliferation: a case report. Pediatr Hematol Oncol 1996; 13: 143–150.

Thompson BJ, Dewhurst S, Gray D. Structure and heterogeneity of the sequences of human herpesvirus 6 strain variants U1102 and Z29 and identification of human telomeric repeat sequences at the genomic termini. J Virol 1994; 68: 3007–3014.

Thomsen DR, Olen NL, Hopkins TA, Knechtel ML, Brideau RJ, Wathen MW, Homa FL. Amino acid changes within conserved region III of the herpes simplex virus and human cytomegalovirus DNA polymerases confer resistance to 4-oxo-dihydroquilolines, a novel class of herpes antiviral agents. J Virol 2003; 77: 1868–1876.

Townsend LB, Devivar RV, Turk SR, Nassiri MR, Drach JC. Design, synthesis and antiviral activity of certain 2,5,6-trihalo-1-(beta-D-ribofuranosyl) benzimadazoles. J Med Chem 1995; 38: 4098–4105.

Ueda K, Kusuhara K, Okada K, Miyazaki C, Hidaka Y, Tokugawa K, Yamanishi K. Primary human herpesvirus 7 infection and exanthema subitum. Pediatr Infect Dis J 1994; 13: 167–168.

Wang LH, Peck RW, Yin Y, Allanson J, Wiggs R, Wire MB. Phase I safety and pharmacokinetic trials of 1263W94, a novel oral anti-human cytomegalovirus agent, in healthy and human immunodeficiency virus-infected subjects. Antimicrob Agents Chemother 2003; 47: 1334–1342.

Ward KN. The natural history and laboratory diagnosis of human herpesviruses-6 and -7 infections in the immunocompetent. J Clin Virol 2005; 32: 183–193.

Ward KN, Andrews NJ, Verity CM, Miller E, Ross EM. Human herpesviruses-6 and -7 each cause significant neurological morbidity in Britain and Ireland. Arch Dis Child 2005; 90: 619–623.

Weinberg A, Enomoto L, Li S, Shen D, Coll J, Shpall EJ. Risk of transmission of herpesviruses through cord blood transplantation. Biol Blood Marrow Transplant 2005; 11: 35–38.

A. Ansari, A. Weinberg

Wilborn F, Schmidt CA, Brinkmann V, Jendroska K, Oettle H, Siegert W. A potential role for human herpesvirus type 6 in nervous system disease. J Neuroimmunol 1994; 49: 213–214.

Williams-Aziz SL, Hartlin CB, Harden EA, Daily SL, Prichard MN, Kushner NL, Beadle JR, Wan WB, Hostetler KY, Kern ER. Comparative activities of lipid esters of cidofovir and cyclic cidofovir against replication of herpesviruses *in vitro*. Antimicrob Agents Chemother 2005; 49: 3724–3733.

Yalcin S, Mukai T, Kondo K, Ami Y, Okawa T, Kojima A, Kurata T, Yamanishi K. Experimental infection of cynomolgus and African green monkeys with human herpesvirus 6. J Gen Virol 1992; 73: 1673–1677.

Yamanishi K, Okuno T, Shiraki T, Takahashi M, Kondo T, Asano Y, Kurata T. Identification of human herpesvirus-6 as a causal agent for exanthem subitum. Lancet 1988; 1: 1065–1067.

Yoshikawa T, Ihira M, Suzuki K, Kito H, Iwasaki T, Kurata T, Tanaka T, Saita Y, Asano Y. Fatal acute myocarditis in an infant with human herpesvirus 6 infection. J Clin Pathol 2001; 54: 792–795.

Yoshikawa T, Suzuki K, Umemura K, Akimoto S, Miyake F, Usui C, Fujita A, Suga S, Asano Y. Atypical clinical features of a human herpesvirus-6 infection in a neonate. J Med Virol 2004; 74: 463–466.

Zahorsky J. Roseola infantum. Arch Pediatr 1954; 71: 124–128.

Zerr DM, Meier AS, Selke SS, Frenkel LM, Huang ML, Wald A, Rhoads MP, Nguy L, Bornemann R, Morrow RA, Corey L. A population-based study of primary human herpesvirus 6 infection. N Engl J Med 2005; 352: 768–776.

Congenital and Other Related Infectious
Diseases of the Newborn
Isa K. Mushahwar (Editor)
© 2007 Elsevier B.V. All rights reserved
DOI 10.1016/S0168-7069(06)13004-9

Varicella-Zoster Virus Infections during Pregnancy

Andreas Sauerbrei

Institute of Virology and Antiviral Therapy, Friedrich-Schiller University, Jena, Germany

Abstract

Chickenpox is rare in pregnancy. However, the disease must be considered to lead occasionally to disastrous maternal, fetal, and neonatal diseases. By contrast, the appearance of normal zoster is not associated with special problems during pregnancy and perinatal period. Pregnant women who contract varicella are at risk of severe pneumonia and death. At any stage during pregnancy, chickenpox may cause intrauterine infection. The consequences for the infant depend on the time of maternal disease. During the first two trimesters, maternal varicella may result in congenital varicella syndrome which has been reported in nearly 2%. Maternal infection near term is associated with a substantial risk of intrauterine acquired neonatal chickenpox in the newborn infant, who can develop the clinical picture of serious disseminated varicella with visceral involvement. The present paper reviews the clinical consequences as well as the current possibilities of diagnosis, prevention and therapy of varicella-zoster virus infections during pregnancy.

Varicella-zoster virus

Chickenpox (varicella) was rarely recognized until the sixteenth century. The name is thought to be derived from the Old English *gican*, meaning "itch". While shingles (herpes zoster) has been recognized as a unique clinical entity, varicella was differentiated from smallpox by the English physician Heberden in 1767. The relationship between chickenpox and shingles was first noted in 1898 by the Hungarian pediatrician Bokay. In 1952, the American virologists Weller and Stoddard first isolated the etiologic agent of varicella and zoster, the varicella-zoster virus (VZV), in cell cultures from varicella vesicle fluid. Weller had been able to establish in 1958 that there were no biologic and immunologic differences between the viruses isolated from patients with varicella and subsequent zoster. In 1974, a live-attenuated varicella vaccine was established by a Japanese group under Takahashi after isolating and attenuating the virus from a child with chickenpox named Oka. Straus proved in 1984 the identity of viral DNA by using the restriction endonuclease analysis.

The VZV is a member of the *Alphaherpesvirinae* subfamily within the family *Herpesviridae*. The spherical, 120–300 nm large particle of virus consists of a linear double-stranded DNA genome with about 125,000 base pairs and an icosahedric capsid composed of 162 capsomers. This nucleocapsid is surrounded by the tegument made up of glycoproteins as well as a trilaminar glycoprotein- and lipid-containing envelope. VZV cannot be distinguished from other herpesviruses electron microscopically. Some VZV genes have homologues in the genome of herpes simplex virus (HSV). Anti-VZV drugs such as aciclovir act on the virus-encoded thymidine kinase and DNA polymerase. There is only one serotype of VZV, and little antigenic variations have been noted between different isolates. VZV particles are exceedingly labile. Growth is highly cell-associated and almost exclusively restricted to cells of human and simian origin.

Epidemiology and consequences of varicella-zoster virus infections during pregnancy

Seroepidemiology

VZV is spread by respiratory transmission or direct contact with infectious lesions. Seronegative persons are at risk of primary infection manifest as varicella. According to a seroepidemiological study in Germany, the prevalence of VZV-specific IgG class antibodies increases from 7 to 61% after the first to fifth year and reaches 94% among the 8–9 years olds. Among the more than 40 years olds, only isolated individuals are susceptible to VZV (Wutzler et al., 2001). Seroepidemiological studies performed between 1973 and 2002 in different industrial countries revealed that up to 26% of women of reproductive age do not possess VZV-specific IgG class antibodies (Table 1). Women from tropical and subtropical areas are more likely to be seronegative for VZV IgG and are, therefore, more susceptible to the development of chickenpox (Garnett et al., 1993). However, although only 3–4% of women of child-bearing age in Germany were found to be susceptible to primary VZV infection (Wutzler et al., 2001), the number of women, who become pregnant without any protection against chickenpox, is about 20,000–30,000 per year (Sauerbrei and Wutzler, 2004a). In early reports, the average incidence of varicella in pregnant women was calculated as 0.7 per 1000 pregnancies (Sever and White, 1968; Stagno and Whitley, 1985), but the current rates appear to be higher (2–3 per 1000 pregnancies) (Enders and Miller, 2000). Even though chickenpox is a rare event during pregnancy, the disease must be considered to lead occasionally to disastrous maternal and fetal diseases (Table 2).

Table 1

Seroprevalence of varicella-zoster virus (VZV) in women of reproductive age

Country	Year of the study	Age of women (years)	Prevalence of VZV-specific antibodies (%)	Reference
United States	1975	Parturient women	91	Gershon et al. (1976)
Israel	1973/1976	17–40	74.1–81.3	Leventon-Kriss et al. (1978)
Czechoslovakia	1972/1981	15–19	93.8	
		Adults	97.5–100	Trlifajová et al. (1989)
Germany	1982/1983	18–39	93.3	Schneweis et al. (1985)
Germany	1984	16–40	94.8	Enders (1984)
Germany	1990	17–36	93.2	Sauerbrei et al. (1990)
St Lucia, Carribean island	1993	18–39 (adults)	18–60	Garnett et al. (1993)
United Kingdom	1991	15–40	> 90–> 97	Fairley and Miller (1996)
Australia	1995	20–34	78–97	Chant et al. (1998)
Germany	1995/1998	18–39	96.7	Wutzler et al. (2001)
Spain	1996	15–34	95.3	Salleras et al. (2001)
Belgium	1999/2000	25–34	94.9	Thiry et al. (2002)
Finland	2000	Parturient women	96.2	Alanen et al. (2005)
Ireland	2002	Pregnant women	83.9–88.7	Knowles et al. (2004)

Maternal varicella

At any stage during pregnancy, chickenpox may cause intrauterine infection. Maternal varicella resulting in viremia may transmit the virus into the fetus by either transplacental spread, or by ascending infection from lesions in the birth canal (Birch et al., 2003). Furthermore, direct contact or respiratory droplet can lead to infection after birth. The consequences for the infant depend on the time of maternal disease. They range from asymptomatic infection to fetal loss especially in case of severe maternal disease. Pregnant women who contract varicella are at risk

Table 2

Varicella-zoster virus infections and their potential consequences during pregnancy

Maternal disease	Timing during pregnancy	Consequences for mother, fetus, term neonate
Varicella	At any stage	Intrauterine death, neonatal or infantile zoster
	5–20th (24th) weeks	Congenital varicella syndrome (risk: 2%, mortality: 30%)
	At any stage, especially in the 3rd trimester	Maternal pneumonia (risk: 10–20%, mortality: 10–45%)
	Near term: $\geqslant 5$ days before delivery	Neonatal varicella at ages 10 (–12) days (risk: 20–50%, mortality: 0%)
	Near term: $\leqslant 4$–5 days before to 2 days after delivery	Neonatal varicella 0–4 days after birth (risk: 20–50%, mortality: 0–3%); neonatal varicella 5–10 (–12) days delivery after birth (risk: 20–50%, mortality: 20–25%)
Normal zoster	At any stage	No risk for severe maternal, fetal or neonatal infections

of pneumonia associated with life-threatening ventilatory compromise and death. The disease seems to occur more often in the third trimester (Smego and Asperille, 1991). However, gestational age at onset of maternal disease was not identified as a significant risk factor for VZV pneumonia in a recently published multivariable logistic regression analysis (Harger et al., 2002a). In principle, varicella pneumonia is the most common serious maternal complication in pregnancy. Since no reliable prospective studies on the incidence of VZV pneumonia in pregnant women are available, the frequency of this complication remains largely unknown. On the basis of retrospective hospital-based studies, an incidence of 10–20% among adults with chickenpox was reported (Smego and Asperille, 1991; Baren et al., 1996). But data from population-based studies suggest that the risk of hospitalization for VZV pneumonia in adults is below 8% (Guess et al., 1986; Choo et al., 1995).

According to data from the literature, primary VZV infection during the first two trimesters of pregnancy may result in intrauterine infection in up to a quarter of the cases (Paryani and Arvin, 1986; Prober et al., 1990; Enders et al., 1994; Liesnard et al., 1994). As result, spontaneous abortions have been reported. But the rate of abortion following acute varicella did not exceed the rate of abortion in pregnant women without chickenpox (Paryani and Arvin, 1986; Pastuszak et al., 1994). Thus, the observed abortions do not necessarily result from maternal chickenpox. A congenital varicella syndrome (CVS) can be expected in about 12% of infected fetuses (Prober et al., 1990). On the basis of prospective studies in Europe and North America, the incidence of embryopathy and fetopathy after maternal varicella infection in the first 20 weeks of pregnancy is estimated to be about 1–2%

(Enders et al., 1994; Pastuszak et al., 1994). The latest prospective study from the United States has confirmed this low frequency of the CVS (Harger et al., 2002b).

Neonatal varicella can be expected if a mother contracts chickenpox during the last 3 weeks of pregnancy. After maternal varicella between 4 and 5 days before and 2 days after delivery, generalized neonatal varicella leading to death in up to 20% of the cases may occur, since these infants have not acquired protecting antibodies (Sauerbrei and Wutzler, 2001).

Maternal and infantile herpes zoster

On the basis of current knowledge, zoster during pregnancy is not associated with birth defects (Enders et al., 1994; Sauerbrei and Wutzler, 2000). In addition, maternal zoster during the perinatal period does not cause problems for newborn infants (Miller et al., 1989) as the infants possess specific maternal IgG class antibodies and there is usually no longer viremic spread of VZV unless the women is immunocompromised.

Nearly 20% of infants with intrauterine-acquired VZV primary infection develop neonatal or infantile zoster, usually with uncomplicated course (Sauerbrei and Wutzler, 2003). The disease is thought to represent reactivation of the virus after primary infection *in utero*. The relatively short viral latency period may be explained by the immature cell-mediated immune response in young children.

Varicella pneumonia

Although chickenpox is much less common in adults than in children, the infection is associated with greater morbidity, namely pneumonia, hepatitis, and encephalitis. The varicella pneumonia in pregnancy must be regarded as a medical emergency (Frangidis and Pneumatikos, 2004). The clinical course is unpredictable and may rapidly progress to hypoxia and life-threatening respiratory failure. Retrospective studies suggest that varicella pneumonia may be more severe, although not more frequent, in pregnant compared to non-pregnant women (Harris and Rhoades, 1965). A case control study of 18 pregnant women with varicella pneumonia and 72 pregnant controls with varicella but no pneumonia found that smoking and the occurrence of at least 100 skin lesions were risk factors for the development of pneumonia (Harger et al., 2002a).

The disease usually develops within 3–5 days of the rash. Predominant signs and symptoms are cough, dyspnea, fever, and tachypnea. Additionally, cyanosis, pleuritic pain in the chest, and hemoptysis have been observed. Secondary bacterial infections occur frequently. The chest X-ray findings include a diffuse or miliary/nodular infiltrative pattern often in the peribronchial distribution involving both lungs (Haake et al., 1990). In the general population, varicella pneumonia has a mortality of 10–20%. However, in untreated pregnant women the mortality rate is in excess of 45%. These data may reflect a bias toward reporting of more severe cases during pregnancy (Nathwani et al., 1998). More recent studies suggest that the mortality of varicella pneumonia has decreased to 10–11% for both non-pregnant and pregnant patients most likely due to the effects of antiviral therapy and better respiratory management (Chandra et al., 1998). Nevertheless, the risk of fatal varicella appears to be about fivefold higher in pregnant than in non-pregnant immunocompetent adults. The estimated case fatality rate in pregnancy is 1 per 2000 (Enders and Miller, 2000).

In case of suspected varicella pneumonia, a laboratory diagnosis is necessary for reason of differential diagnosis. As method of choice, the polymerase chain reaction (PCR) should be used to detect viral DNA in broncho-alveolar lavage.

Congenital varicella syndrome

Definition, frequency, and pathogenesis

After reviewing the literature, the CVS has not been so rarely reported as formerly assumed. This syndrome has been variously referred to as "fetal varicella syndrome", "congenital varicella-zoster syndrome", "varicella embryo-fetopathy", "varicella embryopathy" and "varicella fetopathy". Finally, the term "fetal varicella-zoster syndrome" has been proposed in view of the pathogenesis of this condition as well as for the clear differentiation from "congenital varicella" occasionally used for intrauterine-acquired "neonatal varicella" (Higa et al., 1987; Birthistle and Carrington, 1998).

Since the first report by Laforet and Lynch (1947), nearly 130 infants born with signs of CVS have been described in the English, German, and French literature (Boumahni et al., 2005; Sauerbrei and Wutzler, 2005). Because most cases of CVS have been reported during the last 10–15 years, it can be concluded that many cases of this syndrome were formerly not seen in connection with chickenpox during pregnancy. On the basis of the described data about the incidence of varicella and the risk of CVS, there are at least 10 infants with varicella embryo-fetopathy to be expected in Germany per year. Mustonen et al. (2001) reported four neonates with neurological manifestations of apparent congenital VZV infection but with no maternal clinical disease during pregnancy. The diagnosis was made serologically, whereas both the antigen detection and the PCR were negative.

CVS has generally to be expected after maternal chickenpox between the 5th and 24th gestational weeks. Nearly 80% of all cases have been observed between the 9th and 20th weeks of gestation. Before the 5th and after the 24th gestational weeks, the probability of CVS is extremely low.

The route of fetal infection is considered to be transplacental. Ascending infection from the epithelium of the cervix uteri is also conceivable (Birch et al., 2003). Pathogenic mechanisms leading to several organ injuries of CVS are in close relationship with the neurotropic nature of VZV and the immature immune system of the unborn infant. On the basis of the segmental distribution of some of the signs, especially the skin lesions, it was postulated that the CVS is not the immediate consequence of intrauterine varicella, but caused by intrauterine zoster-like VZV reactivations with accompanying encephalitis (Higa et al., 1987). In a recently published case report, a widespread non-productive VZV infection has been described in non-neural fetal tissues within 2 weeks following the onset of chickenpox in the mother (Nikkels et al., 2005). Immunologic studies suggest that the fetus is not able to mount a VZV-specific cell-mediated immune response (Grose, 1989).

Clinical picture

The characteristic clinical findings consist of skin lesions in dermatomal distribution (Fig. 1), neurological defects, eye diseases, and/or limb hypoplasia (Table 3). Less-frequent abnormalities include muscle hypoplasia, affections of the internal organs as well as gastrointestinal, genitourinary, and cardiovascular manifestations. There were only small differences regarding the dependence of symptoms on the onset of maternal chickenpox. In early infection, neurological defects and limb hypoplasia have been more frequently described than skin lesions and eye diseases which were dominant when maternal disease occurred later. No relationship has been reported in the literature between the number of clinical features, the gestational age of maternal varicella and the immune response in the infant (Enders and Miller, 2000). Nearly 30% of infants born with signs of CVS died during the first months of life. A follow-up report in the literature demonstrates that in spite of initially poor prognosis a good long-term outcome can be observed in patients with CVS (Schulze and Dietzsch, 2000).

Diagnosis

Most cases of CVS have been only reported on the basis of clinical symptoms including skin lesions, neurological defects, eye diseases, and limb hypoplasia

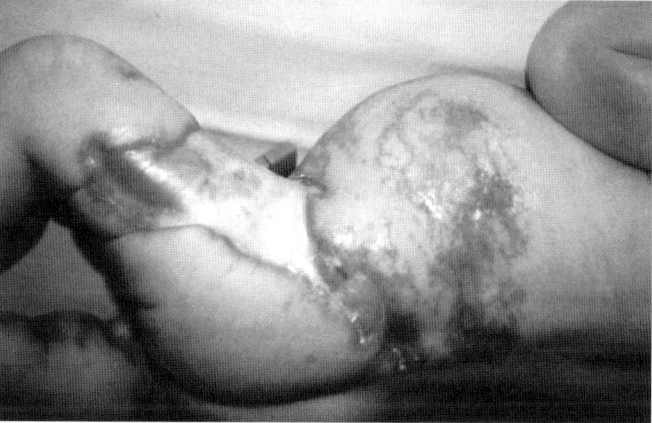

Fig. 1 Female stillborn with cicatricial skin lesions involving the left side of chest, axilla, and shoulder as well as hypoplasia of the left upper limb after maternal varicella between the 13th and 15th gestational weeks (for color version: see color section on page 265).

Table 3

Main symptoms of infants with congenital varicella syndrome cited in the literature

Symptoms	Children (n = 125)	
	n	%
Skin lesions (cicatrical scars, skin loss)	90	72
Neurological defects or diseases (cortical atrophy, spinal cord atrophy, limb paresis, seizures, microcephaly, Horner's syndrome, encephalitis, dysphagia)	78	62
Eye diseases (microphthalmia, enophthalmia, chorioretinitis, cataract, nystagmus, anisocoria, optic atrophy)	66	53
Limb hypoplasia and other skeletal anomalies	55	44
Intrauterine retardation	28	22
Gastrointestinal abnormalities	25	20
Muscle hypoplasia	24	19
Genitourinary abnormalities	15	12
Affections of internal organs	15	12
Developmental delay	14	11
Defects of the cardiovascular system	9	7
Defects of other organs	9	7

without laboratory evidence of intrauterine infection (Table 4). However, the causal relationship between maternal varicella infection and congenital abnormalities would be most convincingly verified by detection of the virus, viral antigens or viral DNA in the infant. With the use of PCR and nucleic acid hybridization assays, VZV DNA can be detected in fetal or infantile tissue samples, fetal blood, cerebrospinal fluid, and/or amniotic fluid (Scharf et al., 1990; Michie et al., 1992; Sauerbrei et al., 1996). At present, molecular biological methods should be regularly included in the diagnosis of CVS. In particular, cases presented with rare malformations or after subclinical maternal VZV infection need confirmation by virological methods, otherwise the causal relationship between maternal infection and congenital abnormalities remains doubtful (Al-Katawee et al., 2005). Cytomorphological methods for identifying VZV infections (Tzanck stain) need considerable experience for interpretation and do not differentiate between HSV and VZV (Sauerbrei et al., 1999). The detection of virus-specific antibodies in newborns may usually also confirm a suspected prenatal infection with VZV. Serologic diagnosis is mostly based on the persistence of VZV-specific IgG class antibodies beyond 7 months of life when maternal antibodies should normally have disappeared (Gershon et al., 1976; Akisu et al., 2003). The presence of virus-specific IgM has only been reported in about one quarter of the CVS cases (Sauerbrei and Wutzler, 2000). Although IgM seems to be produced in small amounts by the fetus, the detection rate depends significantly on sensitivity of enzyme immunoassays,

Table 4

Evidence of intrauterine varicella-zoster virus (VZV) infection in cases of congenital varicella syndrome cited in the literature

Diagnostic criteria	Children ($n = 128$[a])	
	n	%
Persistence of VZV-specific IgG	30	23
VZV-specific IgM	28	22
Zoster in early infancy	22	17
Viral DNA and/or antigens in fetal tissues	6	5
Viral DNA in cerebrospinal fluid	5	4
Viral DNA in amniotic fluid	2	2
No laboratory evidence of intrauterine VZV infection	51	40

[a]In 13 (10%) cases, more than one diagnostic criterion has been used for evidence of *in utero* VZV infection.

which are most frequently used to detect VZV-specific IgM. Unlike in cases of intrauterine rubella or cytomegalovirus infection, VZV has not been isolated in cell cultures from any infant with CVS. To establish a relationship between maternal VZV infection and congenital anomalies of infant, the following criteria should be used:

(i) Appearance of maternal varicella during pregnancy
(ii) Neonate or fetus with
  • congenital skin lesions in dermatomal distribution and/or
  • neurological defects
  • eye diseases
  • limb hypoplasia
(iii) Proof of intrauterine VZV infection by
  • detection of viral DNA using PCR and/or
  • presence of specific IgM/persistence of IgG beyond 7 months of age
  • appearance of zoster during early infancy.

Concerning differential diagnosis, a variety of defects and clinical symptoms described in infants with CVS may also occur in other congenital infections which should therefore be excluded by means of virological, serological, and cytogenetic studies. Neurological defects and eye diseases are typical of congenital infections caused by rubella virus, cytomegalovirus, and *Toxoplasma gondii* (Koskimies et al., 1978). Symptoms, especially skin lesions, similar to CVS can also be diagnosed after primary HSV infections during early pregnancy (Johansson et al., 2004). Intrauterine transmission of coxsackie viruses during the late pregnancy may lead to varicella-like congenital skin lesions (Sauerbrei et al., 2000). Congenital skin defects in dermatomal distribution and microphthalmia represent the cardinal symptoms of a specific genetic disorder called MIDAS (Microphthalmus, Dermal Aplasia, Sclerokornea) syndrome. It is due to a partial deletion of the short arm from chromosome X, with consecutive monosomy Xp22.3 (Spranger et al., 1998).

Zoster and congenital malformations

Concerning a relationship between maternal zoster and CVS, there are some reports of infants with congenital malformations being born to mothers with a history of zoster during the first 12 weeks of pregnancy (Webster and Smith, 1977; Brazin et al., 1979). But, in none of these cases was the diagnosis of shingles proven by laboratory investigation, and no case showed laboratory evidence of intrauterine infection with VZV. In a large prospective study of 366 pregnant women with zoster in pregnancy, no infants had clinical evidence of intrauterine infection (Enders et al., 1994). This confirmed the expert opinion: zoster in pregnancy does not cause fetal sequelae.

Neonatal varicella

Definition, frequency, and pathogenesis

During the perinatal period, maternal varicella can infect the baby by (i) transplacental viremia, (ii) ascending infection during birth, or (iii) respiratory droplet/direct contact with infectious lesions after birth. Chickenpox occurring in the first 12 days of life is described as intrauterine-acquired neonatal varicella. The disease can be expected if a mother contracts chickenpox during the last 3 weeks of pregnancy. Intrauterine-transmitted neonatal chickenpox has been occasionally referred to as "congenital varicella" or "neonatal varicella syndrome" (Sauerbrei and Wutzler, 2001). These terms should be avoided, since they do not allow a clear differentiation from the CVS caused by maternal chickenpox in the first two trimesters.

Varicella within the first 12 days of life has to be caused by intrauterine transmission of VZV because of the incubation period which is usually calculated as 14–16 days; however, it can range from 10 to 21 days. Clinical observations suggest that the incubation period of intrauterine-transmitted varicella from the beginning of maternal varicella rash to the onset of rash in the newborn infant is about 12 days, but it can be reduced to few days (Meyers, 1974; Enders and Miller, 2000). On the basis of these data, chickenpox after the 10th (–12th) day of the neonatal period is most likely not transmitted by intrauterine infection, but it is acquired by postnatal VZV infection.

Neonatal varicella was first recognized by Hubbard (1878). To date, hundreds of cases have been reported (Sauerbrei and Wutzler, 2001). After maternal varicella between 2 weeks ante partum and 2 days post partum, the risk of neonatal chickenpox is generally calculated as 20–50% (Hanngren et al., 1985; Prober et al.,

1990). On the basis of this data and the described incidence of varicella, there is a maximum of 30 neonatal chickenpox cases to be expected in Germany per year.

Clinical course

The severity of intrauterine-acquired neonatal chickenpox is closely related to the time of onset of maternal infection as transplacentally transmitted antibodies may reduce the severity of symptoms in the newborn. Generalized neonatal varicella leading to death is much more likely to occur if mothers develop the varicella rash between 4 (–5) days before and 2 days after delivery (Meyers, 1974; Sterner et al., 1990; Sauerbrei and Wutzler, 2001). After maternal varicella during this period, a fatal outcome (Fig. 2) has been reported in about 20% of the cases (Table 5). These

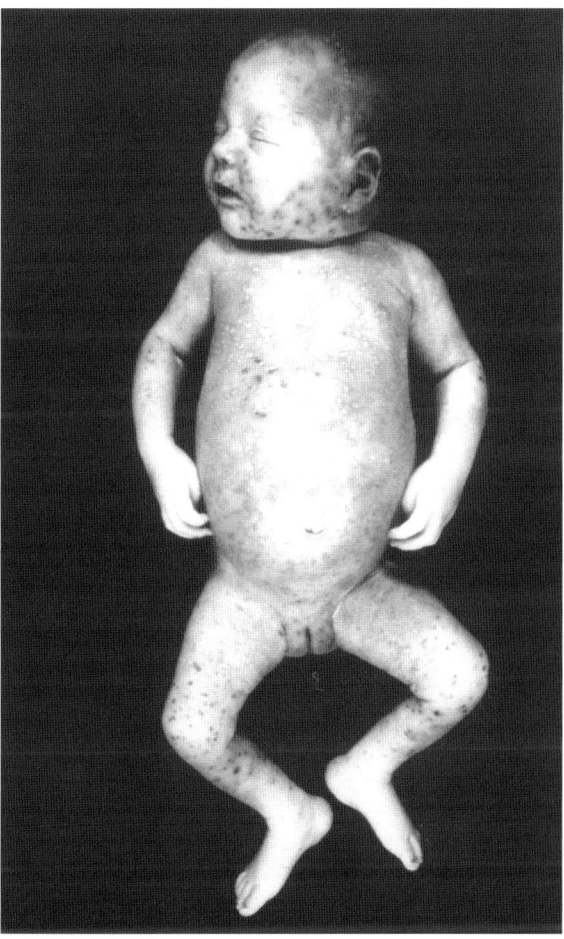

Fig. 2 Female neonate with lethal neonatal varicella (for color version: see color section on page 266).

Table 5

Prognosis of neonatal varicella without antiviral treatment in 136 term infants cited in the literature
(Sauerbrei and Wutzler, 2001)

Day of rash onset		Cases	
		Non-fatal (%)	Fatal (%)
Mother			
$\geqslant 5^a$	($n = 57$)	57 (100)	0
4^a—2^b	($n = 79$)	65 (82)	14 (18)
Neonate[c]			
0–4[d]	($n = 35$)	34 (97)	1 (3)
5–10[d]	($n = 47$)	36 (77)	11 (23)

[a]Days before delivery.
[b]Days after delivery.
[c]Data of 54 neonates have not been described.
[d]Days after birth.

infants have been exposed to maternal viremia without having acquired protecting antibodies. In addition, the cell-mediated immune response of the neonate is likely insufficient to retard the hematogeneous dissemination of VZV after transplacental spread (Baba et al., 1982).

Furthermore, there is a close relationship between the prognosis of intrauterine-acquired neonatal varicella and the onset of disease in the newborn infant. A fatal outcome is thus more likely if the neonatal disease occurs between 5 and 10 (–12) days after delivery. To our knowledge, 23% of the infants reported in the literature died from a disseminated and fulminant infection (Table 5). In comparison, neo-natal varicella within the first 4 days after birth has usually been found to be comparatively mild. Its mortality is calculated as 3% (Sauerbrei and Wutzler, 2001).

Fetuses exposed to VZV between 20 and 6 days before delivery may also de-velop neonatal chickenpox however with non-fatal course. These infants get ma-ternal antibodies and have therefore a lower risk of complications.

Neonatal varicella acquired by postnatal infection has a low morbidity rate (Heidl, 1985) as most neonates are protected by maternally derived antibodies. Complications are rarely observed. However, premature infants younger than 28 weeks gestation or below 1000 g birth weight are at an increased risk for severe varicella during the first 6 weeks after birth (Advisory committee on immunization practices, 1996; Deutsche Gesellschaft für Pädiatrische Infektiologie, 2003). It has been suggested that they have got no protecting maternal antibodies because of the reduced gestation period. However, transplacental IgG antibody transfer has been documented before 28 weeks gestation in several studies (Van der Zwet et al., 2002; Leineweber et al., 2004). Neonatal VZV IgG titers were predominantly predicted by maternal VZV IgG titers (Van der Zwet et al., 2002).

Diagnosis

The diagnosis of neonatal varicella is usually based on the typical clinical picture. In case of intrauterine-acquired neonatal varicella, the characteristic point in time and the maternal history of chickenpox during the last weeks of pregnancy have to be considered. Serological methods have been widely used to confirm the clinical diagnosis of neonatal varicella. However, the detection of virus-specific antibodies is not useful for early diagnosis. In addition, cross-reactions to HSV have to be considered in most antibody assays with VZV-infected cells as antigen, probably based on the known antigenic cross-reactivity of VZV and HSV glycoproteins B (Krah, 1996). Therefore, PCR should be used as method of choice for laboratory diagnosis of VZV infection (Sauerbrei et al., 1999). Where molecular biological methods are not available, immunofluorescent VZV-specific antigen staining in vesicle specimens can be recommended (Dahl et al., 1997). As patient materials serve skin swabs or biopsies, liquor specimens, and tissue samples. The differential diagnosis includes HSV and enterovirus infections (Gershon, 1998; Sauerbrei et al., 2000).

Prophylaxis and therapy

Varicella occurring at every time of pregnancy

An effective prophylaxis of chickenpox in pregnant women is only possible by active immunization of seronegative women before pregnancy. A live-attenuated varicella vaccine has been shown to be safe and effective in preventing chickenpox in adults (Gershon and Steinberg, 1990). Varicella vaccine, as all live-attenuated vaccines, is contraindicated in pregnant women. Pregnancy has to be avoided for at least 4 weeks following vaccination. Seronegative women undergoing infertility treatment or those presenting for preconceptual counseling may be offered vaccination in the United States and some European countries (Royal College of Obstetricians and Gynecologists, 2001). The Pregnancy Registry, managed by the Merck Research Laboratories (United States) in collaboration with the Centers for Disease Control and Prevention (United States), records women who exposed to varicella vaccine during pregnancy or within 3 months before conception. Preliminary results show no hints to any birth defects related to vaccine exposure (Shields et al., 2001). In a case report was documented that the varicella vaccine virus was transmitted from a vaccinated 12-month-old boy to his pregnant mother who subsequently developed chickenpox. After an elective abortion between the seventh and eighth weeks of gestation, no virus was detected in the fetal tissue (Salzman et al., 1997). The pregnancy of a mother has also not been regarded as contraindication for the vaccination of her non-protected child (Robert Koch-Institut, 2005).

Vaccinated persons can develop mild varicella that occurs 42 days after vaccination and represents wild virus infection. These cases have been referred to as breakthrough. The rates vary between 1 and 4% per year independent of time since immunization (Watson, 2002). Most breakthrough diseases are very mild, the infectivity is relatively low and there is a low or no risk for complications (Vázquez and Shapiro, 2005). Therefore, the risk for CVS from breakthrough varicella can be regarded as considerably lower than that for CVS in unvaccinated women with varicella. However, since data about the risk for CVS after breakthrough varicella are not available to date, measures should be considered as in unvaccinated women who develop varicella. But the atypical presentation makes it difficult to diagnose isolated breakthrough cases clinically.

Pregnant women have to be advised to avoid exposure to chickenpox and zoster if the individual is non-immune or has an uncertain serologic status. VZV-specific IgG antibodies should be measured without delay in pregnant women exposed significantly to VZV and with a negative or indeterminate history of varicella (Fig. 3). Significant exposure means: (i) household contact, (ii) face-to-face contact for at least 5 min, or (iii) indoors contact for more than 15 min (Royal College of Obstetricians and Gynecologists, 2001). A woman has to be regarded as susceptible, if no antibodies can be detected or there is an indeterminate or unknown status of immunity. Antibodies detected within 7–10 days of contact must have been acquired before exposure. In case of negative, indeterminate or unknown serologic status, the administration of varicella-zoster immune globulin (VZIG) within 72 (–96) h has been recommended (Royal College of Obstetricians and Gynecologists, 2001; Robert Koch-Institut, 2004). The prescribed dose administered intramuscularly is 125 U/

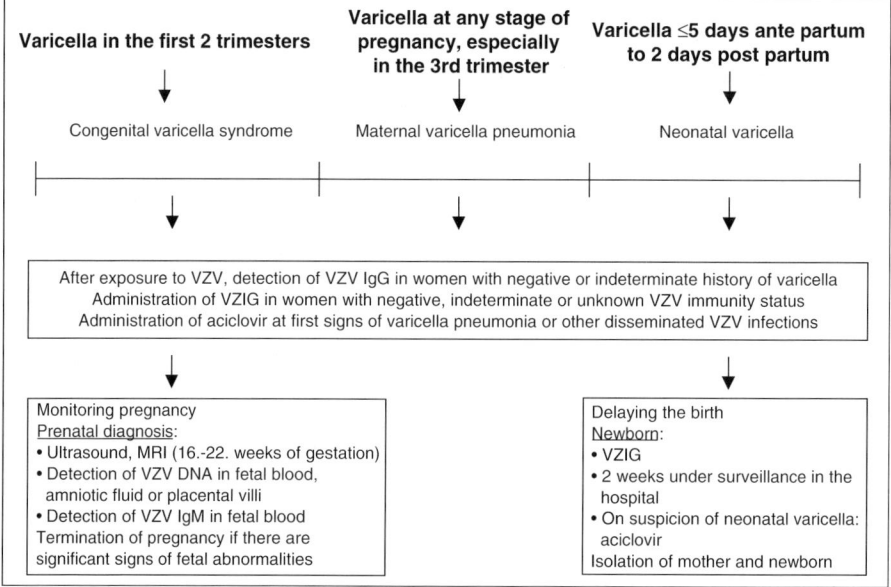

Fig. 3 Measures in case of varicella during pregnancy depending on point of time of infection. MRI, magnetic resonance imaging, VZIG, varicella-zoster immune globulin, VZV, varicella-zoster virus.

10 kg of body weight, up to a maximum of 625 U (Advisory committee on immunization practices, 1996) or 0.5 ml/kg of body weight (Sauerbrei and Wutzler, 2004b). As alternative, 1 ml/kg of body weight can be administered intravenously (Sauerbrei and Wutzler, 2004b). This cost-intensive prophylactic measure has not been undisputed in the literature (Unger-Köppel et al., 1985). Although passive immunization may theoretically reduce the risk of fetal infection, there is no evidence that this prevents fetal viremia or CVS. In a prospective study, there was no case of CVS or zoster during infancy in 97 pregnancies where maternal varicella occurred despite VZIG administration to the mother post exposure before 36 weeks of gestation (Enders et al., 1994). However, there is a case report of CVS in a woman who received VZIG (Pastuszak et al., 1994). But in this case, VZIG was administered 4 days following exposure where neither the dosage nor the antibody concentration of the VZIG preparation were mentioned by the authors. Therefore, the primary reason for VZIG is to prevent severe chickenpox and complications in the mother. If there is a definitive past history of chickenpox, it is reasonable to assume that the woman is immune to varicella.

Pregnant women, who were adequately vaccinated with two doses should be regarded as immune to varicella because 99% of persons become seropositive after the second dose of vaccination (Kuter et al., 1995). Thus, following exposure, routine serologic testing and administration of VZIG are not considered necessary. Furthermore, currently used enzyme immunoassays may be too insensitive to detect vaccine-induced VZV-specific IgG antibodies (Sauerbrei and Wutzler, 2004c). On the other hand, sensitive fluorescent antibody to membrane antigen (FAMA) assay or tests for the determination of the cell-mediated immune response are too laborious and/or time-consuming for daily routine. Nevertheless, if a vaccinated pregnant woman was tested VZV IgG-negative, she should be managed as an vaccinated seronegative pregnant woman without varicella vaccination. However, in most cases, seronegative vaccinees should have acquired VZV-specific cell-mediated immunity.

The administration of VZIG will not uniformly prevent chickenpox in susceptible contacts who have significant exposure. But it will attenuate the severity of disease and prevent complications (Ogilvie, 1998). VZIG has no therapeutic benefit once chickenpox has developed. Women who have had exposure to chickenpox regardless of whether or not they have received VZIG should contact their doctor as soon as possible if a rash develops (Nathwani et al., 1998). Indications for referral to hospital include the development of chest symptoms, neurological symptoms, hemorrhagic rash or bleeding, a dense rash with or without mucosal lesions, and significant immunosuppression (Royal College of Obstetricians and Gynecologists, 2001). If there are risk factors for the development of pneumonia (Harger et al., 2002a), hospital assessment should be considered. At first signs of varicella pneumonia or other disseminated infections, an antiviral treatment has immediately to be introduced.

As the only therapeutic agent, aciclovir (10 mg/kg every 8 h intravenously for 10 days) is indicated in pregnant women. The United Kingdom Advisory Group on

Chickenpox recommends that oral aciclovir be prescribed for pregnant women with chickenpox if they present within 24 h of the onset of the rash and if they are more than 20 weeks of gestation (Royal College of Obstetricians and Gynecologists, 2001). Results from the aciclovir-in-pregnancy registry do not show teratogenic effects of the drug (Andrews, 1994). Comparable data have been reported for the oral administration of valaciclovir (Enders and Miller, 2000), whereas no data about other nucleoside analogous compounds such as famciclovir and brivudin during pregnancy are available. As aciclovir is not officially approved for the treatment of pregnant women, patients should be informed about the limited information and give consent before the drug is used. To date, there are no controlled studies concerning antiviral chemotherapy in preventing CVS.

Varicella occurring at the first and second trimester

Mothers with varicella during the first or second trimester should be carefully monitored because an intrauterine infection may lead to CVS. Fetal ultrasound at 16–22 weeks gestational age or 5 weeks after infection can identify signs of CVS (Pretorius et al., 1992) (Fig. 3). Most lesions of thoracic, abdominal and retroperitoneal viscera, limb involvement, and even dermatologic features have been described to be apparent on ultrasonography (Verstraelen et al., 2003). However, involvement of the central nervous system, including cerebellar hypoplasia, was not apparent on ultrasound examination, but was clearly demonstrated by prenatal magnetic resonance imaging (MRI). Therefore, MRI should be included into prenatal diagnosis of CVS. Laboratory investigations for VZV DNA in placental villi, fetal blood, or amniotic fluid and for VZV IgM in fetal blood are only indicated if suspicious fetal abnormalities can be seen on ultrasound or MRI (Pretorius et al., 1992). In one observational study, 9 (8.4%) out of 107 women who developed chickenpox before 24 weeks gestation had VZV DNA detected in the amniotic fluid (Mouly et al., 1997). Five of these 9 women subsequently delivered normal infants. No case of CVS occurred when amniocentesis was negative for VZV DNA. Thus, one should be aware that the presence of VZV DNA does not necessarily correlate with fetal disease. The question of how severely the fetus is affected cannot yet be answered definitely. This and the low risk of CVS should be considered in counseling women with varicella in early pregnancy. Termination of pregnancy is only indicated if there are definitive signs of serious fetal abnormalities.

An antiviral treatment of neonates with CVS has been described in few cases (Wutzler et al., 1990–1991, Sauerbrei et al., 2003; Schulze-Oechtering et al., 2004). According to clinical observations, aciclovir therapy may be helpful especially to stop the progression of eye diseases or to prevent neurological diseases after VZV reactivations.

Varicella during the perinatal period

After maternal chickenpox during the last weeks of gestation longer than 5 days before the delivery, neonatal varicella may occur, however, the newborns do usually not develop any complications. For this reason, passive immunization or antiviral treatment are mostly not necessary in these cases. If maternal chickenpox is observed between 4 (–5) days before and 2 days after delivery, there is a risk of severe varicella for the neonate within the first 12 days of life. To reduce the mortality from neonatal chickenpox, the date of delivery may be postponed for several days by means of tocolysis to allow maternal antibodies to pass the placental barrier (Fig. 3). However, there are only few published case reports which describe successfully the delay of labor when neonatal varicella must be expected (Paulman and McLellan, 1990; Zieger et al., 1994). Tocolytic treatment is possible by means of intravenous medication of fenoterolhydrobromide or atosiban. But, an efficacy cannot always be achieved if the treatment is performed after beginning of labor.

VZIG given intravenously at a dosage of 1 ml/kg (Deutsche Gesellschaft für Pädiatrische Infektiologie, 2003) or intramuscularly at a dosage of 125 U (Advisory committee on immunization practices, 1996) or 0.2 (–0.5) ml/kg, maximally 5 ml (Deutsche Gesellschaft für Pädiatrische Infektiologie, 2003) is indicated for neonates whose mothers have signs and symptoms of varicella between 5 days pre partum and 2 days post partum. The Department of Health Joint Committee on Vaccination and Immunisation (United Kingdom) recommends passive immunization for a period between 7 days before and 2 days after delivery (Miller, 1994) and the Committee on Infectious Diseases of the American Academy of Pediatrics (United States) recommends VZIG for infants whose mothers develop chickenpox between 5 days before and 3 days after delivery (Prober et al., 1990). However, VZIG is probably not necessary for neonates whose mothers have sings of varicella > 5 days before or > 2 days after delivery, because those infants are not at risk of severe neonatal varicella. Hospitalized-premature infants, younger than 28 weeks gestation or below 1000 g birth weight, who are exposed to VZV, have to receive VZIG, regardless of the maternal history of chickenpox as these infants may not have acquired maternal antibodies (Advisory committee on immunization practices, 1996). Following treatment, these newborns should be under surveillance in the hospital for 2 weeks, i.e. to the end of incubation period (Prober et al., 1990; Deutsche Gesellschaft für Pädiatrische Infektiologie, 2003). When a neonate who has received VZIG is discharged home, it must be made clear to the parents that prompt hospital review should be undertaken if the baby becomes unwell or develops rash. It is generally accepted that passive immunization of the newborn can modify beneficially the clinical course of neonatal varicella but it does not prevent the disease and, although decreased, the risk of death is not eliminated (Holland et al., 1986; King et al., 1986; Sauerbrei, 1998). Normal immunoglobulin preparations for intravenous use (IVIG) also provide sufficient amount of antibodies against VZV. Hence, IVIG could be used for the purpose if VZIG is not available (Huang et al., 2002).

On suspicion of neonatal chickenpox, aciclovir therapy should be administered promptly at a dosage of 10–15 mg/kg every 8 h intravenously for 5–7 days. Prophylactic intravenous aciclovir can prevent neonatal varicella or reduce the severity of the disease markedly (Carter et al., 1986). To date, well-controlled studies on the use of aciclovir in newborns have not been reported. Mothers and newborns suffering from or being at risk of varicella have to be isolated on maternity wards.

References

Advisory committee on immunization practices (ACIP). Prevention of varicella. MMWR 1996; 45: 1.

Akisu M, Yalaz M, Aksu G, Arslanoglu S, Genel F, Kutukculer N, Kultursay N. Maternally acquired varicella-zoster virus antibodies disappear at 6 months of age in prematurely born children. Panminerva Med 2003; 45: 155.

Alanen A, Kahala K, Vahlberg T, Koskela P, Vainionpää R. Seroprevalence, incidence of prenatal infections and reliability of maternal history of varicella zoster virus, cytomegalovirus, herpes simplex virus and parvovirus B19 infection in South-Western Finland. BJOG 2005; 112: 50.

Al-Katawee YA, Al-Hassoun YA, Taha MN, Al-Moslem K. Congenital varicella-zoster virus infection. A rare case of severe brain and ocular malformations without limb or cutaneous involvement in a newborn after maternal subclinical infection. Saudi Med J 2005; 26: 869.

Andrews EB. Acyclovir does not increase risk in pregnancy. Am Pharm 1994; NS34: 6.

Baba K, Yabuuchi H, Takahashi M, Ogra PL. Immunologic and epidemiologic aspects of varicella infection acqired during infancy and early childhood. J Pediatr 1982; 100: 881.

Baren JM, Nenneman PL, Lewis RJ. Primary varicella in adults: pneumonia, pregnancy, and hospital admission. Ann Emerg Med 1996; 28: 165.

Birch CJ, Druce JD, Catton MC, MacGregor L, Read T. Detection of varicella-zoster virus in genital specimens using a multiplex polymerase chain reaction. Sex Transm Infect 2003; 79: 298.

Birthistle K, Carrington D. Fetal varicella syndrome—a reappraisal of literature. J Infection 1998; 36: 25.

Boumahni B, Kauffmann E, Laffitte A, Randrianaivo H, Fourmaintraux A. Congenital varicella: limits of prenatal diagnosis. Arch Pediatr 2005; 12: 1361.

Brazin SA, Simkowich JW, Johnson T. Herpes zoster during pregnancy. Obstet Gynecol 1979; 53: 175.

Carter PE, Duffty P, Lloyd DJ. Neonatal varicella infection. Lancet 1986; 2: 1459.

Chandra PC, Patel H, Schiavello HJ, Briggs SL. Successful pregnancy outcome after complicated varicella pneumonia. Obstet Gynecol 1998; 92: 680.

Chant KG, Sullivan EA, Burgess MA, Ferson MJ, Forrest JM, Baird LM, Tudehope DI, Tilse M. Varicella-zoster virus infection in Australia. Aust N Z J Public Health 1998; 22: 413.

Choo PW, Donahue JG, Manson JE, Platt R. The epidemiology of varicella and its complications. J Infect Dis 1995; 172: 706.

Dahl H, Marcoccia J, Linde A. Antigen detection: the method of choice in comparison with virus isolation and serology for laboratory diagnosis of herpes zoster in human immunodeficiency virus-infected patients. J Clin Microbiol 1997; 35: 347.

Deutsche Gesellschaft für Pädiatrische Infektiologie. Handbuch 2003: Infektionen im Kindesalter. München: Futuramed; 2003; p. 732.

Enders G, Miller E, Cradock-Watson J, Bolley I, Ridehalgh M. Consequences of varicella and herpes zoster in pregnancy: prospective study of 1739 cases. Lancet 1994; 343: 1548.

Enders G, Miller E. Varicella and herpes zoster in pregnancy and the newborn. In: Varicella-Zoster Virus. Virology and Clinical Management (Arvin AM, Gershon AA, editors). Cambridge: University Press; 2000; p. 317.

Enders G. Varicella-zoster virus infection in pregnancy. Prog Med Virol 1984; 29: 166.

Fairley CK, Miller E. Varicella-zoster virus epidemiology—a changing scene? J Infect Dis 1996; 174(Suppl 3): S314.

Frangidis CY, Pneumatikos I. Varicella-zoster pneumonia in adults: report of 14 cases and review of the literature. Eur J Internal Med 2004; 15: 364.

Garnett GP, Cox MJ, Bundy DA, Didier JM, St Catharine J. The age of infection with varicella-zoster virus in St Lucia, West Indies. Epidemiol Infect 1993; 110: 361.

Gershon AA, Raker R, Steinberg S, Topf-Olstein B, Drusin LM. Antibody to varicella-zoster virus in parturient women and their offspring during the first year of life. Pediatrics 1976; 58: 692.

Gershon AA, Steinberg SP. The National Institute of Allergy and Infectious Disease Varicella Vaccine Collaborative Study Group. Live attenuated varicella vaccine: protection in healthy adults compared with leukemic children. J Infect Dis 1990; 158: 661.

Gershon AA. Varicella-zoster virus. In: Textbook of Pediatric Infectious Diseases (Feigin RD, Cherry JD, editors). 4th ed. Philadelphia: W. B. Saunders Company; 1998; p. 1769.

Grose C. Congenital varicella-zoster virus infection and the failure to establish virus-specific cell-mediated immunity. Mol Biol Med 1989; 6: 453.

Guess HA, Broughton DD, Melton III LJ, Kurland LT. Population-based studies of varicella complications. Pediatrics 1986; 78: 723.

Haake DA, Zakowski PC, Haake DL, Bryson XJ. Early treatment with acyclovir for varicella pneumonia in otherwise healthy adults: retrospective controlled study and review. Rev Infect Dis 1990; 12: 788.

Hanngren K, Grandien M, Granström G. Effect of zoster immunoglobulin for varicella prophylaxis in the newborn. Scand J Infect Dis 1985; 17: 343.

Harger JH, Ernest JM, Thurnau GR, Moawad A, Momirova V, Landon MB, Paul R, Miodovnik M, Dombrowski M, Sibai B, Van Dorsten P, National Institute of Child Health and Human Development, Network of Maternal-Fetal Medicine Units. Risk factors and outcome of varicella-zoster virus pneumonia in pregnant women. J Infect Dis 2002a; 185: 422.

Harger JH, Ernest JM, Thurnau GR, Moawad A, Thom E, Paul R, Miodovnik M, Dombrowski M, Sibai B, Van Dorsten P, McNellis D, National Institute of Child Health and Human Development, Network of Maternal-Fetal Medicine Units. Frequency of congenital varicella syndrome in a prospective cohort of 347 pregnant women. Obstet Gynecol 2002b; 100: 260.

Harris RE, Rhoades ER. Varicella pneumonia complicating pregnancy. Report of a case and review of literature. Obstet Gynecol 1965; 25: 734.

Heidl M. Varicella-Zoster-Virus-Infektion in der Schwangerschaft, beim Neugeborenen und jungen Säugling. Z Klin Med 1985; 40: 245.

Higa K, Dan K, Manabe H. Varicella-zoster virus infections during pregnancy: hypothesis concerning the mechanisms of congenital malformation. Obstet Gynecol 1987; 69: 214.

Holland P, Isaacs D, Moxon ER. Fatal neonatal varicella infection. Lancet 1986; 2: 1156.

Huang YC, Lin TY, Lin YJ, Lien RI, Chou YH. Prophylaxis of intravenous immunoglobulin and acyclovir in perinatal varicella. Eur J Pediatr 2002; 160: 91.

Hubbard TW. Varicella occurring in an infant twenty four hours after birth. BMJ 1878; 1: 822.

Johansson AB, Rassart A, Blum D, Van Beers D, Liesnard C. Lower-limb hypoplasia due to intrauterine infection with herpes simplex virus type 2: possible confusion with intrauterine varicella-zoster syndrome. Clin Infect Dis 2004; 38: e57.

King SM, Gorensek M, Ford-Jones EL, Read SE. Fatal varicella-zoster infection in a newborn treated with varicella-zoster immunoglobulin. Pediatr Infect Dis 1986; 5: 588.

Knowles SJ, Grundy K, Cahill I, Cafferkey MT. Susceptibility to infectious rash illness in pregnant women from diverse geographical regions. Commun Dis Public Health 2004; 7: 344.

Koskimies O, Lapinleimu K, Saxén L. Infections and other maternal factors as risk indicators for congenital malformations: a case-control study with paired serum samples. Pediatrics 1978; 61: 832.

Krah DL. Assays for antibodies to varicella-zoster virus. Infect Dis Clin North Am 1996; 10: 507.

Kuter BJ, Ngai A, Patterson CM, Staehle BO, Cho I, Matthews H, Provost PJ, White CJ. Safety, tolerability, and immunogenicity of two regimens of Oka/Merck varicella vaccine (Varivax®) in healthy adolescents and adults. Vaccine 1995; 13: 967.

Laforet EG, Lynch Jr. CJ. Multiple congenital defects following maternal varicella. N Engl J Med 1947; 236: 534.

Leineweber B, Grote V, Schaad UB, Heininger U. Transplacentally acquired immunoglobulin G antibodies against measles, mumps, rubella and varicella-zoster virus in preterm and full term newborns. Pediatr Infect Dis 2004; 23: 361.

Liesnard C, Donner C, Brancart F, Rodesch F. Varicella in pregnancy. Lancet 1994; 344: 350.

Leventon-Kriss S, Yoffe R, Rannon L, Modan M. Seroepidemiologic aspects of varicella-zoster virus infections in an Israeli Jewish population. Israel J Med Sci 1978; 14: 766.

Meyers JD. Congenital varicella in term infants: risk reconsidered. J Infect Dis 1974; 129: 215.

Michie CA, Acolet D, Charlton R, Stevens JP, Happerfield LC, Bobrow LG, Kangro H, Gau G, Modi N. Varicella-zoster contracted in the second trimester of pregnancy. Pediatr Infect Dis J 1992; 11: 1050.

Miller E. Varicella-zoster virus infection in pregnancy. Arch DisChild 1994; 70: F157.

Miller E, Cradock-Watson JE, Ridehalgh MK. Outcome in newborn babies given anti-varicella-zoster immunoglobulin after perinatal maternal infection with varicella-zoster virus. Lancet 1989; 2: 371.

Mouly F, Mirlesse V, Meritet JF, Rozenberg F, Poissonier MH, Lebon P, Daffos F. Prenatal diagnosis of fetal varicella-zoster virus infection with polymerase chain reaction of amniotic fluid in 107 cases. Am J Obstet Gynecol 1997; 177: 894.

Mustonen K, Mustakangas P, Valanne L, Haltia M, Koskiniemi M. Congenital varicella-zoster virus infection after maternal subclinical infection: clinical and neuropathological findings. J Perinatol 2001; 21: 141.

Nathwani D, Maclean A, Conway S, Carrington D. Varicella infections in pregnancy and the newborn. J Infect 1998; 36(Suppl 1): 59.

Nikkels A, Delbecque K, Pierard GE, Wienkötter P, Schalasta G, Enders M. Distribution of varicella-zoster virus DNA and gene products in tissues of a first-trimester varicella-infected fetus. J Infect Dis 2005; 191: 540.

Ogilvie NM. Antiviral prophylaxis and treatment in chickenpox. A review prepared for the UK Advisory Group on chickenpox on behalf of the British Society for the Study of Infection. J Infect 1998; 36(Suppl 1): 31.

Paryani SG, Arvin AM. Intrauterine infection with varicella-zoster virus after maternal varicella. N Engl J Med 1986; 314: 1542.

Pastuszak AL, Levy M, Schick B, Zuber C, Feldkamp M, Gladstone J, Bar-Levy F, Jackson E, Donnenfeld A, Meschino W, Koren G. Outcome after maternal varicella infection in the first 20 weeks of pregnancy. N Engl J Med 1994; 330: 901.

Paulman PM, McLellan R. Varicella during pregnancy: the timing of effective treatment. J Am Board Fam Pract 1990; 3: 121.

Pretorius DH, Hayward I, Jones KL, Stamm E. Sonographic evaluation of pregnancies with maternal varicella infection. J Ultrasound Med 1992; 11: 459.

Prober CG, Gershon AA, Grose C, McCracken GH, Nelson JD. Consensus: varicella-zoster infections in pregnancy and the perinatal period. Pediatr Infect Dis J 1990; 9: 865.

Robert Koch-Institut. Empfehlungen der Ständigen Impfkommission (STIKO) am Robert Koch-Institut/Stand: Juli 2004. Epidemiol Bull 2004; 30: 235.

Robert Koch-Institut. Neuerungen in den aktuellen Impfempfehlungen der STIKO. Epidemiol Bull 2005; 31: 273.

Royal College of Obstetricians and Gynecologists. Chickenpox in pregnancy, 2001; Guideline No. 13.

Salleras L, Dominguez À, Vidal J, Plans P, Salleras M, Taberner JL. Seroepidemiology of varicella-zoster virus infection in Catalonia (Spain). Rationale for universal vaccination programmes. Vaccine 2001; 19: 183.

Salzman MB, Sharrar RG, Steinberg S, LaRussa P. Transmission of varicella-vaccine virus from a healthy 12-month-old child to his pregnant mother. J Pediatr 1997; 131: 151.

Sauerbrei A. Varicella-zoster virus infections in pregnancy. Intervirology 1998; 41: 191.

Sauerbrei A, Eichhorn U, Schacke M, Wutzler P. Laboratory diagnosis of herpes zoster. J Clin Virol 1999; 14: 31.

Sauerbrei A, Glück B, Jung K, Bittrich H, Wutzler P. Congenital skin lesions caused by intrauterine coxsackievirus B3 infection: a case report. Infection 2000; 28: 326.

Sauerbrei A, Müller D, Eichhorn U, Wutzler P. Detection of varicella-zoster virus in congenital varicella syndrome: a case report. Obstet Gynecol 1996; 88: 687.

Sauerbrei A, Pawlak J, Luger C, Wutzler P. Intracerebral VZV reactivation in congenital varicella syndrome? A case report. Dev Med Child Neurol 2003; 45: 837.

Sauerbrei A, Sonntag S, Wutzler P. Durchseuchung von Schwangeren mit dem Varicella-Zoster-Virus. Zentbl Gynaekol 1990; 112: 223.

Sauerbrei A, Wutzler P. The congenital varicella syndrome. J Perinatol 2000; 20: 548.

Sauerbrei A, Wutzler P. Neonatal varicella. J Perinatol 2001; 21: 545.

Sauerbrei A, Wutzler P. Das fetale Varizellensyndrom. Monatsschr Kinderheilkd 2003; 151: 209.

Sauerbrei A, Wutzler P. Varicella during pregnancy. Part 1: epidemiology and clinical symptoms. Dtsch Med Wochenschr 2004a; 129: 1983.

Sauerbrei A, Wutzler P. Varicella-Zoster-Virus-Infektionen: Aktuelle Prophylaxe und Therapie. Bremen: Uni-Med; 2004b; p. 43.

Sauerbrei A, Wutzler P. Labordiagnostik der Varizellen. Kinderärztl Prax 2004c; Sonderheft Impfen; 18.

Sauerbrei A, Wutzler P. Varicella-zoster virus infections during pregnancy: epidemiology, clinical symptoms, diagnosis, prevention and therapy. Curr Pediat Rev 2005; 1: 205.

Scharf A, Scherr O, Enders G, Helftenbein E. Virus detection in the fetal tissue of a premature delivery with congenital varicella syndrome: a case report. J Perinatol Med 1990; 18: 317.

Schneweis KE, Krentler C, Wolff MH. Durchseuchung mit dem Varicella-Zoster-Virus und serologische Feststellung der Erstinfektionsimmunität. Dtsch Med Wschr 1985; 110: 453.

Schulze A, Dietzsch HJ. The natural history of varicella embryopathy: a 25-year follow-up. J Pediatr 2000; 137: 871.

Schulze-Oechtering F, Roth B, Enders G, Grosser R. Kongenitales Varizellensyndrom—besteht eine Infektionsgefahr für die Umgebung? Dtsch Med Wochenschr 2004; 208: 25.

Sever J, White LR. Intrauterine viral infections. Ann Rev Med 1968; 19: 471.

Shields KE, Galil K, Seward J, Sharrar RG, Cordero JF, Slater E. Varicella vaccine exposure during pregnancy: data from the first 5 years of the pregnancy registry. Obstet Gynecol 2001; 98: 14.

Smego Jr. RA, Asperille MO. Use of acyclovir for varicella pneumonia during pregnancy. Obstet Gynecol 1991; 78: 1112.

Spranger S, Stute H, Blankenagel A, Jauch A, Hager D, Tariverdian G. MIDAS-Syndrom—Eine X-chromosomale Erkrankung. Differenzialdiagnose zum kongenitalen Varizellensyndrom. Monatsschr Kinderheilkd 1998; 146: 761.

Stagno S, Whitley RJ. Herpesvirus infections of pregnancy. Part II: herpes simplex virus and varicella-zoster virus infections. N Engl J Med 1985; 313: 1327.

Sterner G, Forsgren M, Enocksson E, Grandien M, Granström G. Varicella-zoster infections in late pregnancy. Scand J Infect Dis 1990; 71: 30.

Thiry N, Beutels B, Shkedy Z, Vranckx R, Vandermeulen C, Wielen MV, Damme PV. The seroepidemiology of primary varicella-zoster virus infection in Flanders (Belgium). Eur J Pediatr 2002; 161: 588.

Trlifajová J, Švandová E, Pokorný J, Pokorný J. A laboratory study of age-related varicella incidence and prevalence in the Czech Socialist Republic. Acta Virol 1989; 33: 183.

Unger-Köppel J, Kilcher P, Tönz O. Varizellenfetopathie. Helv Paediat Acta 1985; 40: 399.

Van der Zwet WC, Vandenbroucke-Grauls C, Elburg RM, Cranendonk A, Zaaijer HL. Neonatal antibody titers against varicella-zoster virus in relation to gestational age, birth weight, and maternal titer. Pediatrics 2002; 109: 79.

Vázquez M, Shapiro ED. Varicella vaccine and infection with varicella-zoster virus. N Engl J Med 2005; 352: 439.

Verstraelen H, Vanzieleghem B, Deroort P, Vanhaesebrouck P, Temmerman M. Prenatal ultrasound and magnetic resonance imaging in fetal varicella syndrome: correlation with pathology findings. Prenat Diagn 2003; 23: 705.

Watson B. Varicella: a vaccine preventable disease? J Infect 2002; 44: 220.

Webster MH, Smith CS. Congenital abnormalities and maternal herpes zoster. BMJ 1977; 2: 1193.

Wutzler P, Färber I, Wagenpfeil S, Bisanz H, Tischer A. Seroprevalence of varicella-zoster virus in the German population. Vaccine 2001; 20: 121.

Wutzler P, Sauerbrei A, Scholz H, Müller D, Wiedersberg H. Varicella-Zoster-Virusinfektionen in der Schwangerschaft. Paediat Prax 1990–1991; 41: 213.

Zieger W, Friese K, Weigel M, Becker KP, Melchert F. Varizellen-Infektion am Geburtstermin. Z Geburtsh Perinatol 1994; 198: 134.

Congenital and Other Related Infectious
Diseases of the Newborn
Isa K. Mushahwar (Editor)
© 2007 Elsevier B.V. All rights reserved
DOI 10.1016/S0168-7069(06)13005-0

Human Immunodeficiency Viruses: Molecular Virology, Pathogenesis, Diagnosis and Treatment

Isa K. Mushahwar

Abbott Laboratories, Congenital Infectious Diseases,
Abbott Park, IL 60064, USA

Introduction

Acquired immunodeficiency syndrome (AIDS) was first reported in the United States in 1981, and has established a worldwide epidemic. AIDS is caused by human immunodeficiency virus (HIV), which selectively kills cells of the immune system that are important to prevent disease due to infectious agents. There are more than 40 million people now living with HIV worldwide. There were 3 million HIV-related deaths in 2003, indicating that HIV has emerged as a major cause of death due to an infectious agent.

Etiologic agent

There are two major subtypes of HIV, HIV-1 and HIV-2. It is believed that HIV-1 arose from a strain of SIV in chimpanzees (SIV cpz) while HIV-2 arose from a strain of SIV from the sooty mangabey monkey (SIV-SM). Both HIV-1 and HIV-2 are members of the genus Lentivirinae of the family Retroviridae. Retroviruses are spherical enveloped, positive strand RNA viruses with diameters of about 80–120 nm. The infectious virions contain two copies of a single-stranded genomic RNA about 7–11 kb in length. The RNA is surrounded by viral enzymes and structural proteins forming a nucleocapsid and a matrix shell. A lipid envelope derived from the host cell membrane and studded with viral proteins lies to the outside of the matrix shell. Viral glycoprotein (gp) oligomers are found inserted into the membrane. This helps mediate absorption to receptors located on a suitable host cell and penetration of the host membrane (Schupbach and Gallo, 2000).

The HIV-1 genome is comprised of nine genes, three of which are common to other retroviruses and six of which are unique to HIV-1. The common genes include 5'-gag-pol-env-3'. The gag gene directs the synthesis and assembly of the structural precursor protein gag that is processed via the protease gene to form inner structural proteins (nucleocapsid, matrix and capsid proteins) that are present in the mature infectious virions. The pol gene encodes the enzymatic proteins including protease (PR), reverse transcriptase (RT) and integrase (IN). These enzymes are required to generate mature inner structural proteins by processing of the gag precursor protein (PR), to produce viral DNA from RNA template (RT) and to allow the double-stranded (ds) viral DNA to integrate into the host genome prior to the transcription of viral mRNA (IN). The envelop gene encodes for a precursor protein (gp160) that is processed by cellular proteases to yield the surface (SU) lipoprotein gp120 that determines cell tropism (by attaching to CD4 receptors and other co-receptors) and the gp41 protein that is a transmembrane protein that is also involved in viral entry into cells, and play a role in cellular fusion.

Pathogenesis

Following infection with HIV, a flu-like syndrome may develop within days to weeks, although some individuals may be asymptomatic. Primary HIV infection includes fever, fatigue, lympadenopathy and sometimes a macular rash. Symptoms may last for days to several weeks. Most individuals are asymptomatic for several months to several years following the primary infection. Despite this apparent latency, there is continuous viral replication and over time, progressive reduction in the T-helper lymphocytes.

The natural history of HIV-1 infection involves a continuous process wherein immune dysfunction and the loss of CD4-bearing cells begin at infection and progressively increase over time (Dawson and Mushahwar, 2005). Eventually, the immune system is impaired and the individual becomes susceptible to opportunistic infections. The time for infection to the development of frank AIDS may range from several months to 15 or more years. Typically patients with high levels of HIV-1 replication and a high viral load experience more rapid disease progression than those in whom viral replication is contained.

HIV enters susceptible cells by the specific affinity interaction between the outer envelope gp120 of HIV and the CD4 molecule present on the surface of both T helper/inducer lymphocytes and monocytes (Phupuakrat et al., 2005) Alternatively, HIV may gain entry into cells by phagocytosis, independent of CD4 on the cell surface. Following entry, reverse transcriptase (RT) catalyzes the synthesis of double-stranded HIV DNA, which enters the nucleus and integrates into the host cellular DNA. The virus may then initiate replication or, alternatively, assume a latent state. Latently infected cells may later be activated in the presence of certain cytokines.

The first HIV genes to be expressed are those that encode for regulatory functions that enhance RNA transcription and affect the transport of spliced transcripts into the cytoplasm (Green, 1991). These transcripts encode for the HIV structural and enzymatic proteins necessary for the production of infectious progeny. As the replication cycle is completed, the HIV-infected cell may be destroyed as a direct result of the viral products, or because of the effects of viral building on the cellular membrane, completing of gp120 and CD4 molecules intracellularly, or the accumulation of toxic viral products such as unintegrated viral DNA (Rosenberg and Fauci, 1991; Panteleo and Fauci, 1996). Alternatively, CD4 cells may be killed indirectly by antibody dependent cellular cytotoxicity, complement-mediated cell lysis, or vial syncytial formation with other CD4-bearing cells (Rosenberg and Fauci, 1991).

Among the factors that allow HIV to persist are the heterogeneity of the virus, both within a given individual and between populations of infected individuals (Panteleo and Fauci, 1996) and the ability of HIV to evade the host immune system by establishing a latent infection (Levy et al., 1987), or by replicating in monocyte/macrophage cells after being organized (Robinson et al,. 1988).

The key event in the initiation and progression of HIV disease is the selective destruction of CD4 bearing T cells (T helper/inducer cells). The T helper/inducer CD4+lymphocyte population may be reduced from approximately 1000×10^6 cells/ml to approximately 200–400 10^6 cells/ml (Panteleo and Fauci, 1996). As the numbers of T helper cells decrease, an immune impairment ensues that renders the host susceptible to disease caused by organisms usually held in check by the host's immune system. Most of the illnesses and death attributed to HIV infection are due to opportunistic infectious by organisms such as *Pneumocystis carinii* (pneumonia), *Toxoplasma gondii* (toxoplasmosis), *Crpytococcus neoformans* (cryptococcal meningitis), *Mycobacterium avium* (pneumonia, lymphadenopathy, diarrhea), Cytomegalovirus (retinitis, espophagitis), and *Histoplasma capsulatum* (histoplasmosis, pulmonary infection, disseminated infections).

Infection with HIV-2 may also lead to the development of AIDS (Clavel, 1987; D'Aquila, 1996). However, the immunologic impairment in HIV-2 infected individuals appears to be less severe than with HIV-1, and the disease progression is much slower.

Recent studies (Derdeyn and Silvestri, 2005) suggest that the pathogenesis of HIV infection and AIDS involved two distinct phases. During acute infection, massive depletion of CD4+, CCR5 memory T cells with the mucosal associated lymphoid tissue lead to major and potentially irreversible damage to CD4+T-cell-mediated immune functions. The emergence of potent, but ultimately ineffective cell-mediated and humoral response to HIV lead to the chronic phase of infection, which is characterized by partial control of viral replication, chronic immune activation, progressive decline of the naive and memory T cell pool and systemic CD4+T-cell depletion (Derdeyn and Silvestri, 2005).

Current evidence (Almehmi et al., 2005) suggests that HIV infection may impair the hepatic cytochrome oxidase system, which could lead to an aberration in porphyrin metabolism and subsequently cause porphyria.

Transmission

Transmission of HIV occurs by sexual intercourse (via semen or vaginal secretions), by breast-feeding, by parenteral routes (blood transfusion, intravenous drug use, or infusion of blood products by hemophiliacs) and by perinatal exposure (*in utero* or via the colostrum). Worldwide, nearly 4 million children under the age of 15 years of age have been infected with HIV, and in the year 2003 alone an estimated 700,000 children were newly infected, most via mother to child transmission (UNAIDS WHO. Epidemiological Update December 2003. Geneva; UNAIDS WHO, 2003). The time from exposure to the virus until the development of a detectable antibody response is generally believed to be about 6–12 weeks. Following primary infection, individuals may either remain symptomatic or develop mononucleosis-type illness (Panteleo and Fauci, 1996). During this initial phase of infection, HIV-1 frequently produces a viremia resulting in the detection of antigenemia (Paul et al., 1987), concomitant with or preceding the development of IgG class and sometimes IgM class antibodies against HIV proteins.

Current estimates indicate that over 40 million persons have been infected with HIV-1 and nearly 16,000 new infections occur worldwide each day based on World Health Organization (WHO) reports. HIV-1 is the predominant HIV type throughout the world, and HIV-2, a less-spread type and mostly found in West Africa (D'Aquila, 1996; Soriano et al., 2000). Other areas of high prevalence of HIV-2 include parts of India and Portugal. HIV-2 appears to be less pathogenic than HIV-1 with a prolonged period of asymptomatic infection and slower rates of disease progression reflecting a low rate of vertical transmission (D'Aquila, 1996; Reeves and Doms, 2002).

HIV variants

Phylogenetic analyses have classified HIV-1 strains into three different groups: M that is responsible for the HIV-1 pandemic, O (outlier) and N (non-M/non-O). O and N strains are mainly found in West Africa. HIV group M strains are subdivided into 9 different subtypes (subtype A to D, F to H, J and K), and also into at least 15 circulating recombinant forms such as B/F, A/F, G/A, B/D, F/B, A/D (URF), D/A, and A/E (CRF) (Kuiken et al., 2000). In North America and Western Europe, subtype B is the most prevalent HIV-1 variant. However, a rapid spread of non-B variants have been reported in these countries (Holguin et al., 2005). This has been attributed mainly to population movement, such as migration, travel and high-risk behavior of HIV-1 infectious individuals from various parts of the world where these variants are highly prevalent.

The highly genetic variability of HIV-1 is driven by rapid viral turnover in the HIV infected individual, by a high error rate of the RT, and by the presence of viral RNA as a dimer and by selective immune pressure (Heyndrickx et al., 2000).

So far, seven HIV-2 subtypes have been described (Gueudin et al., 2005), namely, A, B, C, D, E, F and G. The average genetic divergence between different subtypes is about 20% of the gag gene, which is higher than those among HIV-1 group M subtypes (Gao, 2005). Only HIV subtypes A and B are prevalent, the others being considered self-limiting infections at the epidemiological level (Gueudin et al., 2005).

Diagnostic and assay technology

The discovery that interleukin-2 activates T-cells and permits their sustained growth in *vitro* (Poiesz et al., 1980) provided the knowledge needed for propagating HIV-1 *in vitro* in a large scale (Barre-Sinoussi et al., 1983). This feat resulted in the development of several useful immunoassays for the detection of antibodies and a variety of antigens to HIV in serum (Dawson et al., 1988), and also for the detection of viral RNA or DNA in serum or in blood samples.

Enzyme-linked immunoassays

The early serologic techniques utilized infected cells (immunofluorescence) or purified virus (Western blots) to determine exposure to HIV. These were followed by first-generation tests utilizing viral lysate proteins to capture antibodies. The detection was based on use of a probe composed of antibodies to human immunoglobulin conjugated to an enzyme such as horseradish peroxidase or alkaline phosphatase. The second-generation assays for the detection of antibodies to HIV used HIV recombinant antigens. Third-generation assays also employed recombinant antigen in a different assay format, an antibody sandwich assay, employing recombinant antigens on the solid-and liquid-phase conjugates consisted of recombinant proteins labeled with enzymes or with chemiluminescent dyes to form an antibody sandwich type of assay format. In later versions of both the second-and-third generation assays, recombinant antigens representing HIV-2 and group O variants were included in order to enhance detection of these variants.

Antigen assays

Utilizing the above-mentioned antibody tests to HIV, it was found that the seroprevalence for HIV infection among US blood donors was between 0.009% and 0.041% in 1986–1987 (Dawson and Mushahwar, 2005). Although at the time the latest generation of antibody tests provided improved sensitivity for detecting antibodies to HIV, the window to seroconversion remained at about 22–25 days. Since it has been known that viral antigens can be detected in serum prior to seroconversion (Paul et al., 1987), and that transmission of HIV by antibody negative, antigen-positive blood donors has been reported (Gilcher et al., 1990). The US Federal Drug Administration licensed in 1997, a new HIV-1 test to detect the p24 HIV antigen. This test reduced the window period to seroconversion from 22 to 25 days with antibody testing alone to about 16–19 days by using both an antibody test and the antigen test.

With the licensure of nucleic acid amplification tests in the US, the FDA has permitted the discontinuation of HIV-1 p24 testing on the basis of data showing that HIV-1 RNA screening is better able to detect infection in the window period shortly after infection and that all p24 antigen-positive donations are also HIV-RNA positive (Stramer et al., 2004).

Combo assays

In order to reduce the diagnostic window period to seroconversion, new fourth-generation diagnostic assays were introduced in 1998 for the simultaneous detection of HIV antigen and antibody. Further generation assays were proven to detect earlier diagnosis of HIV infection with considerable less false-positive results in comparison to third-generation antibody screening assays (Ly et al., 2004). Many such assays are available commercially and some are also automated. Among these are AxSYM HIV, Ag/Ab Combo (Abbott Laboratories, Abbott Park, IL, USA), Enzygnost Integral (Dade-Behring, Pennsburg, Germany), Genscreen Plus HIV Ag/Ab (Bio Rad, Marnes La Coquette, France), Murex HIV Ag/Ab Combo (Abbott-Dartford, Kent, England), VIDAS HIV DUO Ultra (Biomerieux, Marcy L'Etiole, France), and Vironostika HIV Uniform II Ag/Ab (Organon Teknika, Boxel, The Netherlands).

The assay described by Ly et al., (2004) has been shown to be superior to many other commercially available assays when parameters such as specificity, detection of p24 antigen, number of false-positive samples and overall performance were compared.

Rapid HIV diagnostic tests

The ELISA described previously have been useful and reliable in the diagnosis of and screening for HIV infection in industrialized countries. They are widely used, highly sensitive and specific for the detection of HIV antigens and antibodies. In limited resource settings, however, they are expensive, require complex instrumentation and are too complex to use in the field. Other disadvantages of such tests are the need for well-trained technical manpower, need for a constant supply of electricity and refrigeration for storage, which is impossible to control in rural areas of such settings. Thus, rapid screening for HIV infection performed on site by tests that do not require laboratory infrastructure or highly skilled personnel who can help identify patients who are infected with the virus and can facilitate immediate counseling to help prevent the individual from spreading the virus to others by introducing them to risk-reducing behavior (Palmer et al., 1999). Furthermore, with the implementation of perinatal mother to child transmission (MTCT) programs with rapid HIV testing in antenatal clinics, women can learn their HIV status quickly and can receive short-course antiretroviral prophylaxis to dramatically reduce the risk of transmission of HIV to their children (Rouet et al., 2004). For a complete discussion on advantages of rapid HIV tests the reader is referred to the WHO guidelines for use in HIV testing and counseling in resource constrained settings (World Health Organization, 1992, 1997).

Many rapid HIV commercial kits have been introduced to the diagnostic market in the last few years. Among these rapid assays are: the Determine HIV 1/2 assay (Inverness Medical Innovations); the Genie II HIV-1/HIV-2 (Bio-Rad); rapid check HIV-1 and 2 (Nucleo-de Doencas) and Particle Agglutination Assays (Fujirebio).

During field trials, there was a complete agreement among various investigators (Urassa et al., 1994; Arai et al., 1999; Palmer et al., 1999; Lien et al., 2000; Menard et al., 2003) as to the very high sensitivity and specificity, ease of use, reliability and reproducibility of the rapid Determine assay. Because of this, a description of this assay is appropriate.

The Determine assay (Arai et al., 1999) is based on the sandwich immunoassay technique with HIV-1 and HIV-2 antigens conjugated to selenium colloid and a capture site containing HIV-1 and HIV-2 antigens. If a sample contains anti-HIV-1 or anti-HIV-2 antibodies, the antibodies first react with the antigen–selenium colloid conjugates. As the antibody–antigen selenium colloid complex flow past the capture site, the antibodies react with the antigens at the site with the formation of a visible red line within 15 min. For serum or plasma, 50 µl is placed on the sample application pad. For an EDTA coagulated whole blood sample, 50 µl is placed on the pad, followed by the addition of one drop of buffer. The test also contains a procedural control site that confirms the validity of the assay by the formation of a visible red line. Test devices stored at room temperature (30°C) for 12 months had sensitivity equivalent to that of test devices stored at 2–8°C. No difference in sensitivity was observed when the results were generated at room temperatures ranging from 15°C to 40°C.

Nucleic acid amplification tests

Nucleic acid-based assays for plasma HIV-1 RNA are used to accurately predict the clinical outcome of the HIV-infected patients, to assess the efficacy of anti-retroviral therapies to monitor disease progression. Several commercial assays are available for the quantitative determination of HIV-1 in plasma. These assays include: RT-PCR, nucleic acid sequence-based amplification (NASBA) and the branched-DNA (bDNA) and ligase-chain reaction (LCR). The LCx HIV RNA quantitation assay (Abbott Laboratories) uses competitive RT-PCR followed by microparticle enzyme immunoassay and includes an internal control for inhibition and RNA recovery, that is taken through the entire sample preparation procedure (Johanson, et al., 2001). Commercial assays based upon signal amplification include VERSANT HIV-1 RNA (Bayer), target amplification (COBAS AMP-LICOR HIV-Monitor (Roche) and the Nuclisens HIV RT (Bio-Merieux). The performance of these assays in terms of sensitivity, linearity, reproducibility, specificity and detection of HIV-1 subtypes is practically similar.

An increasingly popular approach to an accurate quantitation of viral RNA is real-time PCR, an alternative quantitation method to conventional RT-PCR quantitation. Real-time PCR offers a wider dynamic range of up to 10^7-fold compared to 1000-fold in conventional PCR and thus offers more accurate quantitation of viral loads (Livak et al., 1995). According to Ambion (Ambion TechNotes, 8:1, 2001), "all real-time PCR systems rely upon the detection and quantitation of a fluorescent reporter, the signal of which increases in direct proportion to the amount of PCR product in a reaction. The reporter is the double-stranded DNA-specific dye SYBR Green (Molecular Probes). SYBR Green binds double-stranded DNA, and upon excitation emits light. Thus, as a PCR product accumulate, fluorescence increase."

Ambion has many products useful for real-time PCR and are routinely used for such analysis at Ambion in the ABI PRISM 7700 Sequence Detection Systems. Real-time PCR assays for the quantitation of HIV RNA are supplied commercially by Roche and Abbott Diagnostics.

More affordable assays for non-industrialized countries have been introduced recently. One of these is the NucliSens Easy HIV-1 assay version (BioMerieux). This assay is a real-time NASBA using molecular beacon-based detection technology (deMendoza et al., 2005). The assay consists of two-step process, namely, nucleic acid amplification combined with a homogenous detection step. Overall, good correlation was demonstrated for this affordable assay when compared to Roche Ampliform version 1.5 (deMendoza et al, 2005).

Antivirals

Three distinct classes of drugs for the clinical therapy of HIV have been approved for treating HIV patients. These drugs inhibit HIV RT, protease or virus entry. Among the nucleoside RT inhibitors (NRTI) are zidoviudine (AZT), lamivudine (3T3), stavudine (d4T) and efavirenz (EFV). These NRTI are used by the viral RT in place of the normal nucleotides and prevent further synthesis, thus inhibiting HIV replication. AZT was one of the first NRTI used to treat HIV patients. It has been effective in both prolonging the survival time of treated patients and in reducing the severity of symptoms associated with HIV disease. However, the virus eventually develops resistance to AZT through the appearance of HIV mutants of RT and disease progression continues.

Among the protease inhibitors (PI) besides the well-known norvir are amprenavir (APV), atazanavir (ATV), indinavir (IDV), lopinavir (LPV), nelfinavir (NFV), ritonavir (RTV) and saquinavir (SQV). Protease inhibitors are known to prevent processing of the viral capsid proteins resulting in non-infectious virions.

A combination therapy of NRTI and PI drugs has been very effective in treating HIV patients. The current standard of care in anti-retroviral therapy includes two NRTI plus a potent third drug, usually a PI (Moyle, 1998). This combination therapy provides impressive reductions in viral loads. However, long-term administration of this combination therapy may increase selective pressure against HIV and subsequently induce the emergence of drug-resistant HIV-1 variants (Imamichi, 2004).

The introduction of antiviral for the clinical therapy of HIV-1 has seen the emergence of drug resistance as a major factor limiting drug efficacy. Resistance to antiviral therapy has been observed for each of the well-known antiviral drugs (Burlet et al., 2005). It has been reported that primary resistance accounts for 8–30% of new HIV-1 infections in Western Europe and North America (Wensing and Boucher, 2003), and in a recent study in the former Soviet Union, the overall prevalence of resistance was 13.3% (Vasques de Parga et al., 2005). Thus, the best HIV therapy should improve patient outcomes and should also deter the transmission of drug-resistant strains (Kiessling et al., 2005). HIV-1-infected individuals should therefore undergo genotypic resistance testing in order to select the most suitable drug regimen.

Genotypic resistance testing is accomplished by sequencing of DNA products generated by PCR (Huang et al., 2005); Garcia-Bujalance et al., 2005). Recently, however, a new high throughput assay system was developed to identify drug resistance (Chen et al., 2005). This assay was designed to specifically detect frame-shift mutations in a single virus replication cycle.

Due to viral resistance and emergence of HIV-1 mutants, attempts have been made to design novel antiretroviral drugs (Imamichi, 2004) to suppress the replication of the resistant variants. Among the first drugs to satisfy this need was enfuvirtide. Enfuvirtide belongs to the third family of antiviral (Barbaro et al., 2005), and is an HIV fusion inhibitor (FI). This drug has a unique mechanism of action involving HIV entry at the stage of membrane fusion. Its antiviral activity and favorable safety and tolerability features have been demonstrated in combination with other agents. It is claimed that the drug offers a low potential for cross-resistance with other anti-retroviral drugs and its extracellular distribution means that drug interactions and intracellular metabolic disturbances are unlikely (Lazzarin, 2005).

Currently, a fourth family of HIV antivirals as investigational drugs are being tested in Phase I clinical trials. These are called integrase inhibitors. The enzyme integrase catalyzes the insertion of the viral cDNA and generated by RT of the viral RNA genome into host chromosomes. The integration reaction consists of two consecutive steps: 3′processing and strand transfer (Pommier et al., 2005).

Diketo acids and diketo-like acids are the most promising integrase inhibitors (Pommier et al, 2005). They are referred to as strand transfer inhibitors because they uncouple the two integrase reactions. They can block strand transfer without affecting 3′-processing by chelating divalent cofactors in the integrase active site and by interfering with host (acceptor) DNA binding (Pommier et al., 2005).

Acknowledgments

The input and constructive comments of Dr. George J. Dawson are gratefully acknowledged.

References

Almehmi A, Deliri H, Szego GG, Teague AC, Pfister AK. Porphyria cutanea tarda in a patient with HIV infection. W V Med J 2005; 101: 19–21.

Arai H, Petchclai B, Khupulsup K, Kurimura T, Takeda K. Evaluation of a rapid immuno-chromatographic test for detection of antibodies to human immunodeficiency virus. J Clin Microbiol 1999; 37: 367–370.

Barbaro G, Scozz A, Mastrolorenzo A, Supuran CT. Highly active antiretroviral therapy: current state of the art, new agents and their pharmacological interactions useful for improving therapeutic outcome. Curr Pharm Des 2005; 11: 1805–1843.

Barre-Sinoussi F, Chermann JC, Rey F, Nugeyre MT, Charmaret S, Gruest J, Dauget S, Axler-Blin C, Vezinet-Brun F, Rouzioux C, Rozenbaum W, Montagnier L. Isolation of a T-lymphotropic retrovirus from a patient at risk for AIDS. Science 1983; 220: 868–870.

Burlet S, Petrancosta N, Laras Y, Garino C, Quelever G, Kraus JL. Prospects for the resistance to HIV protease inhibitors: current drug design approaches and perspectives. Curr Pharm Des 2005; 11: 3077–3090.

Chen R, Yokoyama M, Sato H, Reilly C, Mansky LM. Human immunodeficiency virus mutagenesis during antiviral therapy: impact of drug-resistant reverse transcriptase and nucleotide and nonnucleotide reverse transcriptase inhibitors on human immunodeficiency virus type 1 mutation frequencies. J Virol 2005; 79: 12045–12057.

Clavel F. HIV-2, the West African AIDS virus. AIDS 1987; 1: 135–140.

D'Aquila RT. Human immunodeficiency virus type 2: human biology of the other AIDS virus. Curr Clin Top Infect Dis 1996; 16: 84–101.

Dawson GJ, Heller JS, Wood CA, Gutierrez RA, Webber JS, Hunt JC, Hojvat SA, Senn D, Devare S, Decker RH. Reliable detection of individuals seropositive for human immuno-deficiency virus by competitive immunoassays using *E. coli*-expressed HIV structural proteins. J Infect Dis 1988; 157: 149–155.

Dawson GJ, Mushahwar IK. Human retroviruses. In: The Immunoassay Handbook (Wild D, editor). 3rd ed. London: Elsevier; 2005; pp. 771–778.

deMendoza C, Koppleman M, Montes B, Ferre V, Soriano V, Cypers H, Segondy M, Oosterlaken T. Multicenter evaluation of the NucliSens Easy Q HIV-1 v1.5 assay for the quantitative detection of HIV-1 RNA in plasma. J Virol Methods 2005; 127: 54–59.

Derdeyn CA, Silvestri G. Viral and host factors in the pathogenesis of HIV infection. Curr Opin Immunol 2005; 4: 366–373.

Gao F. Detection of HIV-2 by PCR. Methods Mol Biol 2005; 304: 191–120.

Garcia-Bujalance, de Guevara CL, Gonzalez-Garcia J, Arribas JR, Gutierrez A. Comparison between sequence analysis and a line probe assay for testing genotypic resistance of human immunodeficiency virus type 1 to antiretroviral drugs. J Clin Microbiol 2005; 43: 4186–4188.

Gilcher RO, Smith J, Thompson S, Chandler L, Epstein J, Axelrod F. Transfusion associated HIV from anti-HIV non-reactive, antigen-reactive donor blood. In: *Abstracts of the International Society of Blood Transfusion/American Association of Blood Banks Joint Congress*, Los Angeles, November 10–15. American Association of Blood Banks, Arlington, VA; 1990.

Green WC. The molecular biology of human immunodeficiency virus type 1 infection. New Engl J Med 1991; 324: 308–317.

Gueudin M, Damond F, Simon F. Quantitation of proviral DNA load of HIV-2 subtype A and B using real-time PCR. Methods Mol Biol 2005; 304: 215–220.

Heyndrickx L, Janssens W, Zekeng L, Mussanda R, Anagohou S, Aywera GV, Coppers S, Vereeken K, Witte KD, Rampelbergh RV, Kahindo M, Morison L, McCutchen FE, Carr JK, Albert J, Essex M, Goudsmit J, Asjo B, Salminen M, Bure A. Simplified strategy for detection of recombinant human immunodeficiency virus type 1 group M isolates by gag/env heteroduplex mobility assay. J Virol 2000; 741: 363–370.

Holguin A, Alvarez A, Soriano V. Heterogeneous nature of HIV-1 recombinants spreading in Spain. J Med Virol 2005; 75: 374–380.

Huang DD, Bremer JW, Brambilla DJ, Palumbo PE, Aldrovandi G, Eshleman S, Brown C, Fiscus S, Frenkel L, Hamdan H, Hart S, Kovacs A, Krogstadt P, LaRussa P, Sullivan J, Weinberg A, Zhao YO. Model for assessing proficiency of human immunodeficiency virus type 1 sequencing-based genotypic antiretroviral assays. J Clin Microbiol 2005; 43: 3963–3970.

Imamichi T. Action of anti-HIV drugs and resistance: reverse transcriptase inhibitors and protease inhibitors. Curr Pharm Des 2004; 10: 4039–4053.

Johanson J, Abravaya K, Caminiti W, Erickson D, Flanders R, Leckie G, Marshall E, Mullen C, Obhashi Y, Perry R, Ricci J, Salituro J, Smith A, Tang N, Vi M, Robinson J. A new ultrasensitive assay for quantitation of HIV-1 RNA in plasma. J Virol Methods 2001; 95: 81–92.

Kiessling AA, Eyre SJ, Desmarais BD. Detection of drug resistant HIV-1 strains. Methods Mol Biol 2005; 304: 287–313.

Kuiken C, Foley B, Hahn B. HIV Sequence Compendium. Los Alamos, NM: Theoretical Biology and Biophysics Group, Los Alamos National Laboratory; 2000.

Lazzarin A. Enfuviritide: the first HIV fusion inhibitor. Expert Opin Pharmacother 2005; 6: 453–464.

Levy JA, Evans I, Cheng-Mayer C, Pan IZ, Lane A, Staben C, Dina D, Wiley C, Nelson J. Biologic and molecular properties of the AIDS associated retrovirus that affect antiviral therapy. Ann Inst Pasteur 1987; 138: 101–111.

Lien TX, Tien NT, Chanpong GF, Cuc CT, Yen VT, Soderquist R, Laras K, Corwin A. Evaluation of rapid diagnostic tests for the detection of human immunodeficiency virus type 1 and 2, hepatitis B surface antigen, and syphilis in Ho Chi Minh City,Vietnam. Am J Trop Med Hyg 2000; 62: 300–301.

Livak KJ, Flood SJ, Maramoro J, Giusti W, Deetz K. Oligonucleotides with fluorescent dyes at opposite ends provide a quenched probe system useful for detecting PCR product and nucleic acid hybridization. PCR Methods Appl 1995; 4: 357–362.

Ly TD, Laperche S, Brennan C, Vallari A, Ebel A, Hunt J, Martin L, Daghfal D, Schochetman G, Devare S. Evaluation of the sensitivity of six HIV combined p24 antigen and antibody assays. J Virol Methods 2004; 122: 185–194.

Menard D, Marolomade EE, Mandeng MJ, Talarmin A. Advantages of an alternative strategy based on consecutive HIV serological tests for detection of HIV antibodies in Central African Republic. J Virol Methods 2003; 111: 129–134.

Moyle G. The role of combinations of HIV protease inhibitors in the management of persons with HIV infection. Expert Opin Investig Drugs 1998; 7: 413–426.

Palmer CJ, Duban JM, Koenig E, Perez E, Ager A, Jayaweera D, Cuadrado RR, Rivera A, Rubido A, Palmer DA. Field evaluation of the determine rapid human immunodeficiency virus diagnostic test in Honduras and the Dominican Republic. J Clin Microbiol 1999; 37: 3698–3700.

Panteleo G, Fauci AS. Immunopathogenesis of HIV infection. Annu Rev Microbiol 1996; 50: 825–854.

Paul DA, Falk LA, Kessler HA, Chase RM, Blauuw B. Correlation of serum HIV antigen and antibody with clinical status in HIV-infected patients. J Med Virol 1987; 22: 357–363.

Phupuakrat A, Paris RM, Nittayaphan S, Louisirirotchanakul S, Aeuwarakul P. Functional variation of HIV-1 rev response element in a longitudinally studied cohort. J Med Virol 2005; 75: 367–373.

Poiesz BJ, Ruscetti FW, Gazder AF, Bunn PA, Minna JD, Gallo RC. Detection and isolation of type C retrovirus particles from fresh and cultured lymphocytes of a patient with cutaneous T-cell lymphoma. Proc Natl Acad Sci USA 1980; 77: 7415–7418.

Pommier Y, Johnson AA, Marchand C. Integrase inhibitors to treat HIV/AIDS. Nat Rev Drug Discov 2005; 4: 236–248.

Reeves JD, Doms RW. Human immunodeficiency virus type 2. J Gen Virol 2002; 83: 1253–1265.

Robinson WE, Montefiore DC, Mitchell WM. Antibody dependent enhancement of human immunodeficiency virus type 1 infection. Lancet 1988; 1: 790–794.

Rosenberg ZF, Fauci AC. Immunopathogenesis of HIV infection. FASEB J 1991; 5: 2382–2390.

Rouet F, Didier K, Ekouevi DK, Inwoley A, Chaix M-L, Burgard M, Bequet L, Viho I, Leroy V, Simon F, Dabis F, Rouzioux C. Field evaluation of a rapid human immuno-deficiency virus (HIV) serologic testing algorithm for diagnosis and differentiation of HIV Type 1 (HIV-1), HIV-2 and dual HIV-1-HIV-2 infections in West African pregnant women. J Clin Microbiol 2004; 42: 4147–4153.

Schupbach J, Gallo RC. Human retroviruses. In: Virology Manual (Specter S, Hodinka RL, Young SA, editors). 3rd ed. Washington, DC: ASM Press; 2000; pp. 513–560.

Soriano V, Gomes P, Heneine W, Holguin A, Doruana M, Antunes R, Mansinho K, Switzer WM, Araujo C, Shanmugam V, Lourenco H, Gonzalez-Lahoz J, Antunes F. Human immunodeficiency virus type 2 (HIV-2) in Portugal: clinical spectrum, circulating sub-types, virus isolation and plasma viral load. J Med Virol 2000; 61: 111–116.

Stramer SL, Glynn SA, Kleinman SH, Strong M, Caglioti S, Wright DJ, Dodd RY, Busch MP. Detection of HIV-1 and HCV infections among antibody-negative blood donors by nucleic acid amplification testing. N Eng J Med 2004; 351: 760–768.

Urassa W, Bredberg-Raden MF, Biberfeld G. Evaluation of the WHO human immuno-deficiency virus (HIV) antibody testing strategy for the diagnosis of HIV infection. Clin Diagn Virol 1994; 2: 1–6.

Vasques de Parga E, Rakhmanova A, Perez-Alvarez L, Vinogradova A, Delgado E, Thomson MM, Casado G, Sierra M, Mynoz M, Carmona R, Vegn Y, Contreras G, Medrano L, Osmanov S, Najera R. Analysis of drug resistance-associated mutations in treatment-naïve individuals infected with different genetic forms of HIV-1 circulating in countries of the former Soviet Union. J Med Virol 2005; 77: 337–344.

Wensing AM, Boucher CA. Worldwide transmission of drug resistant HIV. AIDS Rev 2003; 5: 140–155.

World Health Organization. WHO recommendation for HIV antibody testing. Wkly Epidemiol Rec 1992; 67: 145.

World Health Organization. Revised recommendation for the selection and use of HIV antibody tests. Wkly Epidem Rec 1997; 72: 81.

Congenital and Other Related Infectious
Diseases of the Newborn
Isa K. Mushahwar (Editor)
© 2007 Elsevier B.V. All rights reserved
DOI 10.1016/S0168-7069(06)13006-2

Mother-to-Child Transmission of Human Immunodeficiency Virus Type 1

Gabriella Scarlatti

Unit of Viral Evolution and Transmission, DIBIT, Fondazione San Raffaele del Monte Tabor, Via Olgettina 58, 20132 Milano, Italy

Abstract

The World Health Organization (WHO) and United Nations Programme on HIV/ AIDS (UNAIDS) estimated that in the year 2005 there were an additional 700,000 new infections in children, who have been infected through mother-to-child transmission (MTCT). MTCT of HIV-1 accounts for a few hundred infected newborns only in those countries where services for large cover of voluntary counseling and testing of pregnant women and supply of antiretroviral drugs throughout pregnancy with elective Cesarian section and avoidance of breastfeeding are fully established. Intrapartum transmission contributes to approximately 20–25% of infected children, whereas *in utero* transmission to 5–10% and postnatal transmission to additional 10–15% of cases. The single-dose nevirapine (NVP) regimen has provided the momentum to start MTCT programs in many resource-limited countries; however, regimens using a combination of antiretroviral drugs may be more effective in reducing MTCT rates and limiting resistant mutation development.

Epidemiology of HIV-1: 2005 update

Despite decreases in the rate of infection in certain countries, in year 2005 the overall number of people living with HIV has continued to increase in all regions of the world except the Caribbean, as declared by the Joint United Nations Programme on HIV/AIDS (UNAIDS) and World Health Organization (WHO) (World Health Organization (WHO) and United Nations Programme on HIV/ AIDS (UNAIDS), 2005). The number of people living with HIV globally has reached its highest level with an estimated 40.3 million people, almost 3 million more than in 2003. According to the report, the steepest increases in HIV infections have occurred in Eastern Europe and Central (25% increase) and East Asia. However, sub-Saharan Africa continues to be the most affected globally with 64% of new infections occurring.

Levels of knowledge of safe sex and HIV remain low in many countries. In many sub-Saharan countries, two-thirds or more of young women aged 15–24 years lacked comprehensive knowledge of HIV transmission. In several southern African countries, more than three-quarters of all young people living with HIV are women; while in sub-Saharan Africa overall, women between 15 and 24 years old are at least three times more likely to be HIV positive than young men.

More than three million people died of AIDS-related illnesses in 2005; of these, more than 500,000 were children. In Africa, the share of under-five mortality due to AIDS rose from 2% in 1990 to 6.5% in 2003. In a recent pooled meta-analysis study, mortality in infected children was about nine-fold greater than that of un-infected children (Newell et al., 2004). By age 1 year, an estimated 35% infected and 4.9% uninfected children will have died; by 2 years of age, 52.5% of infected children will have died.

The targets within the Declaration of Commitment on HIV/AIDS by the United Nations General Assembly include a 25% reduction by 2010 in the per-centage of 15–24-years-old HIV-infected pregnant women and a 20% reduction by 2005 in infant HIV infection and 50% by 2010, with the global aim of achieving as closely as possible universal access to treatment for all those who need it by 2010.

Epidemiology of mother-to-child transmission of HIV-1

In 2005 there were an additional 5 million new infections, of which 700,000 in children who have mostly been infected through mother-to-child transmission (MTCT) (World Health Organization (WHO) and United Nations Programme on HIV/AIDS (UNAIDS), 2005). This estimate may be affected by the lack of ap-propriate and affordable diagnostic tests for HIV-1 infection in the pediatric popu-lation in resource-limited settings. The routine test available in these countries, based on the detection of antibodies against HIV in the serum, is useless in babies younger than 18 months because of the persistence of antibodies from the mother.

Without drug access rates of HIV-1 MTCT differ from 15to 25% in Europe and the United States of America (USA) to 25–40% in some African and Asian studies (World Health Organization/UNAIDS, 1999). Contributing factors to these geo-graphical differences in the rate of transmission include between others frequency of breastfeeding, and possibly concomitant infections in the pregnant women as well as differences in virulence of the virus according to subtype. While MTCT of HIV-1 has been virtually eliminated from industrialized countries, it still falls far short in most of sub-Saharan Africa. Indeed, MTCT of HIV-1 accounts for a few hundred infected newborns only in those countries where services for large cover of voluntary counseling and testing of pregnant women and supply of antiretroviral drugs throughout pregnancy with elective Cesarian section and avoidance of breastfeeding are established (Mayaux et al., 1997). Elective Cesarian section appears to remain an important intervention to reduce MTCT in women with high viral load even in the *era* of highly active antiretroviral therapy (HAART) (European Collaborative Study, 2005).

An accelerated scale-up of adequate services is urgently needed to reduce this unacceptable gap. Prevention of MTCT of HIV-1 is a crucial entry point for primary prevention, treatment, care and support for mothers, their children and families.

Timing of infection

An accurate understanding of the timing of HIV-1 MTCT is very important for the design of intervention strategies. Today it is clear that transmission of HIV-1 infection can occur before, during and after delivery. The relative contribution of each of these routes has been estimated in the last decade by different approaches and studies. Most (approximately 50%) of the transmission events occur close to delivery, whereas pregnancy and breastfeeding, when performed, contribute to a minor although important extend (20% and 30%, respectively) (De Cock et al., 2000). In absolute numbers intrapartum transmission contributes to approximately 20–25% of infected children, whereas *in utero* transmission to 5–10% and postnatal transmission to additional 10–15% of cases. Early breastfeeding transmission occurring within 6–8 weeks after delivery accounts for 5–6% of additional risk (Nduati et al., 2000; Moodley et al., 2003), whereas late postnatal transmission, persistent for the whole period of breastfeeding, can contribute to 23–42% (John-Stewart et al., 2004).

Routes of transmission

Transmission occurs through the placenta or by swallowing of large amounts of infected biological fluids as the amniotic fluid during gestation, or blood and vaginal secretions during delivery and predominantly milk during breastfeeding.

The role of the placenta is still controversial but it possibly acts as a barrier to the transfer of virus as only a limited number of transmission events occur during pregnancy. The transplacental pathway may include passage of maternal infected cells through breaches of the placental tissue or direct infection of placental cells. Indeed, placental cells, trophoblasts and villous Hofbaur cells, were demonstrated *in vivo* to carry virus from early on in gestation (Lewis et al., 1990; Backé et al., 1992). Virus is not found in placental tissue when the pregnant women undergo antiretroviral prophylaxis with zidovudine (ZDV) throughout gestation (Tscherning-Casper et al., 1999), thus, indicating an effect of the drug on placental level. Indeed, *in vitro* and *in vivo* studies support the view that the nucleoside reverse transcriptase inhibitors (NRTI) cross the placenta and produce significant pharmacological concentrations in the amniotic fluid and in the fetal circulation, nevirapine (NVP) reaches the equilibrium between the fetal and maternal concentration, whereas the protease inhibitors have a poor transfer across the placenta

(Chappuy et al., 2004a, b; Pacifici, 2005). Recently, a study based in Thailand reported that short-term prophylaxis (less than 30 days) with ZDV was significantly less efficient in reducing viral expression in placental tissue than treatment lasting at least 60 days (Bhoopat et al., 2005). This study also confirmed previous findings that infection of the placenta does not always result in transmission to the fetus (Menu et al., 1999).

The placenta may be involved in protecting the fetus from infection through a series of mechanisms. *In vitro* experiments showed that HIV can easily transcytose through a trophoblastic barrier of BeWo cells or, alternatively, HIV infected cells can fuse with trophoblastic cells and transmit the virus to underlying receptive cells (Lagaye et al., 2001). However, the same cells do not replicate HIV due to a restriction postentry level (Dolcini et al., 2003). A balance of cytokines and chemokines at placental level may direct the infection of trophoblastic cells (Derrien et al., 2005). Recently it has been reported that the placenta is likely the site for engagement of innate immunity (Winchester et al., 2004). These data are in favor of selective processes occurring at placental level possibly regulated by factors, as cytokine, chemokines, hormones or antibodies. Perturbation of this microenvironment as for example the ones induced by concomitant infections of the placenta, may result in a lack of the selective process.

Evidence for swallowing of maternal-infected body fluids has been since long demonstrated by the detection of HIV-1 in gastric aspirates of neonates (Nielsen et al., 1996). During breastfeeding the child ingests first colostrums and then milk at increasing volumes. Breast milk contains approximately 10^6 cells/ml, including macrophages, lymphocytes and mammary epithelial cells. The mononuclear cells in the milk are constituted by 75–95% of large, lipid-filled macrophages and 5–25% of predominant activated T lymphocytes (Eglinton et al., 1994), which are cells prone to infection with HIV-1. Of note are recent data suggesting that cell-associated HIV may play a more-important role in transmission via breastfeeding than does cell-free virus (Rousseau et al., 2004).

Mucosal surfaces as the lymphoepithelial tissue of the tonsils or the intestinal mucosa may act as portal of entry, although the exact pathways of the virus are still unclear. Ingested infected fluids and cells can easily pass the neonatal stomach, which does not present an acid environment, and reach the lower intestine. *In vivo* relevance of gut infection has been shown in the simian immunodeficiency virus (SIV) model demonstrating the destruction of CD4+ T cells in the *lamina propria* as early as during acute infection (Li et al., 2005; Mattapallil et al., 2005). It can be envisaged that the M cells in the Peyer's plaques of the digestive epithelium, which deliver samples of foreign material directly to the close intraepithelial lymphoid cells, may be involved. Otherwise, HIV-1 may cross the enterocytes, the cells covering the digestive mucosa. Both types of cells have been shown *in vitro* to be competent for the transport of virus through a mechanism of transcytosis by binding with galactosyl ceramide (Bomsel et al., 1998; Fotopoulos et al., 2002). Knowledge on the mechanisms of virus entry will provide insight for preventive means.

Correlates of HIV-1 MTCT: a mean to predict transmission

A high plasma virus load and a low CD4+ T-cell count of the pregnant women were repeatedly demonstrated to be independent risk factors for the transmission of HIV-1 from an untreated mother to her child. Unfortunately, these markers cannot be used as absolute indicators and predictors of MTCT of HIV-1 for individual mothers (Contopoulos-Ioannidis and Ioannidis, 1998).

Viral genotype and phenotype have given little evidence of a specific pattern associated with MTCT of HIV-1. Most maternal isolates are able to use CCR5 as coreceptor alone or in association with CXCR4 or other chemokine receptors, independently from transmission (Scarlatti, 2004), and thus are not useful predictive markers.

The role of the humoral immune response in predicting and/or preventing MTCT has been target of many studies (Scarlatti, 2004). However, investigation on the maternal serum antibody reactivity to HIV-derived peptides or neutralization of autologous or heterologous virus never gave a conclusive response. Evidence of the relevance of the humoral antibody response in MTCT comes from a study in monkeys, which demonstrated that injection of a cocktail of HIV neutralizing human monoclonal antibodies (2F5, 4E10, IgGb12 and 2G12) can prevent transmission of a lentivirus challenge to baby macaques (Baba et al., 2000). On the basis of these results the authors initiated recently a clinical trial in Kenya to prevent postpartum MTCT of HIV-1 with the same combination of antibodies.

During the last few years a series of studies have provided repeatedly the evidence of transmission of HIV-specific cytotoxic T lymphocytes (CTL) epitopes in which escape had occurred in the transmitting mother (Wilson et al., 1999; Goulder et al., 2001). The different escape mutations localized in Gag were restricted by the HLA molecules B57/5801 or B27 (Leslie et al., 2005). Interestingly, the B57/5801 restricted mutation reverted to wild type when transmitted to a B57/5801 negative child. These results suggest a selection process occurring already in the mother and also indicate that the transmitted escape mutant, which reverts, will be an useful epitope for CTL-based vaccine development.

A series of host genetic factors have been studied to identify correlates of protection. A recent large multivariate analysis showed that mother and child concordance at any HLA class I locus but not class II locus is a strong predictor of MTCT (Polycarpou et al., 2002), however, no specific maternal HLA locus was associated with transmission. Other studies instead showed a predictive value of specific HLA genes. In one study, approximately half of the mothers who transmitted low viral loads had HLA-B*1302, B*3501, B*3503, B*4402 or B*5001 alleles (Winchester et al., 2004), whereas in another study, decreased HIV-1 MTCT risk was strongly associated with a functional cluster of related HLA alleles, the A2/6802 supertype (MacDonald et al., 2001).

The 32-basepair deletion of the CCR5 gene of the mother, which affects the expression of the chemokine receptor on the cell surface, does not correlate with transmission; however, the heterozygous mutation of the child appears to exert a protective effect against MTCT in children exposed to a low maternal viral burden of an R5-type isolate (Ometto et al., 2000). The mutated SDF-1 gene was shown to have some effect only in postpartum transmission in an African study (John et al., 2000).

Many other studies analyzed the genome of the child and not that of the mother, and thus cannot be used as predictive markers of transmission. Anyhow, the results of these studies are relevant to identify mechanism involved in transmission. The presence of a mutated allele of the SDF-1 gene, of the CCR5 gene or of the CCR2b gene of the child does not seem to protect against HIV-1 MTCT (Romiti et al., 2000; Tresoldi et al., 2002). A polymorphism of the mannose-binding protein (MBP) gene (at codon 54) of the child does not correlate with MTCT of HIV-1, however, mutations in the promoter of the MBL2 gene, which codify for the MBP, apparently do (Amoroso et al., 1999; Boniotto et al., 2000). A single-nucleotide polymorphism in the 5′-untranslated region of the DEFB1 gene of the child, which probably regulates the gene expression of human beta defensin 1 (hBD-1), was significantly correlated to risk of HIV-1 MTCT, pointing to the importance of innate immunity in HIV-1 infection (Braida et al., 2004).

Thus, it is evident that as of today there is no possibility to assess the absolute risk of MTCT of HIV-1 in the individual pregnant woman. Possibly, the predictive values of a combination of factors may be more relevant than each factor considered singularly.

A decade of clinical trials with antiretroviral drugs to prevent MTCT of HIV-1

In 1994 the first clinical trial on MTCT (ACTG076), a collaboration between USA and France, proofed the concept that antiretroviral therapy could substantially decrease the risk of MTCT of HIV-1 (Centers for Disease Control, 1994). ZDV given to the pregnant women from the second trimester of gestation and to the baby for 1 month reduced transmission by approximately two-thirds compared to the placebo-treated group. During the following years, a series of clinical trials performed in resource-limited countries demonstrated that ZDV prophylaxis with shorter protocols, more appropriate for the local conditions, was safe and could still reduce the transmission though by not more than 50% (Dabis et al., 1999; Wiktor et al., 1999; Lallemant et al., 2000). Furthermore, longer (from 28 weeks of gestation) antepartum treatment was significantly more effective than shorter (from 35 weeks of gestation) therapy (1.6% vs. 5.1% transmission, respectively), showing that a significant proportion of in utero infection occurs during the last trimester of gestation (Lallemant et al., 2000). The Thai study (PHPT-1) also suggested that longer treatment of the infant could not substitute for a longer treatment of the mother.

During the same time period the national guidelines were modified in several European countries and USA, elective Caesarean section started, women were more frequently treated with combination of antiretroviral drugs and the baby treated for 1 week postpartum only. At these conditions, transmission rates dropped to less than 2%.

At the beginning of the new century the results of the first randomized clinical trials were published, which explored whether short-course combination regimens might have improved efficacy (Mofenson and McIntyre, 2000). Indeed, ZDV plus lamivudine (3TC) prophylaxis showed to be more effective than ZDV alone in short-course regimens using drugs during the last weeks of pregnancy, labor and/or delivery (Mandelbrot et al., 2001; Chaisilwattana et al., 2002; The Petra Study Team, 2002).

The question if a similar efficacy to combination prophylaxis could be achieved with alternative drugs that were less expensive and could be used in very simple regimens was cleared by the HIVNET 012 study. A drug regimen as simple as a single dose of NVP to the mother at labor and to the baby close to birth reduced the transmission rate of approximately 50% compared to ZDV only given to the woman at labor and delivery and to the baby for up to 1 week (Guay et al., 1999). In addition, in the SAINT clinical trial single-dose NVP had similar efficacy to short-course regimens with azidothymidine (AZT) and 3TC (Moodley et al., 2003). The use of NVP was immediately adopted by many public health operators and authorities in resource-limited countries due to the low cost and the shortness of this regimen. Indeed, the single-dose NVP regimen has provided the momentum to start MTCT programs in many resource-limited countries, which in turn have provided the experience and the foundation for treatment access programs.

Although, results from the trials individually suggest that regimens using a combination of antiretroviral drugs may be more effective than single-drug regimens in reducing MTCT rates, the formal comparison of the efficacy of these antiretroviral regimens allowing for other MTCT determinants such as maternal plasma viral load, CD4+ T-cell count and infant feeding practices had not been possible. Recently Leroy and colleagues directly compared the 6-weeks peripartum efficacy of five different antiretroviral interventions in different African settings, taking into account heterogeneity between trials in population characteristics (maternal CD4+ cell count, Caesarean section, breastfeeding, gender and birth weight) in a pooled individual patient data analysis (Leroy et al., 2005). Their results demonstrate that a combination of ZDV and 3TC from 36 weeks of pregnancy had greater efficacy in preventing MTCT than the same combination starting during labor and delivery or than antiretroviral mono therapy (short antenatal ZDV or single dose NVP). At similar CD4+ T-cell levels, MTCT rates were higher in west Africa than in east and South Africa within placebo groups. In comparison with single-dose NVP, the longer ZDV and 3TC combination was the only regimen statistically and significantly more efficacious in preventing MTCT.

More recently completed trials (PHPT-2 and DITRAME-Plus) have focused on enhancement of short-course regimens (Lallemant et al., 2004; Dabis et al., 2005). Addition of single-dose NVP to short-course antiretroviral drug regimens appears to improve efficacy in formula- and breast-fed populations. In the Thai study a single dose of NVP to the mother, with or without a dose to the formula-fed infant, added to oral ZDV prophylaxis starting at 28 weeks of gestation, was highly effective in reducing MTCT of HIV-1 to less than 2% (Lallemant et al., 2004). In the DITRAME-Plus study in Ivory Coast in a breastfeeding setting the 6-week transmission probability was 6.5% with ZDV and single-dose NVP (a 72% reduction compared with ZDV alone) and 4.7% with ZDV, 3TC and single-dose NVP (Dabis et al., 2005).

Recently, a randomized control trial in Malawi, the NVAZ study, compared transmission rates in infants administered NVP only at birth or NVP at birth with ZDV for 1 week, in absence of mother's prophylaxis (Taha et al., 2003). The overall transmission rate at 6–8 weeks was 15.3% in 484 babies who received NVP and ZDV and 20.9% in 468 babies who received NVP only. Thus, 1 week of ZDV added to single-dose infant NVP improved efficacy when no maternal intrapartum NVP prophylaxis was administered.

There are a series of questions, which may undermine the success of antiretroviral prophylaxis in HIV-1 MTCT. It was shown that the reduction in transmission rates was lower among pregnant women with more advanced immune deficiency (Leroy et al., 2003). Cumulative postnatal transmission risk of HIV-1 at 2 years of age of the child was higher among ZDV-treated women with CD4+ T-cell counts below 500 cells/ml than among those with CD4+ T-cell counts above 500 cells/ml (rates 22% and 2%, respectively). Analogously, in another study on the efficacy of ZDV given from 36 weeks of gestation and intrapartum the risk of transmission was significantly reduced only in the women with a plasma viral load below 50,000 copies/ml at enrollment (Jamieson et al., 2003). Further studies are needed to continue and expand efforts for the prevention of MTCT while preserving treatment efficacy.

Prevention of transmission through breastfeeding

The Petra study mined the field when demonstrating the complete loss of the benefits achieved with antiretroviral prophylaxis due to breastfeeding transmission (The Petra Study Team, 2002). Transmission rates evaluated at the age of 18–24 months of the child dramatically increase when the baby has been breastfed. Figure 1 is a graphical representation of the transmission rates evaluated during the first 3 months and at 18–24 months of age of breastfed children born under different prophylaxis protocols. The reduction of transmission by breastfeeding remains a challenge. While formula feeding is an obvious alternative in high-income settings, concern was raised about the need for breastfeeding in areas with low-sanitary standards and high risk of diarrheal diseases.

Feeding practices have been suggested to play a crucial role and contribute differently to transmission. Exclusive breastfeeding, i.e. no other liquids than the mother's milk, could be associated with lower rates of transmission than mixed feeding of breast milk with other milk or feeds and with a similar risk to no breastfeeding (Coutsoudis et al., 1999).

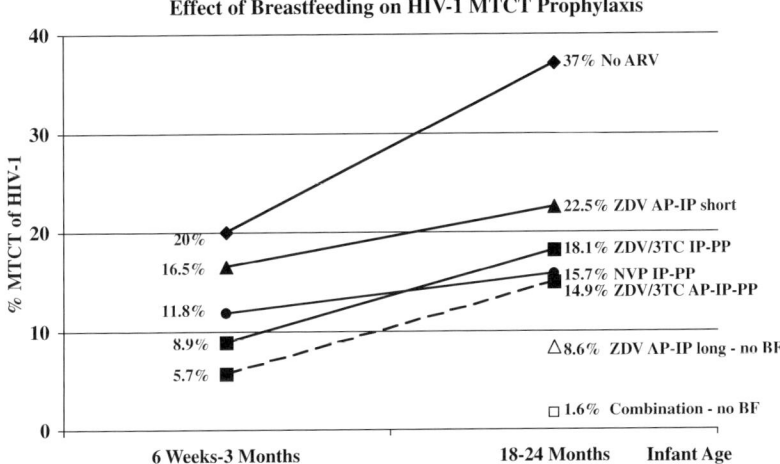

Fig. 1 Effect of breastfeeding on MTCT of HIV-1 in the presence or absence of antiretroviral prophylaxis. The figure indicates the variation in percentages of HIV-1 infection in infants at 6 weeks to 3 months and at 18 to 24 months of age with or without prophylaxis of the women who are breastfeeding in comparison to transmission rates in non-breastfed children born to women with long ZDV or combined antiretroviral prophylaxis. No BF, breastfeeding not performed; No ARV, no antiretroviral prophylaxis given; ZDV, zidovudine; 3TC, lamivudine; NVP, nevirapine; AP, IP, and PP, antepartum, intrapartum, and postpartum, respectively.

Recently, in the context of a trial of postpartum vitamin A supplementation, a program in Zimbabwe provided education and counseling about infant feeding and HIV, prospectively collected information on infant-feeding practices, and measured associated infant infections and deaths (Iliff et al., 2005). Overall postnatal transmission (defined by a positive HIV test after the 6-week negative test) was 12.1%. Compared with exclusive breastfeeding, early mixed breastfeeding was associated with a 4.0%, 3.8% and 2.6% greater risk of postnatal transmission at 6, 12 and 18 months, respectively. Predominant breastfeeding was associated with a 2.6%, 2.7% and 1.6% trend toward greater postnatal transmission risk at 6, 12 and 18 months, compared with exclusive breastfeeding. In the frame of a well-controlled education and counseling program, exclusive breastfeeding may substantially reduce breastfeeding-associated HIV transmission. This same study pointed out that 68.2% of postnatal transmission events occurred after 6 months, which suggests that breastfeeding should be interrupted when the child can take solids safely. Appropriate timing for initiation of weaning is a matter of discussion, however, abrupt weaning should be taken into consideration to avoid mixed breastfeeding.

In a Kenyan study, the use of breast milk substitutes prevented 44% of infant infections and was associated with significantly improved HIV-1-free survival (Nduati et al., 2000). This same study group showed that breastfeeding by HIV-1-infected women might result in adverse outcomes for both mother and infant

(Nduati et al., 2001). Subsequent studies exploring the risks associated to and the feasibility of exclusive breastfeeding practices indicate that either formula or breastfeeding are acceptable and feasible options for HIV-infected women (Rollins et al., 2004).

Alternative methods to prevent HIV transmission through breastfeeding include treatment of the mother's milk. The WHO lists direct boiling, shown to cause significant nutritional damage, and pasteurization, such as Holder pasteurization (62.5 °C for 30 min), which has been reported to inactivate HIV, although retaining most of breast milk's protective elements. A recent pilot study investigated and compared the virologic, nutritional and antimicrobial safety of flash-heating and Pretoria pasteurization, two heat treatments that a mother in a developing country could implement over a fire or in her kitchen (Israel-Ballard et al., 2005). This study shows that flash-heating method would inactive cell-free and cell-associated HIV as well as bacteria in breast milk, but retain nutrients. The problems and doubts on acceptability and feasibility issues because of the stigma that may arise for a mother who is not breastfeeding or who is expressing and heat-treating her milk, however, remain and need to be addressed for the different local realities.

Research for evaluating safety and efficacy of antiretroviral prophylaxis on the risk of early and/or late postnatal transmission has and is actively ongoing. Findings from several clinical trails in breastfeeding populations support the efficacy of short-course antiretroviral prophylaxis of the baby on early postpartum transmission (Guay et al., 1999; Leroy et al., 2002; The Petra Study Team, 2002; Jackson et al., 2003; Moodley et al., 2003). ZDV or NVP mono therapy or ZDV and 3TC together given to the baby either at birth or for 1 week have shown an effect on early transmission rates.

The NVAZ study in Malawi showed that in babies who were HIV negative at birth, and were retested at 6–8 weeks (which accounts for early postnatal transmission) 7.7% of babies who received NVP and ZDV and 12.1% who received NVP only were infected (Taha et al., 2003). Thus, combination therapy had a protective efficacy of 36% on early postnatal transmission in babies born to mothers who were not administered any prophylaxis. This study has now been programmed to investigate if other infant prophylaxis schemes (ZDV only or ZDV with NPV for 16 weeks) increase the efficacy of reducing postnatal transmission rates.

Other ongoing or planned clinical trials will evaluate the efficacy of different regimen and combination of antiretroviral drugs given to the breastfeeding mothers and/or to the breastfed baby from delivery on for varying time periods. Recently, the SIMBA study performed in Rwanda and Uganda, evaluated the effect of NVP or 3TC given from soon after birth until duration of breastfeeding to babies born to mothers treated with AZT and ddI from week 36 of gestation until 1 week postpartum (Giuliano et al., 2005). Overall, transmission rate was 2.4%, with 1.6% early and 0.8% late (above 1 month of age) postnatal transmission events. Transmission rates did not differ between the two arms of treatment (1.1 and 0.6%, respectively).

Resistance to antiretroviral treatment and possible consequences

Drug resistance induced by short-course regimens to prevent MTCT that do not fully suppress the virus has been a concern since early 2000. The factors associated with selection of mutations can be multiple (Fig. 2). Resistance to NVP develops rapidly and has been noted following single doses of NVP until up to 1 year although fading over time (Eshleman et al., 2001; Johnson et al., 2005). Between 15% and 100% of women and their infected children treated with single-dose NVP have one or more non-NRTI (NNRTI) mutations depending on the timing of the sampling and the methodology used for the detection. Real-time polymerase chain reaction reveals a substantial higher percentage of resistance mutations by detecting mutations in two or three times more cases than conventional sequencing techniques do (Johnson et al., 2005; Loubser et al., 2005; Palmer et al., 2005). The *in vivo* relevance of this high frequency of mutations has still to be investigated.

Recent studies suggest that the emergence of NNRTI mutations may be virus subtype dependent. In a multivariate model, subtype and viral load at delivery independently predicted NVP resistance mutations, but maternal age, parity and time between single-dose NVP and the 6–8 week visit did not. The rate of resistance mutations after single-dose NVP was significantly higher in women with HIV-1 subtype C than in women with subtype A or D (69.2%, 19.4% and 36.1%, respectively) (Eshleman et al., 2005b). Analogously, NVP resistance was significantly more frequent in infants with subtype C than with subtypes A and D (87% vs. 50%) (Eshleman et al., 2005c). Studies are needed to assess the clinical significance of the emergence of viral resistance in the different subtypes or recombinant forms induced by NVP prophylaxis.

Factors associated with selection of NNRTI resistance

- Time of sampling after single-dose NVP prophylaxis

- Increased NVP exposure (longer NVP Therapy)

- Number of maternal NVP doses

- Viral subtype (C > D > A)

- High baseline (pre-NVP) HIV-1 RNA load

- Low baseline CD4 + T cell count

- Compartment (eg, breast milk *vs* plasma)

Fig. 2 Factors associated with selection of NNRTI resistance.

The type of resistant mutation detected seems to be dependent upon timing of sampling as well. The NVP mutation Y181C was shown to be the most common occurring at 7 days after NVP administration, whereas the K103N mutation was the most common at 6–8 weeks post-NVP (Eshleman et al., 2004). Furthermore, subtype appeared to influence selection and fading of HIV-1 mutants. At 6–8 weeks post-NVP, the resistant mutations were more frequently detected in women carrying subtype D than in those carrying subtype A viruses (Eshleman et al., 2005a). The explanation appears to be the rate of appearance or disappearance of the NVP mutations. The Y181C mutations faded at greater rate in women with subtype A viruses while the K102N accumulated at greater rate in women with subtype D viruses.

The impact of the resistance development due to single-dose NVP on the following pregnancies is certainly a great concern. As of today, there are few data in this regard. Martinson et al. (2005) showed in a South African study that the effectiveness of single-dose NVP in a second pregnancy is reduced. HIV-1 MTCT rates were substantially higher in women who had been previously exposed to NVP prophylaxis than in those that were naïve to therapy (14% and 4% MTCT rates, respectively). However, the frequency of NNRTI resistant mutations did apparently not differ between the two groups.

The potential impact of these mutations on the efficacy of future NNRTI-based treatment is also of concern. A recent report showed that women exposed to single-dose NVP for MTCT prevention in Thailand experienced a lower but not significant virological success rate of subsequent NNRTI-based therapy compared to non-exposed women (Jourdain et al., 2004). Significant risk factors for a virological failure (i.e. RNA viral load > 50 copies/ml) at 6 months antiretroviral therapy were a viral load at or above median at initiation of therapy, and intrapartum NVP exposure independently of the presence of resistance mutations. However, the timing of treatment initiation postpartum in relation to NVP exposure affected this response: the longer the time the better the response.

For future intervention policies it is important to understand if the selection of NNRTI resistant variants following NVP use for prevention of HIV-1 MTCT can be reduced. Cressey et al. (2005) detected significant NVP concentrations for up to 20 days in the plasma of approximately 55% Thai women following single-dose NVP and suggested that 1 month of additional antiretroviral therapy after delivery should be considered to prevent the emergence of NVP-resistant viruses. In line with this approach, there are several clinical trials. The DITRAME study showed that single-dose NVP associated with short-course treatment during gestation and 3 days postpartum with ZDV and 3TC was more efficient in reducing MTCT rates and in containing the appearance of NVP resistance mutations than a similar treatment with single-dose NVP and short-course ZDV during gestation and 1 week postpartum (NNRTI resistance was 1.14% vs. 28%, and MTCT rates 4.7% vs. 6.5%, respectively) (Dabis et al., 2005). Association of drugs as ZDV and 3TC should be safe as ZDV resistance usually only emerges after several months of partly suppressive therapy. Resistance to 3TC has not been detected when it has been used in combination with ZDV for short periods, but has been detected following longer periods of exposure. Indeed, a recent study did not detect any resistant mutations to ZDV and 3TC used for short-course prophylaxis in any of the 32 treated women (Chokephaibulkit et al., 2005).

Until additional data are available, HIV-infected women and children exposed to single-dose NVP prophylaxis should be considered eligible for NNRTI-based regimens as recommended in the 2003 WHO guidelines for antiretroviral treatment in resource-constrained settings.

WHO recommendations for the prevention of HIV-1 MTCT

The last expert consultation at WHO (June 28–29, 2005, Geneva) agreed that in those settings where full range of antiretroviral drugs are available, pregnant women should be given ZDV from 28 weeks of gestation throughout labor and possibly 7 days postpartum combined with single-dose NVP at labor (World Health Organization (WHO), 2005). Their babies should receive single-dose NVP at birth and ZDV for 1 week. The technical consultation has also made a series of recommendations and provided a full array of circumstances-specific guidelines as to ensure that the largest number of women and their babies benefit from effective MTCT prophylaxis. If single-dose NVP to mother and baby remains the first choice when only minimal range of antiretroviral drug exists, HAART should be initiated as soon as possible when the pregnant woman is in need of this treatment to protect her health and diminish the risk of transmission. To reduce the emergence of NVP-resistant mutations in those settings where the full range of antiretroviral drugs are available, women administered ZDV during pregnancy and single-dose NVP during delivery should be considered to receive ZDV and 3TC combined treatment for 7 days postpartum.

Further, WHO recommendations are that HIV infected women should avoid all breastfeeding only when replacement feeding is acceptable, feasible, affordable, sustainable and safe. Otherwise, exclusive breastfeeding is recommended during the first months of life.

General considerations

The "MTCT-Plus" programmes, which aim to provide lifetime treatment to mothers receiving antiretroviral drugs to prevent neonatal transmission, offer an existing model of intersection between treatment and prevention services. According to WHO in sub-Saharan Africa, a comprehensive prevention and treatment package would avert 55% of the new infections that otherwise could be expected to occur until 2020 (World Health Organization (WHO) and United Nations Programme on HIV/AIDS (UNAIDS), 2005).

Several clinical trails with an array of different drug combinations and intervention regimens have been planned or recently started to respond to unresolved questions on MTCT of HIV-1 during pregnancy, delivery and breastfeeding. An exhaustive list of past, ongoing and future clinical trials is updated on the website www.womenchildrenHIV.org. Questions and problems on MTCT of HIV-1 continuously evolve and are in need of alternative and new solutions according to the setting and available services.

Although triple-combination regimens are widely used in industrialized countries for preventing MTCT in women who do not yet require antiretroviral treatment for their own health, their safety and effectiveness have not been assessed in resource-constrained settings (Thorne and Newell, 2005). There is serious concern about risk to the woman if possible toxicity cannot be carefully monitored.

References

Amoroso A, Berrino M, Boniotto M, Crovella S, Palomba E, Scarlatti G, Serra C, Tovo PA, Vatta S. Polymorphism at codon 54 of mannose-binding protein gene influences AIDS progression but not HIV infection in exposed children. AIDS 1999; 13: 863.

Baba TW, Liska V, Hofmann-Lehmann R, Vlasak J, Xu W, Ayehunie S, Cavacini LA, Posner MR, Katinger H, Stiegler G, Bernacky BJ, Rizvi TA, Schmidt R, Hill LR, Keeling ME, Lu Y, Wright JE, Chou TC, Ruprecht RM. Human neutralizing monoclonal antibodies of the IgG1 subtype protect against mucosal simian-human immunodeficiency virus infection. Nat Med 2000; 6: 200.

Backé E, Jimenez E, Unger M, Schäfer A, Jauniaux E, Vogel M. Demonstration of HIV-1 infected cells in human placenta by *in situ* hybridisation and immunostaining. J Clin Pathol 1992; 45: 871.

Bhoopat L, Khunamornpong S, Lerdsrimongkol P, Sirivatanapa P, Sethavanich S, Limtrakul A, Gomutbuthra V, Kajanavanich S, Thorner PS, Bhoopat T. Effectiveness of short-term and long-term Zidovudine prophylaxis on detection of HIV-1 subtype E in human placenta and vertical transmission. J Acquir Immune Defic Syndr 2005; 40: 545.

Bomsel M, Heyman M, Hocini H, Lagaye S, Belec L, Dupont C, Desgranges C. Intracellular neutralization of HIV transcytosis across tight epithelial barriers by anti-HIV envelope protein dIgA or IgM. Immunity 1998; 9: 277.

Boniotto M, Crovella S, Pirulli D, Scarlatti G, Spano A, Vatta L, Zezlina S, Tovo PA, Palomba E, Amoroso A. Polymorphisms in the MBL2 promoter correlated with risk of HIV-1 vertical transmission and AIDS progression. Genes Immun 2000; 1: 346.

Braida L, Boniotto M, Pontillo A, Tovo PA, Amoroso A, Crovella S. A single-nucleotide polymorphism in the human beta-defensin 1 gene is associated with HIV-1 infection in Italian children. AIDS 2004; 18: 1598.

Centers for Disease Control. Zidovudine for the prevention of HIV transmission from mother to infant. MMWR 1994; 43: 285.

Chaisilwattana P, Chokephaibulkit K, Chalermchockcharoenkit A, Vanprapar N, Sirimai K, Chearskul S, Sutthent R, Opartkiattikul N. Short-course therapy with zidovudine plus lamivudine for prevention of mother-to-child transmission of human immunodeficiency virus type 1 in Thailand. Clin Infect Dis 2002; 35: 1405.

Chappuy H, Treluyer JM, Jullien V, Dimet J, Rey E, Fouche M, Firtion G, Pons G, Mandelbrot L. Maternal–fetal transfer and amniotic fluid accumulation of nucleoside analogue reverse transcriptase inhibitors in human immunodeficiency virus-infected pregnant women. Antimicrob Agents Chemother 2004a; 48: 4332.

Chappuy H, Treluyer JM, Rey E, Dimet J, Fouche M, Firtion G, Pons G, Mandelbrot L. Maternal–fetal transfer and amniotic fluid accumulation of protease inhibitors in pregnant women who are infected with human immunodeficiency virus. Am J Obstet Gynecol 2004b; 191: 558.

Chokephaibulkit K, Chaisilwattana P, Vanprapar N, Phongsamart W, Sutthent R. Lack of resistant mutation development after receiving short-course zidovudine plus lamivudine to prevent mother-to-child transmission. AIDS 2005; 19: 1231.

Contopoulos-Ioannidis DG, Ioannidis JP. Maternal cell-free viremia in the natural history of perinatal HIV-1 transmission: a meta-analysis. J Acquir Immune Defic Syndr 1998; 18: 126.

Coutsoudis A, Pillay K, Spooner E, Kuhn L, Coovadia HM. Influence of infant-feeding patterns on early mother-to-child transmission of HIV-1 in Durban, South Africa: a prospective cohort study. South African vitamin A study group. Lancet 1999; 354: 471.

Cressey TR, Jourdain G, Lallemant MJ, Kunkeaw S, Jackson JB, Musoke P, Capparelli E, Mirochnick M. Persistence of nevirapine exposure during the postpartum period after intrapartum single-dose nevirapine in addition to zidovudine prophylaxis for the prevention of mother-to-child transmission of HIV-1. J Acquir Immune Defic Syndr 2005; 38: 283.

Dabis F, Bequet L, Ekouevi DK, Viho I, Rouet F, Horo A, Sakarovitch C, Becquet R, Fassinou P, Dequae-Merchadou L, Welffens-Ekra C, Rouzioux C, Leroy V. Field efficacy of zidovudine, lamivudine and single-dose nevirapine to prevent peripartum HIV transmission. AIDS 2005; 19: 309.

Dabis F, Msellati P, Meda N, Welffens-Ekra C, You B, Manigart O, Leroy V, Simonon A, Cartoux M, Combe P, Ouangre A, Ramon R, Ky-Zerbo O, Montcho C, Salamon R, Rouzioux C, Van de Perre P, Mandelbrot L. 6-month efficacy, tolerance, and acceptability of a short regimen of oral zidovudine to reduce vertical transmission of HIV in breastfed children in Cote d'Ivoire and Burkina Faso: a double-blind placebo-controlled multicentre trial. DITRAME study group. DIminution de la transmission mere–infant. Lancet 1999; 353: 786.

De Cock KM, Fowler MG, Mercier E, de Vincenzi I, Saba J, Hoff E, Alnwick DJ, Rogers M, Shaffer N. Prevention of mother-to-child HIV transmission in resource-poor countries: translating research into policy and practice. JAMA 2000; 283: 1175.

Derrien M, Faye A, Dolcini G, Chaouat G, Barre-Sinoussi F, Menu E. Impact of the placental cytokine–chemokine balance on regulation of cell–cell contact-induced human immunodeficiency virus type 1 translocation across a trophoblastic barrier *in vitro*. J Virol 2005; 79: 12304.

Dolcini G, Derrien M, Chaouat G, Barre-Sinoussi F, Menu E. Cell-free HIV type 1 infection is restricted in the human trophoblast choriocarcinoma BeWo cell line, even with expression of CD4, CXCR4 and CCR5. AIDS Res Hum Retroviruses 2003; 19: 857.

Eglinton BA, Roberton DM, Cummins AG. Phenotype of T cells, their soluble receptor levels, and cytokine profile of human breast milk. Immunol Cell Biol 1994; 72: 306.

Eshleman SH, Guay LA, Mwatha A, Cunningham SP, Brown ER, Musoke P, Mmiro F, Jackson JB. Comparison of nevirapine (NVP) resistance in Ugandan women 7 days vs. 6–8 weeks after single-dose NVP prophylaxis: HIVNET 012. AIDS Res Hum Retroviruses 2004; 20: 595.

Eshleman SH, Guay LA, Wang J, Mwatha A, Brown ER, Musoke P, Mmiro F, Jackson JB. Distinct patterns of emergence and fading of K103N and Y181C in women with subtype A vs. D after single-dose nevirapine: HIVNET 012. J Acquir Immune Defic Syndr 2005a; 40: 24.

Eshleman SH, Hoover DR, Chen S, Hudelson SE, Guay LA, Mwatha A, Fiscus SA, Mmiro
    F, Musoke P, Jackson JB, Kumwenda N, Taha T. Nevirapine (NVP) resistance in women
    with HIV-1 subtype C, compared with subtypes A and D, after the administration of
    single-dose NVP. J Infect Dis 2005b; 192: 30.
Eshleman SH, Hoover DR, Chen S, Hudelson SE, Guay LA, Mwatha A, Fiscus SA, Mmiro
    F, Musoke P, Jackson JB, Kumwenda N, Taha T. Resistance after single-dose nevirapine
    prophylaxis emerges in a high proportion of Malawian newborns. AIDS 2005c; 19: 2167.
Eshleman SH, Mracna M, Guay LA, Deseyve M, Cunningham S, Mirochnick M, Musoke
    P, Fleming T, Glenn Fowler M, Mofenson LM, Mmiro F, Jackson JB. Selection
    and fading of resistance mutations in women and infants receiving nevirapine to prevent
    HIV-1 vertical transmission (HIVNET 012). AIDS 2001; 15: 1951.
European Collaborative Study. Mother-to-child transmission of HIV infection in the era of
    highly active antiretroviral therapy. Clin Infect Dis 2005; 40: 458.
Fotopoulos G, Harari A, Michetti P, Trono D, Pantaleo G, Kraehenbuhl JP. Transepithelial
    transport of HIV-1 by M cells is receptor mediated. Proc Natl Acad Sci USA 2002; 99: 9410.
GiulianoM, Galluzzo C, Germinario E, Amici R, Pirillo M, Bassani L, Vyankandondera J,
    Mmiro F, Okong P. Vella S. Selection of resistance mutations in children receiving
    prophylaxis with lamivudine or nevirapine for the prevention of postnatal transmission of
    HIV. 12th Conference on Retroviruses and Opportunistic Infections. Boston, MA, USA;
    2005; 99.
Goulder PJ, Brander C, Tang Y, Tremblay C, Colbert RA, Addo MM, Rosenberg ES,
    Nguyen T, Allen R, Trocha A, Altfeld M, He S, Bunce M, Funkhouser R, Pelton SI,
    Burchett SK, McIntosh K, Korber BT, Walker BD. Evolution and transmission of stable
    CTL escape mutations in HIV infection. Nature 2001; 412: 334.
Guay LA, Musoke P, Fleming T, Bagenda D, Allen M, Nakabiito C, Sherman J, Bakaki P,
    Ducar C, Deseyve M, Emel L, Mirochnick M, Fowler MG, Mofenson L, Miotti P,
    Dransfield K, Bray D, Mmiro F, Jackson JB. Intrapartum and neonatal single-dose ne-
    virapine compared with zidovudine for prevention of mother-to-child transmission of
    HIV-1 in Kampala, Uganda: HIVNET 012 randomised trial. Lancet 1999; 354: 795.
Iliff PJ, Piwoz EG, Tavengwa NV, Zunguza CD, Marinda ET, Nathoo KJ, Moulton LH,
    Ward BJ, Humphrey JH. Early exclusive breastfeeding reduces the risk of postnatal HIV-
    1 transmission and increases HIV-free survival. AIDS 2005; 19: 699.
Israel-Ballard K, Chantry C, Dewey K, Lonnerdal B, Sheppard H, Donovan R, Carlson J,
    Sage A, Abrams B. Viral, nutritional, and bacterial safety of flash-heated and pretoria-
    pasteurized breast milk to prevent mother-to-child transmission of HIV in resource-poor
    countries: a pilot study. J Acquir Immune Defic Syndr 2005; 40: 175.
Jackson JB, Musoke P, Fleming T, Guay LA, Bagenda D, Allen M, Nakabiito C, Sherman
    J, Bakaki P, Owor M, Ducar C, Deseyve M, Mwatha A, Emel L, Duefield C, Mirochnick
    M, Fowler MG, Mofenson L, Miotti P, Gigliotti M, Bray D, Mmiro F. Intrapartum and
    neonatal single-dose nevirapine compared with zidovudine for prevention of mother-to-
    child transmission of HIV-1 in Kampala, Uganda: 18-month follow-up of the HIVNET
    012 randomised trial. Lancet 2003; 362: 859.
Jamieson DJ, Sibailly TS, Sadek R, Roels TH, Ekpini ER, Boni-Ouattara E, Karon JM,
    Nkengasong J, Greenberg AE, Wiktor SZ. HIV-1 viral load and other risk factors for
    mother-to-child transmission of HIV-1 in a breast-feeding population in Cote d'Ivoire.
    J Acquir Immune Defic Syndr 2003; 34: 430.

John GC, Rousseau C, Dong T, Rowland-Jones S, Nduati R, Mbori-Ngacha D, Rostron T, Kreiss JK, Richardson BA, Overbaugh J. Maternal SDF1 3′a polymorphism is associated with increased perinatal human immunodeficiency virus type 1 transmission. J Virol 2000; 74: 5736.

John-Stewart G, Mbori-Ngacha D, Ekpini R, Janoff EN, Nkengasong J, Read JS, Van de Perre P, Newell ML. Breast-feeding and transmission of HIV-1. J Acquir Immune Defic Syndr 2004; 35: 196.

Johnson JA, Li JF, Morris L, Martinson N, Gray G, McIntyre J, Heneine W. Emergence of drug-resistant HIV-1 after intrapartum administration of single-dose nevirapine is substantially underestimated. J Infect Dis 2005; 192: 16.

Jourdain G, Ngo-Giang-Huong N, Le Coeur S, Bowonwatanuwong C, Kantipong P, Leechanachai P, Ariyadej S, Leenasirimakul P, Hammer S, Lallemant M. Intrapartum exposure to nevirapine and subsequent maternal responses to nevirapine-based antiretroviral therapy. N Engl J Med 2004; 351: 229.

Lagaye S, Derrien M, Menu E, Coito C, Tresoldi E, Mauclere P, Scarlatti G, Chaouat G, Barre-Sinoussi F, Bomsel M. Cell-to-Cell contact results in a selective translocation of maternal human immunodeficiency virus type 1 quasispecies across a trophoblastic barrier by both transcytosis and infection. J Virol 2001; 75: 4780.

Lallemant M, Jourdain G, Le Coeur S, Kim S, Koetsawang S, Comeau AM, Phoolcharoen W, Essex M, McIntosh K, Vithayasai V. A trial of shortened zidovudine regimens to prevent mother-to-child transmission of human immunodeficiency virus type 1. Perinatal HIV prevention trail (Thailand) investigators. N Engl J Med 2000; 343: 982.

Lallemant M, Jourdain G, Le Coeur S, Mary JY, Ngo-Giang-Huong N, Koetsawang S, Kanshana S, McIntosh K, Thaineua V. Single-dose perinatal nevirapine plus standard zidovudine to prevent mother-to-child transmission of HIV-1 in Thailand. N Engl J Med 2004; 351: 217.

Leroy V, Karon JM, Alioum A, Ekpini ER, Meda N, Greenberg AE, Msellati P, Hudgens M, Dabis F, Wiktor SZ. Twenty-four month efficacy of a maternal short-course zidovudine regimen to prevent mother-to-child transmission of HIV-1 in west Africa. AIDS 2002; 16: 631.

Leroy V, Karon JM, Alioum A, Ekpini ER, van de Perre P, Greenberg AE, Msellati P, Hudgens M, Dabis F, Wiktor SZ. Postnatal transmission of HIV-1 after a maternal short-course zidovudine peripartum regimen in west Africa. AIDS 2003; 17: 1493.

Leroy V, Sakarovitch C, Cortina-Borja M, McIntyre J, Coovadia H, Dabis F, Newell ML, Saba J, Gray G, Ndugwa C, Kilewo C, Massawe A, Kituuka P, Okong P, Grulich A, von Briesen H, Goudsmit J, Biberfeld G, Haverkamp G, Weverling GJ, Lange JM. Is there a difference in the efficacy of peripartum antiretroviral regimens in reducing mother-to-child transmission of HIV in Africa? AIDS 2005; 19: 1865.

Leslie A, Kavanagh D, Honeyborne I, Pfafferott K, Edwards C, Pillay T, Hilton L, Thobakgale C, Ramduth D, Draenert R, Le Gall S, Luzzi G, Edwards A, Brander C, Sewell AK, Moore S, Mullins J, Moore C, Mallal S, Bhardwaj N, Yusim K, Phillips R, Klenerman P, Korber B, Kiepiela P, Walker B, Goulder P. Transmission and accumulation of CTL escape variants drive negative associations between HIV polymorphisms and HLA. J Exp Med 2005; 201: 891.

Lewis SH, Reynolds-Kohler C, Fox HE, Nelson JA. HIV-1 in trophoblastic and villous Hofbauer cells, and hematologic precursors in eight week fetuses. Lancet 1990; 335: 565.

Li Q, Duan L, Estes JD, Ma ZM, Rourke T, Wang Y, Reilly C, Carlis J, Miller CJ, Haase
    AT. Peak SIV replication in resting memory CD4+ T cells depletes gut lamina propria
    CD4+ T cells. Nature 2005; 434: 1148.
Loubser S, Balfe P, Sherman G, Jones S, Cohen S, Kuhn L, Hammer S, Morris L. Sensitive
    real-time PCR quantification of 103N resistance mutants following single-dose treatment
    with nevirapine. 12th Conference on Retroviruses and Opportunistic Infections. Boston,
    MA, USA; 2005; 102.
MacDonald KS, Embree JE, Nagelkerke NJ, Castillo J, Ramhadin S, Njenga S, Oyug J,
    Ndinya-Achola J, Barber BH, Bwayo JJ, Plummer FA. The HLA A2/6802 supertype is
    associated with reduced risk of perinatal human immunodeficiency virus type 1 trans-
    mission. J Infect Dis 2001; 183: 503.
Mandelbrot L, Landreau-Mascaro A, Rekacewicz C, Berrebi A, Benifla JL, Burgard M,
    Lachassine E, Barret B, Chaix ML, Bongain A, Ciraru-Vigneron N, Crenn-Hebert C,
    Delfraissy JF, Rouzioux C, Mayaux MJ, Blanche S. Lamivudine–zidovudine combination
    for prevention of maternal–infant transmission of HIV-1. JAMA 2001; 285: 2083.
Martinson N, Pumla L, Morris L, Ntsala M, Puren A, Chezzi C, Dhlamini P, Cohen S, Gray
    G, Steyn J, McIntyre J. Effectiveness of single-dose nevirapine in a second pregnancy.
    12th Conference on Retroviruses and Opportunistic Infections. Boston, MA, USA; 2005;
    103.
Mattapallil JJ, Douek DC, Hill B, Nishimura Y, Martin M, Roederer M. Massive infection
    and loss of memory CD4+ T cells in multiple tissues during acute SIV infection. Nature
    2005; 434: 1093.
Mayaux MJ, Teglas JP, Mandelbrot L, Berrebi A, Gallais H, Matheron S, Ciraru-Vigneron
    N, Parnet-Mathieu F, Bongain A, Rouzioux C, Delfraissy JF, Blanche S. Acceptability
    and impact of zidovudine for prevention of mother-to-child human immunodeficiency
    virus-1 transmission in France. J Pediatr 1997; 131: 857.
Menu E, Mbopi-Keou FX, Lagaye S, Pissard S, Mauclere P, Scarlatti G, Martin J, Goossens
    M, Chaouat G, Barre-Sinoussi F, M'Bopi Keou FX. Selection of maternal human
    immunodeficiency virus type 1 variants in human placenta. European Network for
    In Utero Transmission of HIV-1 [published erratum appears in J Infect Dis 1999; 179(4):
    1053]. J Infect Dis 1999; 179: 44.
Mofenson LM, McIntyre JA. Advances and research directions in the prevention of mother-
    to-child HIV-1 transmission. Lancet 2000; 355: 2237.
Moodley D, Moodley J, Coovadia H, Gray G, McIntyre J, Hofmyer J, Nikodem C, Hall D,
    Gigliotti M, Robinson P, Boshoff L, Sullivan JL. A multicenter randomized controlled
    trial of nevirapine versus a combination of zidovudine and lamivudine to reduce intra-
    partum and early postpartum mother-to-child transmission of human immunodeficiency
    virus type 1. J Infect Dis 2003; 187: 725.
Nduati R, John G, Mbori-Ngacha D, Richardson B, Overbaugh J, Mwatha A, Ndinya-
    Achola J, Bwayo J, Onyango FE, Hughes J, Kreiss J. Effect of breastfeeding and formula
    feeding on transmission of HIV-1: a randomized clinical trial. JAMA 2000; 283: 1167.
Nduati R, Richardson BA, John G, Mbori-Ngacha D, Mwatha A, Ndinya-Achola J, Bwayo
    J, Onyango FE, Kreiss J. Effect of breastfeeding on mortality among HIV-1 infected
    women: a randomised trial. Lancet 2001; 357: 1651.
Newell ML, Coovadia H, Cortina-Borja M, Rollins N, Gaillard P, Dabis F. Mortality of
    infected and uninfected infants born to HIV-infected mothers in Africa: a pooled analysis.
    Lancet 2004; 364: 1236.

Nielsen K, Boyer P, Dillon M, Wafer D, Wei LS, Garratty E, Dickover RE, Bryson YJ. Presence of human immunodeficiency virus (HIV) type 1 and HIV-1-specific antibodies in cervicovaginal secretions of infected mothers and in the gastric aspirates of their infants. J Infect Dis 1996; 173: 1001.

Ometto L, Zanchetta M, Mainardi M, De Salvo GL, Garcia-Rodriguez MC, Gray L, Newell ML, Chieco-Bianchi L, De Rossi A. Co-receptor usage of HIV-1 primary isolates, viral burden, and CCR5 genotype in mother-to-child HIV-1 transmission. AIDS 2000; 14: 1721.

Pacifici GM. Transfer of antivirals across the human placenta. Early Hum Dev 2005; 81: 647.

Palmer S, Boltz V, Maldarelli F, Martinson N, Gray G, McIntyre J, Mellors JW, Morris L, Coffin JM. Persistence of NNRTI-r resistant variants after single-dose nevirapine in HIV-1 subtype-C-infected women. 12th Conference on Retroviruses and Opportunistic Infections. Boston, MA, USA; 2005; 101.

Polycarpou A, Ntais C, Korber BT, Elrich HA, Winchester R, Krogstad P, Wolinsky S, Rostron T, Rowland-Jones SL, Ammann AJ, Ioannidis JP. Association between maternal and infant class I and II HLA alleles and of their concordance with the risk of perinatal HIV type 1 transmission. AIDS Res Hum Retroviruses 2002; 18: 741.

Rollins N, Meda N, Becquet R, Coutsoudis A, Humphrey J, Jeffrey B, Kanshana S, Kuhn L, Leroy V, Mbori-Ngacha D, McIntyre J, Newell ML. Preventing postnatal transmission of HIV-1 through breast-feeding: modifying infant feeding practices. J Acquir Immune Defic Syndr 2004; 35: 188.

Romiti ML, Colognesi C, Cancrini C, Mas A, Berrino M, Salvatori F, Orlandi P, Jansson M, Palomba E, Plebani A, Bertran JM, Hernandez M, de Martino M, Amoroso A, Tovo PA, Rossi P, Espanol T, Scarlatti G. Prognostic value of a CCR5 defective allele in pediatric HIV-1 infection. Mol Med 2000; 6: 28.

Rousseau CM, Nduati RW, Richardson BA, John-Stewart GC, Mbori-Ngacha DA, Kreiss JK, Overbaugh J. Association of levels of HIV-1-infected breast milk cells and risk of mother-to-child transmission. J Infect Dis 2004; 190: 1880.

Scarlatti G. Mother-to-child transmission of HIV-1: advances and controversies of the twentieth centuries. AIDS Rev 2004; 6: 67.

Taha TE, Kumwenda NI, Gibbons A, Broadhead RL, Fiscus S, Lema V, Liomba G, Nkhoma C, Miotti PG, Hoover DR. Short postexposure prophylaxis in newborn babies to reduce mother-to-child transmission of HIV-1: NVAZ randomised clinical trial. Lancet 2003; 362: 1171.

The Petra Study Team. Efficacy of three short-course regimens of zidovudine and lamivudine in preventing early and late transmission of HIV-1 from mother to child in Tanzania, South Africa, and Uganda (Petra study): a randomised, double-blind, placebo-controlled trial. Lancet 2002; 359: 1178.

Thorne C, Newell ML. The safety of antiretroviral drugs in pregnancy. Expert Opin Drug Saf 2005; 4: 323.

Tresoldi E, Romiti ML, Boniotto M, Crovella S, Salvatori F, Palomba E, Pastore A, Cancrini C, de Martino M, Plebani A, Castelli G, Rossi P, Tovo PA, Amoroso A, Scarlatti G. Prognostic value of the stromal cell-derived factor 1 3'A mutation in pediatric human immunodeficiency virus type 1 infection. J Infect Dis 2002; 185: 696.

Tscherning-Casper C, Papadogiannakis N, Anvret M, Stolpe L, Lindgren S, Bohlin AB, Albert J, Fenyo EM. The trophoblastic epithelial barrier is not infected in full-term placentae of human immunodeficiency virus-seropositive mothers undergoing antiretroviral therapy. J Virol 1999; 73: 9673.

Wiktor SZ, Ekpini E, Karon JM, Nkengasong J, Maurice C, Severin ST, Roels TH, Kouassi MK, Lackritz EM, Coulibaly IM, Greenberg AE. Short-course oral zidovudine for prevention of mother-to-child transmission of HIV-1 in Abidjan, Cote d'Ivoire: a randomised trial. Lancet 1999; 353: 781.

Wilson CC, Brown RC, Korber BT, Wilkes BM, Ruhl DJ, Sakamoto D, Kunstman K, Luzuriaga K, Hanson IC, Widmayer SM, Wiznia A, Clapp S, Ammann AJ, Koup RA, Wolinsky SM, Walker BD. Frequent detection of escape from cytotoxic T-lymphocyte recognition in perinatal human immunodeficiency virus (HIV) type 1 transmission: the ariel project for the prevention of transmission of HIV from mother to infant. J Virol 1999; 73: 3975.

Winchester R, Pitt J, Charurat M, Magder LS, Goring HH, Landay A, Read JS, Shearer W, Handelsman E, Luzuriaga K, Hillyer GV, Blattner W. Mother-to-child transmission of HIV-1: strong association with certain maternal HLA-B alleles independent of viral load implicates innate immune mechanisms. J Acquir Immune Defic Syndr 2004; 36: 659.

World Health Organization (WHO) Antiretroviral drugs and the prevention of mother-to-child transmission of HIV infection in resource-limited settings. Recommendations for a publlic health approach (2005 revision) Expert consultation, Geneva; 2005; 28–29 June. www.whoint/3by5/arv_pmtct/en/.

World Health Organization/UNAIDS HIV in pregnancy: a review. WHO, UNAIDS Occasional Paper; 1999.

World Health Organization (WHO) and United Nations Programme on HIV/AIDS (UNAIDS) AIDS epidemic update 2005; 2005. www.unaids.org.

Congenital and Other Related Infectious
Diseases of the Newborn
Isa K. Mushahwar (Editor)
DOI 10.1016/S0168-7069(06)13007-4

Hepatitis B Virus and Hepatitis C Virus: Molecular Biology and Diagnosis

Vicente Carreño, Javier Bartolomé, Inmaculada Castillo

Fundación para el Estudio de las Hepatitis Virales, Madrid, Spain

Abstract

Hepatitis B virus (HBV) and hepatitis C virus (HCV) are noncytopathic viruses that cause acute and chronic liver diseases. Infection by HBV and HCV represents a major health problem as it is estimated that 500 million people worldwide are persistently infected by these viruses. Although the biology of HBV and HCV is well known, there are still critical steps in their viral life cycle, such as the mechanisms by which these viruses enter into the hepatocytes that are not well understood. Serological markers are key elements for the diagnosis of HBV and HCV infections. Nowadays, highly specific and sensitive assays are commercially available for this purpose, including tests for the detection of HBV and HCV genomes in serum and plasma samples.

Hepatitis B virus

Hepatitis B virus (HBV) is a hepatotropic, noncytopathic virus that causes acute and chronic liver diseases that may end in liver cirrhosis and hepatocellular carcinoma (Pan and Zhang, 2005). HBV is transmitted parenterally, sexually and from infected mothers to their babies at birth. The age at which the virus is acquired determines the outcome of the infection. Thus, while around 95% of perinatal HBV infections become chronic, this only occurs in 3–5% of patients infected in the adult age (McMahon et al., 1985).

Molecular biology of HBV

Human HBV is the prototype member of the family of viruses termed Hepadnaviridae, which also includes viruses infecting other mammals, such as ground squirrel (ground squirrel hepatitis virus) (Marion et al., 1980), woodchucks (wood-chuck hepatitis virus) (Summers et al., 1978), Arctic ground squirrels (Arctic squirrel hepatitis virus) (Testut et al., 1996) and wolly monkeys (Landford et al., 1998). Other hepadnaviruses have been isolated from birds, such as Pekin ducks (duck hepatitis B virus) (Mason et al., 1980), gray herons (heron hepatitis B virus) (Sprengel et al., 1988) and storks (stork hepatitis B virus) (Pult et al., 2001). Owing to the homology in DNA sequences and genome organization, hepadnaviruses-infecting mammals are grouped into the genus Ortohepadnavirus, while those found in birds are grouped into the genus Avihepadnavirus.

Prior to the definition of HBV genotypes, there were nine HBsAg subtypes, namely, ayw1, ayw2, ayw3, ayw4, ayr, adw2, dw4q–, adrq+ and adrq–. The molecular bases for the d/y and w/r variations were both shown to depend on Lys/Arg substitutions at residues 122 and 160, respectively (Okamoto et al., 1987). In 1988, HBV was classified into several genotypes by a sequence divergence in the entire genome exceeding 8%. At present (Norder et al., 2004), there are nine HBV genotypes (A–H). These genotypes have an uneven geographical distribution, and only a few of them are prevalent in a given area of the world.

The HBV genome (Fig. 1) consists of a circular, partially double-stranded DNA molecule of 3.2 kb in length with a nick at a unique site in the long strand of DNA (Galibert et al., 1979). The HBV-DNA presents a length asymmetry in the two strands: one DNA strand is unit length, while the complementary strand is less than unit length. The complete strand is complementary to the viral mRNA and is designated to be of minus polarity, and so, the shorter strand is termed the "plus strand". The 5' position of the plus strand is fixed and the 3' end is at variable positions and the circularity of the HBV genome is maintained by a 5' cohesive terminus of 224 base pair (Sattler and Robinson, 1979). Furthermore, the minus strand has a protein covalently linked to its 5' end (Gerlich and Robinson, 1980), whereas the plus strand contains an oligoribonucleotide attached at this position (Summers et al., 1978).

The HBV-DNA contains four overlapping open reading frames (ORFs) and the regulatory sequences are embedded in the coding regions (Miller et al., 1989) (Fig. 1). This compact organization of the viral genome implies that every nucleotide in the HBV-DNA is in at least one coding region and that 50% of the sequence can be read in more than one frame.

The four overlapping OFRs in the HBV genome are termed ORF S, C, P and X. The ORF S contains three in frame initiation codons (Pre S1, Pre S2 and S) and encodes the three polypeptides (Large-L-, Middle-M- and Small-S-) that form the outer envelope of the virus. These three proteins have a common carboxy terminus and display progressive amino terminal extensions. The Small protein contains the hepatitis B surface antigen (HBsAg). The Middle protein contains the small en-velope product plus the preS2 antigen and the Large envelope protein contains the Small and the Middle proteins plus the preS1 antigen. If the large envelope protein is over expressed, it forms filamentous particles that accumulate into the he-patocytes giving to these cells the "ground-glass" appearance that is characteristic

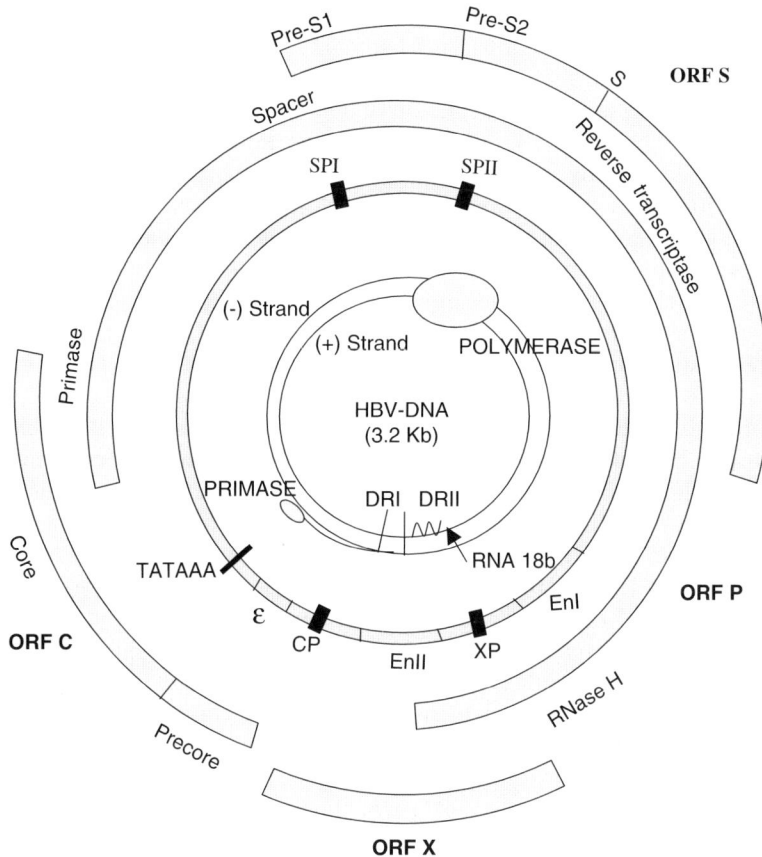

Fig. 1 Organization of the HBV genome. The four open reading frames and the structure of the viral DNA are shown. SPI and SPII: surface promoters I and II; XP, X promoter; CP, core promoter; En I and En II, enhancers I and II; ε, epsilon signal; DRI and DRII, direct repeat regions I and II.

in the liver of patients with chronic hepatitis B (Hadziyannis et al., 1973). The 42-nm-diameter infectious viral particles or Dane particles (Dane et al., 1970) contains the three envelope proteins (Heerman et al., 1987). Apart from virions, the small and the large envelope proteins also form spherical and filamentous void particles that are produced by the infected cells in 10^3–10^5 fold excess over virions.

The ORF C has two in frame initiation codons (PreC and C). When translation initiates at the C codon, the hepatitis B core antigen (HBcAg) is synthesized. The HBcAg forms heterodimers that self-assemble to form the viral nucleocapsid (Chang et al., 1994). If translation initiates at the PreC ATG codon, the produced protein contains the complete HBcAg plus a leader sequence that directs the nascent polypeptide to the endoplasmic reticulum where it is cleaved and secreted as a soluble antigen, termed hepatitis B e antigen (HBeAg), into the blood stream

V. Carreño et al.

(Ou et al., 1986). Detection of HBeAg in serum is associated with high viral replication and infectivity (Magnius and Espmark, 1972; Magnius et al., 1975), although its exact role in the viral life cycle is not fully understood. Studies in mice suggest that HBeAg may cause depletion of Th1 helper cells that would allow viral persistence (Milich et al., 1990, 1998). Apart from this, HBeAg may modulate the nucleocapsid stability by forming heterodimers with the HBcAg (Lamberts et al., 1993; Guidotti et al., 1996).

The ORF P encodes the viral polymerase that has two major domains separated by a spacer region (Bavand et al., 1989) The amino-terminal domain is indispensable for the packaging of the pregenomic RNA and in the priming of minus strand DNA (it is the protein attached at the 5′ end of this DNA strand), while the carboxy-terminal domain is the reverse transcriptase with RNase H activity (Landford et al., 1999).

The fourth ORF, the ORF X, encodes a protein termed X (HBx) which function in natural infections is not well known, although studies performed in woodchucks have shown that the woodchuck HBx is necessary for the establishment of chronic infection (Zoulim et al., 1994). HBx is a transcriptional transactivator of viral and cellular transcription elements and stimulates cytoplasmic signal transduction pathways (Bonchard and Schneider, 2004).

Transcription of the four ORFs is controlled by four independent promoters and a unique polyadenylation signal, producing four overlapping mRNAs of 3.5, 2.4, 2.1 and 0.7 kb in length. The 0.7 kb transcript produces the HBx, while the 3.5 kb mRNA produces the polymerase, precore and core proteins and it is also used as the pregenomic RNA, that is reverse transcribed during replication of the viral genome. The 2.4 kb transcript is the mRNA of the L and M surface proteins, while the 2.1 kb transcript is the mRNA of the S protein (Fig. 2).

The mechanism by which HBV enters into the hepatocytes is not well known. It is thought that the PreS1 region of the large envelope protein mediates the

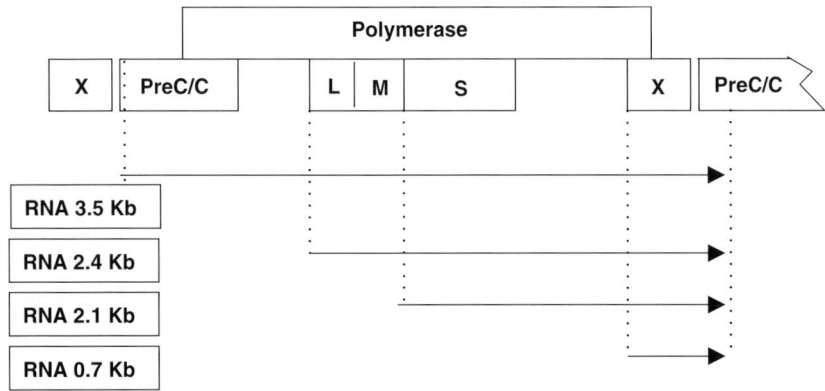

Fig. 2 HBV transcripts.

attachment of the virus with the viral receptor or receptors in the hepatocyte membrane (Machida et al., 1983; Franco et al., 1992; Hertogs et al., 1993; Mehdi et al., 1994; McGwire et al., 1997; Tong et al., 1999). Once into the cell, the virus is uncoated by an unknown mechanism, the synthesis of the plus-strand DNA is completed and the viral DNA is delivered to the cell nucleus. The viral DNA enters the hepatocyte nucleus in a relaxed circular form and it is converted into a covalently closed-circular DNA (cccDNA) molecule by unknown DNA repair enzymes. This cccDNA is the template for the transcription of viral mRNAs, including the pregenomic RNA (Summers and Mason, 1982).

As mentioned above, replication of the viral genome occurs through the reverse transcription of the pregenomic RNA. Pregenomic RNA is packaged into viral nucleocapsids together with the viral polymerase that binds to an RNA stem-loop structure termed Epsilon located at the 5′ end of the pregenomic RNA (Pollack and Ganem, 1993; Wang et al., 1994). The viral polymerase itself functions as a protein primer in the initiation of the synthesis of the minus-strand, being the template of the reaction a bulge of the Epsilon signal (Pollack and Ganem, 1994; Zoulim and Seeger, 1994). After the synthesis of only four nucleotides, the nascent DNA strand is translocated, by an unknown mechanism, to a homologous region in the direct repeat 1 region at the 3′ end of the pregenomic RNA. The synthesis of the plus-strand DNA is primed by an RNA oligomer derived from the 5′ end of the pre-genomic RNA, which is produced after degradation of the remaining pregenomic RNA by the RNase H activity of the viral polymerase (Radziwill et al., 1990). This oligoribonucleotide is translocated to the direct repeat 2 region of the previously synthesized minus-strand DNA which is the template for the synthesis of the plus-strand DNA. Once the synthesis of the plus-strand is initiated, the capsids containing the partially double-stranded viral DNA migrate bidirectionally within the cytoplasm. A fraction of the capsids migrates to the endoplasmic reticulum where it interacts with the envelope proteins to form virions that are transported out of the cell. The other fraction migrates to the nucleus to amplify the pool of cccDNA (Fig. 3).

Natural history of HBV infection

Perinatal or horizontal infection early in life are the main routes of HBV transmission in high endemic areas, whereas in low endemic areas HBV infection occurs in adolescents and adults due to injection drug use or to high sexual activity. In acute HBV infections, HBsAg is first detected in serum after 4–10 weeks of incubation period, followed by antibodies against core antigen (anti-HBc) of IgM type. At the time of detection of HBsAg, viremia is already established and HBV-DNA is detected in serum at very high titers (Hoofnagle, 1981). HBeAg is also detectable in most cases. When acute infection is self-limited, HBsAg and HBeAg disappear and antibodies against HBsAg (anti-HBs) and HBeAg (anti-HBe) become detectable. At this time, HBV-DNA is also undetectable by molecular

　　　　　　　　　V. Carreño et al.

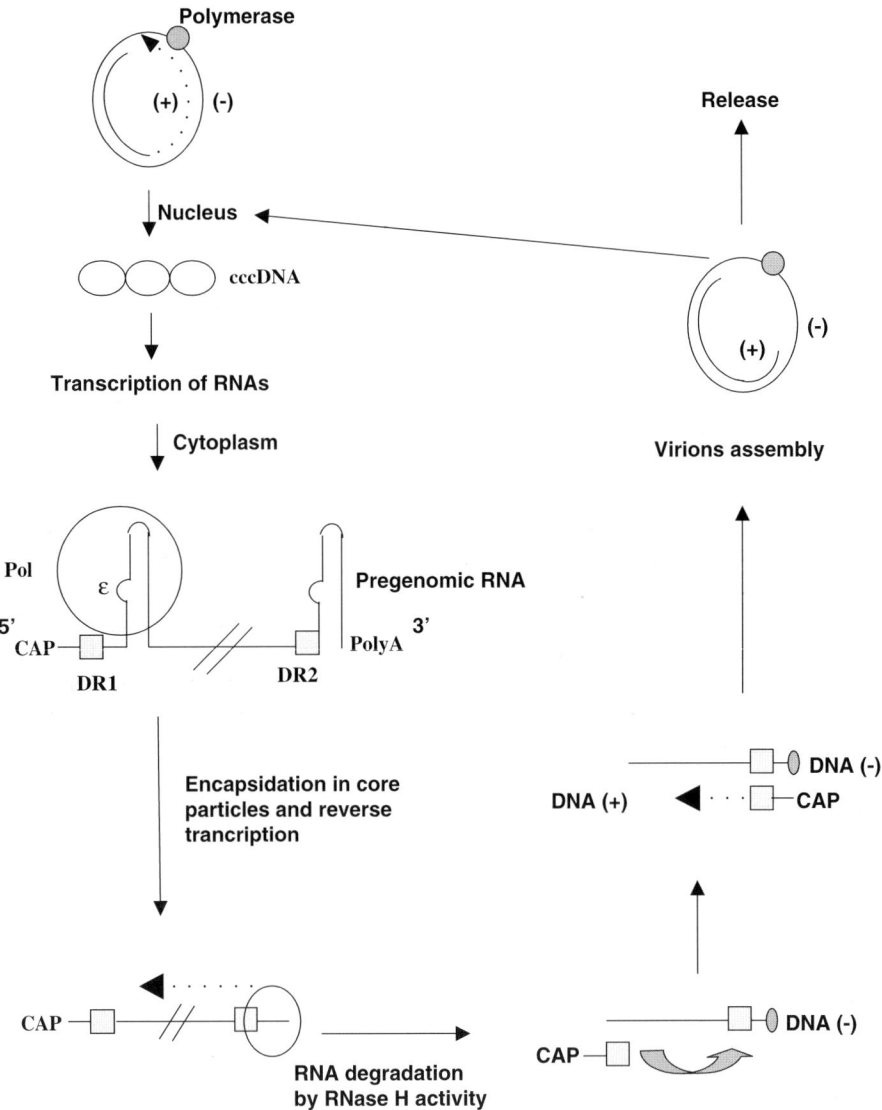

Fig. 3 Schematic representation of HBV replication. cccDNA, covalently closed-circular DNA; DRI and DRII, direct repeat regions I and II; ε, epsilon signal.

hybridization techniques. This fact leads to the notion that the disappearance of HBsAg with the development of anti-HBs and the absence of serum HBV-DNA tested by molecular hybridization techniques implied the complete clearance of the infection. However, with the development of the polymerase chain reaction (PCR) it has became evident that HBV-DNA may persist in serum, liver and peripheral blood mononuclear cells long years after the apparent resolution of the acute HBV infection (Michalak et al., 1994; Cabrerizo et al., 1997; Yotsuyanagi et al., 1998). The clinical significance of this viral persistence (called occult HBV infection) after a self-limited acute HBV infection remains to be established.

In around 95% of adults with an acute hepatitis B, the infection is clinically resolved with the development of anti-HBs. However, in 1–5% of the cases, HBsAg, HBeAg and high serum HBV-DNA levels persist and when this occurs for more than 6 months it is considered that the patients have become chronically infected by the virus. In patients with chronic HBV infection, HBsAg and anti-HBc (IgG class) are always positive, while HBeAg and anti-HBe may be positive or negative. In HBeAg chronic hepatitis, HBV-DNA levels, although lower than in acute phase, are still high enough to be detected by conventional hybridization techniques. The clinical course of this phase of the infection depends on the age at infection. When the virus is acquired at birth or early in childhood, the disease activity is generally mild with normal or near normal serum aminotransferase levels. However, if the infection is acquired in the adolescence or adulthood, the disease activity is usually high with elevated serum aminotransferase levels.

A key event in the evolution in the natural history of chronic hepatitis B is the seroconversion from the HBeAg-positive status to the anti-HBe positive status. Seroconversion is associated with the improvement of disease activity and with a marked decrease in HBV replication and so, in serum HBV-DNA levels that may be undetectable by molecular hybridization techniques, but these viral DNA levels are still detectable by PCR. In most patients, seroconversion into anti-HBe is the initial step to inactive HBsAg carrier state. However, in a fraction of anti-HBe-positive patients, serum HBV-DNA levels remain high. These patients are infected by naturally occurring HBV mutants that are unable to produce HBeAg due to mutations in the precore region or in the core promoter (Carman et al., 1989; Okamoto et al., 1994). These mutants appear during the natural course of the chronic HBV infection and become the predominant viral population during seroconversion into anti-HBe (Lok and McMahon, 2001).

The inactive HBsAg carrier state, also known as healthy or asymptomatic carrier state, is characterized by detectable HBsAg and anti-HBe in serum, normal serum aminotransferase levels and low or undetectable circulating HBV-DNA. The prognosis of this type of patients is usually good but up to 30% of the cases may experience a reactivation of the infection and may develop a progressive liver disease (Hsu et al., 2002). Finally, some carriers may spontaneously lose the HBsAg and develop anti-HBs. Classically, it has been considered that these patients are cured of the HBV infection. However, as occurs with the patients that resolved an acute HBV infection, these patients may have low levels of HBV-DNA in serum and/or in liver (occult HBV infection) (Tanaka et al., 1990; Loriot et al., 1992), but the clinical impact of this viral persistence remains unknown.

The interpretation of HBV serological markers is summarized in Table 1.

Table 1

Interpretation of hepatitis B virus serological markers

HBsAg	Anti-HBs	Anti-HBc	Anti-HBc IgM	HBeAg	Anti-HBe	HBV-DNA	Interpretation
+	−	+	+	+	−	+	Acute infection
+	−	+	−	+	−	+	Chronic infection (active phase)
+	−	+	−	−	+	−	Chronic infection (inactive phase)
+	−	+	−	−	+	+	Chronic infection (pre-core or core mutants)
−	+/−	+	−	−	−	−	Resolution of infection
−	+/−	+	−	−	−	+	Occult infection
−	+	−	−	−	−	−	Successfully vaccinated

Diagnosis of HBV infection

HBV antigens

The two antigens that can be detected in serum or plasma by commercially available enzyme immunoassays (EIA) are HBsAg and HBeAg. HBsAg is the sentinel marker for the confirmation of acute HBV infection as it can be detected as early as 6 weeks after exposure. Furthermore, it is also the viral marker that indicates the establishment of a chronic HBV infection, as this clinical situation is defined by the persistence of HBsAg for at least 6 months after exposure (Lok and McMahon, 2001). HBeAg is detected in the circulation in both acute and chronic infections. Its presence is associated with high serum HBV-DNA levels. However, as mentioned above, in patients infected with viral mutants unable to produce HBeAg, HBV-DNA levels in serum may be also high and so HBeAg is not a reliable marker of HBV replication.

Antibodies against HBV proteins

The anti-HBV antibodies that can be detected by commercial EIA tests are anti-HBc (total and IgM class), anti-HBe and anti-HBs.

Total anti-HBc is detected early after infection and remains detectable for life, independently of the outcome of the infection. Total anti-HBc can be detected in the presence or absence of HBsAg and anti-HBs and it is the only HBV marker that is present in sera of patients who resolve the infection but who do not develop anti-HBs. Anti-HBc of IgM class is present during acute HBV infection at high titers. These titers decline as the acute infection is resolved and the anti-HBc IgM becomes undetectable after the appearance of anti-HBs. Very low titers of anti-HBc IgM can also be detected during chronic infections by means of very sensitive EIA (Brunetto et al., 1993).

Anti-HBe appears after disappearance of HBeAg and, in patients infected with the wild-type HBV, its detection is associated with the decline in viral replication, but in patients infected with mutants unable to produce HBeAg, anti-HBe may be detected in the presence of high viral replication levels.

Anti-HBs appears either after HBV vaccination or after resolution of an acute HBV infection in association with the disappearance of HBsAg and it is considered a marker of the resolution of the infection (although as stated earlier, HBV-DNA may persist in liver and/or in serum of anti-HBs positive patients). Anti-HBs may also appear, although rarely, in chronic HBV carriers who resolved the infection either spontaneously or after a successful antiviral therapy. Anti-HBs usually persists for life but it may become undetectable along time.

HBV-DNA detection

Testing for serum HBV-DNA is the best way to determine viral replication and persistence, although HBV-DNA assays are not recommended at present for the routine evaluation of patients with chronic HBV infection. Serum HBV-DNA is detected few days after infection and reaches the peak at the time at which clinical symptoms of acute hepatitis appears (Whalley et al., 2001). When infection is self-limited, HBV-DNA titers decrease dramatically although viral DNA may remain detectable in serum by PCR long years after the resolution of acute infection (Michalak et al., 1994; Cabrerizo et al., 1997; Yotsuyanagi et al., 1998). In patients with chronic HBV infection, viral DNA levels are high (detectable by hybridization-based techniques) in the HBeAg-positive phase and decline at the time of anti-HBe seroconversion, except in patients infected with precore or core promoter mutants. However, it must be stressed that HBV-DNA may remain detectable in serum by PCR even in those patients that resolve a chronic HBV infection with the disappearance of HBsAg and with the development of anti-HBs.

In early years, HBV-DNA detection in serum was performed by conventional molecular hybridization techniques (Berninger et al., 1982; Valentine-Thon et al., 1991), which had a detection limit of around 10^4 genome copies per reaction. Nowadays, these techniques are not used in the clinical practice since more sensitive commercial available tests have been developed. The main drawback of these tests is that HBV-DNA units used in the various assays do not represent the same amount of viral DNA. However, the establishment by the World Health Organization of an international HBV reference standard and the definition of an HBV-DNA international unit (IU) (Saldanha et al., 2001) allows the comparison of the results obtained with the different assays. These new tests can be divided into two groups: those based on signal amplification following molecular hybridization and those based on target amplification (PCR).

The assays based on signal amplification relay on enhancing a signal instead of the amplification of a nucleic acid target. This implies that strict procedures to prevent contamination (as occurs in PCR-based techniques) are not needed. However, these tests have a lower sensitivity than PCR-based tests.

The first available test for HBV-DNA detection based on signal amplification was the Digene Hybrid Capture assay (De Lamballerie et al., 1995). In this test, denatured HBV-DNA is hybridized with an HBV-RNA probe and the DNA–RNA hybrids are captured by and anti-DNA–RNA antibody immobilized in tubes. Further amplifications lead to the generation of chemiluminescence, which is proportional to the amount of HBV-DNA in a given serum sample. The detection limit of this assay is around 1.4×10^5 copies/ml.

A more sensitive assay, based on signal amplification, is the VERSANT HBV DNA 3.0 assay (Yao et al., 2004). In this test, viral DNA is hybridized with a set of specific oligonucleotides fixed in microtiter wells. Then, a series of sequential hybridizations allows the formation of a branched DNA complex to which, multiple copies of an alkaline phosphatase-labeled probe are hybridized. Finally, detection is performed using an alkaline phosphatase chemiluminescent substrate and the intensity of the light emission is directly related to the HBV-DNA amount on each sample. The HBV-DNA concentration is calculated from a standard curve derived from internal DNA standard. The limit of detection of this assay is 3.6×10^3 copies/ml.

Regarding assays based on target amplification, the first commercially available test was the Amplicor HBV Monitor (Gerken et al., 1998), which was followed by a semiautomatic version (COBAS Amplicor HBV Monitor) of this assay (Lopez et al., 2002). These assays have a lower detection limit (2×10^2 copies/ml) and quantitation of the amount of HBV-DNA relies on the co-amplification of a standard of known concentration. The main drawback of this test is its narrow linear range (from 2×10^2 to 2×10^5 copies/ml). This fact is due to reagent exhaustion and saturation effects due to high template loads.

The problem of the linear range of the PCR-based assays has been solved with the development of the real-time PCR. In this technique, by using fluorochrome labeling, the accumulation of PCR products is measured during the exponential phase of amplification in real time. Regarding the commercial assays based on real-time PCR, the COBAS Taq-Man HBV test employs a dual fluorophore-labeled probe that hybridizes with the PCR product. The linear range of this assay goes from 30 to 1.1×10^8 IU/ml (Gordillo et al., 2005). Another test based on real-time PCR is the Artus realArt HBV PCR Kits that has been developed for different real-time platforms (Stelzl et al., 2004). The linear range of these assays for the different instruments is from 20 to 10^8 IU/ml.

Hepatitis C virus

HCV is the causal agent of chronic liver infection originally identified as non-A, non-B hepatitis. HCV was identified by expression cloning of the genome from a serum sample of a chimpanzee and using for the detection antibodies isolated from the serum of a patient with acute non-A and non-B hepatitis (Choo et al., 1989). The global prevalence of HCV infection is around 3% (170 million people) (Lauer and Walker, 2001) and is the leading cause of liver transplantation in the United States and other countries (Terrault, 2000). The main route of HCV transmission is exposure to infected blood via intravenous drug use or unscreened transfusions (Lauer and Walker, 2001). Nosocomial transmission during hemodialysis, colonoscopy and surgery has been also reported (Duckworth et al., 1999; Kokubo et al., 2002; Tallis et al., 2003). HCV may be also transmitted perinatally and sexually but with a low frequency, except if the HCV-infected mother or the sexual partner is also infected with the human immunodeficiency virus (Everhart et al., 1990; Eyster et al., 1991; Roudot-Thoraval et al., 1993; Zanetti et al., 1995).

Molecular biology of HCV

HCV belongs to the genus Hepacivirus in the Flaviviridae family of viruses, together with Pestiviruses and Flaviviruses (Ohba et al., 1996). HCV genome is a 9.6 kb uncapped, linear, single-stranded RNA molecule of positive polarity (Kato et al., 1990; Takamizawa et al., 1991) that serves as template for both translation and replication. The HCV-RNA contains two untranslated regions at the 5' and 3' ends and a single ORF that encodes for a 3010–3030 amino acid polyprotein that is processed post-transcriptionally by host- and virus-encoded proteinases to produce the structural (core, E1 and E2) and nonstructural (p7, NS2–NS5) viral proteins (Fig. 4). Translation of viral proteins depends on an internal ribosome entry site (IRES) in the 5' untranslated region (5' UTR), which has a complex RNA structure that directly interacts with the 40S ribosomal subunit during translation initiation (Pestova et al., 1998).

Comparison of nucleotide sequences of HCV variants isolated from different geographical regions has revealed the existence of six major genetic groups (genotypes)

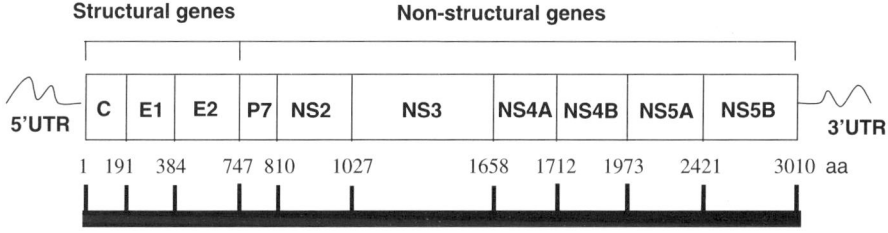

Fig. 4 Organization of the HCV genome.

and more than 30 subtypes throughout the world (Bukh et al., 1995). The importance of the genomic heterogeneity lays in the fact that the response to interferon treatment in patients with chronic HCV infection depends on the infecting HCV genotype (Brechot, 1997). Apart from this genetic diversity of HCV, there is also a high variability of individual HCV variants because of the lack of proof-reading activity of the viral polymerase, which produces mutation rate of the HCV genome of 10^{-3} per nucleotide per year (Ogata et al., 1991). This fact accounts for HCV circulation in a single patient as a population of closely related but heterogeneous sequences or quasispecies (Martell et al., 1992). Although these mutations take place throughout the HCV genome, the highest mutation rate occurs in the E2 protein-coding region in which two hypervariable sequences (HVR1 and 2) are located at the 5' end of this domain. In contrast, the 5'UTR is highly conserved among different isolates.

As mentioned above, the HCV genome contains two long UTRs at its 5' and 3' ends. The 5'UTR has extensive secondary structures (Brown et al., 1992) that provide a structure able to engage the ribosome for translation initiation at the IRES (Hellen and Pestova, 1999). As the 5'UTR is the most conserved region of the HCV genome it is used for the detection of HCV-RNA by PCR in infected patients and for determining the HCV genotype. Regarding the 3'UTR, early studies suggested that this 3' end of the HCV genome was a polyA (Han et al., 1991) or polyU (Chen et al., 1992) tract. However, later studies have shown that the 3'UTR is a tripartite structure comprising the conventional 3' end, a polyU tract and a highly conserved sequenced termed 3'X tail (Kolykhalov et al., 1996; Tanaka et al., 1996; Yonagi et al., 1999). The 3'UTR interacts with cellular hosts proteins (Luo, 1999) and it is essential for both translation and replication of HCV genome (Ito et al., 1998; Yanagi et al., 1999; Kolykhalov et al., 2000).

As previously mentioned, the viral polyprotein is processed by a set of host and viral proteinases into structural proteins and NS enzymes. The structural proteins are located at the carboxy-terminus of the polyprotein, while the NS proteins implicated in viral replication, are located at the amino-terminal portion of the polyprotein.

The core protein is a highly basic protein of 191 amino acids which is cleaved from the polyprotein by host-encoded proteases and that forms the viral nucleocapsid (Santolini et al., 1994). Apart from its ability to interact with genomic HCV-RNA to form nucleocapsids, the core protein modulates several cellular signaling pathways (Ray et al., 1995; Shrivastava et al., 1998; You et al., 1999). In addition, *in vitro* studies suggest that the core protein may modulate the host immune response (Large et al., 1999; De Lucas et al., 2005).

The envelope proteins E1 and E2 are the major structural viral proteins. Both are glycoproteins that are released from the polyprotein by the action of host-encoded signal peptidases. E1 and E2 proteins are essential for cell infection as they bind to cell receptor/s and induce fusion with host-cell membrane (Bartosch et al., 2003a). E2 is the most variable region of the HCV genome (Weiner et al., 1991) and contains two hypervariable regions (HVR1 and 2). HVR1 contains the only neutralization epitope identified in HCV (Farci et al., 1996) and its variability is likely due to antibody selection of immune-escape variants as demonstrated by the lack of variability in this region in an HCV-infected agammaglobulinemic patient after 5 years (Kumar et al., 1994). HVR2 comprises 7 amino acids of the E2 proteins that may have up to 100% of the sequence variability. HVR1 together with HVR2 seem to be implicated in the binding of E2 to the putative HCV receptor in the cell membrane (Roccasecca et al., 2003). Apart from its structural function, the E2 glycoprotein may be implicated in the HCV resistance to interferon by inhibiting the interferon-inducible protein kinase R (PKR) (Taylor et al., 1999).

The p7 polypeptide is a membrane protein of 63 amino acids that is cleaved from the precursor polyprotein by host signal peptidases. The p7 polypeptide has ion-channel activity (Griffin et al., 2003) and although its exact role in viral life cycle is unknown, it seems that it is essential for infectivity (Sakai et al., 2003).

The NS2 is a transmembrane protein with the only known function of participating in the cleavage of the polyprotein at the NS2–NS3 junction (Pieroni et al., 1997).

The NS3 protein is a 70 kDa protein and is a key enzyme in the virus life cycle. This protein has at least two biochemical functions: the first 189 amino-terminal amino acids have a serine protease activity that is responsible of the proteolytic processing of the polyprotein at NS3/NS4a, NS4a/NS4b, NS4b/NS5a and NS5a/NS5b junctions (Gallinari et al., 1998). The 442 carboxy-terminal amino acids of the protein have an RNA helicase function that unwinds RNA for replication and translation (Tai et al., 1996).

The NS4 region of the polyprotein contains two proteins termed NS4a and NS4b. These proteins are cleaved from the polyprotein by the NS3 serine protease (*cis* cleavage at the NS3/NS4a junction and *trans* cleavage at the NS4a/NS4b junction). The NS4a protein is a cofactor of the NS3 serine protease (Sali et al., 1998), while the NS4b is implicated in the formation of the membranous web in which HCV replication takes place (see below) (Egger et al., 2002).

As in the case of NS4, the NS5 region of the polyprotein contains two proteins, NS5a and NS5b, which are released from the polyprotein by the NS3 protease together with NS4a. The actual role of NS5a in the viral life cycle is unknown at present. The fact that adaptive mutations that appear in the replicon system (see below) are clustered in the central region of the NS5a (Blight et al., 2000), suggests that this protein is involved in the viral replication process. However, against this hypothesis is the fact that mutant genomes carrying the mutations that confer replication advantage in the replicon system are unable to initiate productive infections *in vivo* (Bukh et al., 2002). *In vitro* studies have shown that the NS5a protein inhibits the activity of the interferon-inducible PKR (Gale et al., 1998) suggesting that NS5 protein may be involved (together with the core and E2 proteins) in the HCV resistance to interferon. In relation with this, Japanese studies have postulated the existence of a region of 40 amino acids inside the NS5a protein termed "interferon sensitivity-determining region" (ISDR) that modulates the response to interferon alpha therapy *in vivo* (Enomoto et al., 1995, 1996). However, other studies performed outside Japan have not confirmed the existence of the ISDR (Khorsi et al., 1997; Zeuzem et al., 1997) and *in vitro* studies have shown that the NS5A-mediated resistance to interferon is not regulated (at least exclusively) by the ISDR (Paterson et al., 1999).

The sequence of the NS5b protein is highly conserved between the different HCV genotypes. It contains the GDD motif, which is characteristic of all viral RNA-dependent RNA polymerases (Kamer and Argos, 1984). Thus, the NS5b protein is the HCV polymerase and its biochemical properties have been extensively characterized (Behrens et al., 1996; Lohmann et al., 1997).

Regarding HCV virions, virus-like particles of 55–65 nm have been visualized by electron microscopy in plasma from infected patients (Kaito et al., 1994) as well as in the liver of a chimpanzee with acute HCV infection (Shimizu et al., 1996). HCV particles circulate in serum as virions bound to very-low and low-density lipoproteins, virions bound to immunoglobulins and as free virions (Thomssen et al., 1992, 1993; Hijikata et al., 1993). Apart from this, viral particles with characteristics of naked nucleocapsids have been also found in plasma (Maillard et al., 2001). The infectious virion fraction is at present unknown, although it has been suggested that the lipoprotein fraction is more infectious than the antibody-coated fraction (Kanto et al., 1994; Bartosch et al., 2005). The lack of a reliable cell culture system for HCV has hindered the characterization of critical steps of the viral cycle such viral entry into cells. In spite of this, several putative viral receptors have been identified including the low-density lipoproteins receptor (Agnello et al., 1999), the type C lectins DC-SIGN and L-SIGN (Pöhlmann et al., 2003), the tetraspanin CD81 (Pileri et al., 1998) and the scavenger receptor BI (SR-BI) (Scarselli et al., 2002). *In vitro* studies suggest that SR-BI is required for HCV infection of cells that express CD81 or low-density lipoprotein receptor, although other liver specific co-factors seem to be also necessary (Bartosch et al., 2003b).

Hepatitis C virus is mainly hepatotropic. However, patients with chronic HCV infection frequently present several extrahepatic manifestations (Hadziyannis, 1997). In relation with this, HCV-RNA and/or proteins have been detected in several extrahepatic compartments such as peripheral blood mononuclear cells (PBMC), heart, brain, kidney, skin, oral mucosa, salivary glands, sweat glands, pancreas, bone marrow or spleen (Zignego et al., 1992; Laskus et al., 1998; Arrieta et al., 2000; Matsumori et al., 2000; Rodriguez-Iñigo et al., 2000; Yan et al., 2000; Arrieta et al., 2001; Lazaro et al., 2002; Ortiz-Movilla et al., 2002; Radkowski et al., 2002). However, it is unclear at present whether or not these extrahepatic manifestations are directly related with the presence of the virus in the different tissues.

Regarding HCV replication, it is believed that it takes place throughout a RNA intermediate of negative polarity (negative HCV-RNA strand) as occurs in other Flaviviruses (Chambers et al., 1990). In fact, the detection of the negative HCV-RNA strand in a given tissue is considered as an indicator of an ongoing HCV replication in the tissue (Fong et al., 1991; Navas et al., 1994). The development of the HCV replicon system has allowed the study of the molecular aspects of HCV replication. The HCV replicons consist in genomic HCV-RNA that are able to replicate in a specific hepatoma cell line termed Huh-7. The first replicon developed consisted in bicistronic constructs with a selectable gene (neomycin-resistance) downstream the HCV IRES, followed by the encephalomyocarditis virus IRES controlling the translation of the second cistron, consisting in the NS genes NS3–NS5. The latest replicons include in the second cistron the complete HCV ORF (Pietschmann and Bartenschlager, 2001). Using this system, it has been shown that HCV replication occurs via the HCV-RNA negative-strand within a membranous compartment in cell cytoplasm called membranous web (Egger et al., 2002; Gosert et al., 2003). Furthermore, analyses of Huh-7 cells harboring the HCV replicon have demonstrated that HCV replication is coupled with the cell cycle (Pietschmann et al., 2001), as it was previously suggested based on the dependence of the HCV IRES activity on cell cycle (Honda et al., 2000).

The main drawback of the replicon system is that, although it is able to express HCV proteins and to persist for years in the cells, no encapsidation or secretion of viral particles to the culture medium has been observed with this model. However, the recent development of *in vitro* systems that permit the formation and release of HCV particles (Heller et al., 2005; Lindenbach et al., 2005) will allow the study of the molecular mechanisms governing the complete viral life cycle.

Natural history of HCV infection

Clinically, acute hepatitis C is similar to other forms of acute viral hepatitis. The incubation period, from infection to the onset of the symptoms, ranges from 7 to 20 weeks (Alter et al., 1989). The first marker of HCV infection that appears in serum is HCV-RNA that can be detected within 1–2 weeks after exposure (Hino et al., 1994). Later on, serum aminotransferase levels increase followed by appearance of antibodies to HCV (anti-HCV). In general, the first anti-HCV antibodies detected are of IgM class (Quiroga et al., 1991) but in some cases, the appearance of anti-HCV IgM coincides with that of anti-HCV IgG (Brillanti et al., 1993).

If acute HCV infection resolves, the HCV-RNA and the anti-HCV IgM become undetectable in serum, while titers of the anti-HCV IgG decrease and, in some cases, may become undetectable several years after the resolution of the acute infection (Takaki et al., 2000).

In 70–80% of patients acutely infected with HCV, the infection becomes chronic (Puoti et al., 1992; Seeff et al., 2001). In these patients, serum aminotransferase levels remain elevated while HCV-RNA, anti-HCV IgG and IgM are detectable in serum. Around 25% of chronic HCV carriers may have normal aminotransferase levels (Alberti et al., 1992). These so-called healthy carriers do not differ from the chronic carries with abnormal aminotransferase levels in clinical or virological characteristics (Naito et al., 1994; Jamal et al., 1999), but the histological damage is milder and the progression of the liver lesion is slower than in chronic carriers with elevated aminotransferase levels (Shindo et al., 1995; Mathurin et al., 1998).

Recently, a new form of HCV infection called "occult HCV infection" has been described in patients with abnormal liver function tests of unknown etiology (patients were anti-HCV and serum HCV-RNA negative, did not have markers of HBV infection and did not have clinical or biochemical evidences of autoimmunity, genetic or metabolic disorders, alcohol intake or drug toxicity). By analyzing liver biopsies from 100 patients with the above mentioned characteristics, Castillo et al. (2004) found HCV-RNA in the liver of 57 of the cases. Furthermore, the negative HCV-RNA strand was detected in 48 out of the 57 cases (84.2%), indicating that the virus was replicating in the liver of patients with occult HCV infection. The clinical importance of this finding lays in the fact that the percentage of patients with occult HCV infection who had necroinflammation and fibrosis in the liver biopsy was statistically higher than that of patients without detectable HCV-RNA in liver. In fact, 5% of patients with occult HCV infection had liver cirrhosis, while cirrhosis was not seen in patients without occult HCV infection. In 70% of patients with occult HCV infection, HCV-RNA is also detected in PBMC (Castillo et al., 2004) and, as occurs in the liver, the virus also replicates in these cells (Castillo et al., 2005). As mentioned above, patients with occult HCV infection are anti-HCV and serum HCV-RNA negative, but the viral RNA may be detected in a small percentage of them (14%) using whole blood instead of serum to perform the analysis (Carreño et al., 2004). In any case, the only way to identify all cases of occult HCV infection is to test for the presence of HCV-RNA in livers of patients.

HCV-RNA in liver in the absence of viral RNA in serum has also been reported in patients with chronic hepatitis C with a sustained virological response, years after the end of treatment (Pham et al., 2004; Carreño et al., 2005; Radkowski et al., 2005a). Moreover, it has been demonstrated that HCV is also replicating in the liver of these sustained virological responders (Carreño et al., 2005). As occurs in patients with occult HCV infection, testing for HCV-RNA in liver is the only way to determine if HCV persists in the hepatic tissue of patients with chronic hepatitis C who respond to the antiviral therapy with disappearance of HCV-RNA from serum and normalization of aminotransferase values. The clinical relevance of this HCV persistence must be further studied, but this situation should be taken into account in special circumstances (cytotoxic or immunosuppressive therapy), as it has been reported in a patient with chronic hepatitis C who cleared serum HCV-RNA with normalization of aminotransferase levels and persisted so during 8.5 years, the reemergence of HCV infection following prednisone therapy (Lee et al., 2005).

Diagnosis of HCV infection

Screening assays for HCV antibodies

The primary antibody response in patients with an acute HCV infection is an IgM class anti-HCV against the core antigen, which is rapidly followed by the IgG response. However, anti-HCV IgM antibodies are not limited to the acute phase of the disease. Thus, these antibodies can be detected in 50–93% of patients with acute HCV infection and in 50–70% of chronic cases. Because of this, anti-HCV IgM is not a reliable marker of acute infection (Pawlotsky, 1999).

The initial test for routine diagnosis of HCV infection is detection in serum or plasma of anti-HCV IgG class. There are several available tests for this purpose but the most commonly used are EIA or enzyme-linked immunosorbent assays (ELISA), which are rapid, easy to perform and suitable for testing large number of samples. The first-generation EIAs used the c100-3 epitope of the NS4 (Kuo et al., 1989). These assays had a low sensitivity (80%) and specificity (30%) (Gretch, 1997). Thus, second-generation EIAs were developed incorporating additional antigens from core (c22-3) and from NS3 proteins (c33c). These new assays led to a greater sensitivity (95%) and specificity (90%) and detected anti-HCV antibodies 30–90 days sooner than first-generation assays (Alter, 1992; Gretch, 1997). Third-generation immunoassays incorporated an additional antigen (NS5) to the second-generation assays, showing a better sensitivity and specificity (97%) as compared with previous assays (Kao et al., 1996). Finally, a fourth-generation enzyme immunoassay has also been developed using antigens (core, NS3, NS4A, NS4B and NS5A) from the HCV genotypes 1a, 1b, 2 and 3a, which has increased both the sensitivity and specificity (99%) (Neville et al., 1997; Cramp et al., 1999).

Confirmatory tests for anti-HCV

To confer specificity on positive EIA results other assays were introduced based on immunoblotting. The third-generation assays (RIBA, SIA or Inno-LIA) have, applied as separate lines to the solid phase, recombinant or synthetic peptides from the core, NS3, NS4 and NS5 of HCV genome. In addition, Inno-Lia uses also the E2 antigen. All these assays contain human superoxide dismutase or streptavidin in another line to detect nonspecific antibodies (false-positive results on EIAs). As third- and fourth-generation EIAs has remarkably increased the specificity of anti-HCV detection, these confirmatory tests are not necessary when screening high-risk population but they must be used to confirm positive-EIA results in low-risk populations (i.e. healthy blood donors).

HCV core antigen detection

An EIA has been developed to detect and quantitate HCV core antigen in serum or plasma. This assay has an initial immune complex dissociation step that removes bound anticore antibodies prior to the antigen detection with a monoclonal antibody (Bouvier-Alias et al., 2002). The clinical usefulness of this test is limited as HCV-RNA detection methods are more sensitive.

Serum HCV-RNA detection

The most reliable marker for the diagnosis of HCV infection and for assessing antiviral response to treatment is detection of viral RNA in serum or plasma

(Houghton et al., 1991). HCV-RNA can be detected 1–2 weeks after exposure to the virus and weeks before the increase in aminotransferase levels and appearance of anti-HCV (Farci et al., 1991). In some patients, the presence of HCV-RNA may be the only evidence of HCV infection. However, a single negative viral RNA result does not exclude HCV infection as HCV-RNA may be degradated due to improper collection and/or storage of samples (Wang et al., 1992).

Serum HCV-RNA can be detected with several commercially available kits but, due to the limited amount of HCV-RNA in infected persons, a target or signal amplification method is always mandatory. Reverse transcription PCR (RT-PCR) and transcription-mediated amplification (TMA) are target amplification methods, while branched DNA (bDNA) is a signal amplification technique. The 5′ UTR of HCV genome is the template for HCV-RNA detection because it is the most conserved region among all HCV isolates (Han et al., 1991). The commercially available HCV-RNA tests are divided into two categories: qualitative assays (presence or absence of viral RNA in blood) and quantitative assays (amount of virus in 1 ml of blood).

Qualitative HCV-RNA assays. The qualitatitve tests are currently the most sensitive methods for detecting the presence of HCV-RNA and thus, they are used to confirm or to diagnose an HCV infection and to assess complete viral clearance from blood during treatment or post-treatment period. These tests can detect as low as 5 IU/ml (Table 2) and their specificities are estimated to be greater than 99.5%.

Quantitative HCV-RNA assays. These assays quantitate HCV-RNA in blood by comparison with a standard curve established in each run by quantifying known amounts of standard sequences. Initially, the units of expression of HCV-RNA load differed among these assays and so, results obtained were not comparable. Nowadays, these tests have been standardized and viral load is expressed in IU per ml of serum (Table 2) (Saldanha et al., 1999). These assays are used to establish

Table 2

Qualitative and quantitative tests for HCV-RNA detection

	Method	Dynamic range (IU/ml)
Qualitative tests		
Amplicor HCV Test 2.0	PCR	⩾ 50
Cobas Amplicor HCV Test 2.0	PCR	⩾ 50
Versant HCV RNA assay	TMA	⩾ 5
Quantitative tests		
Amplicor HCV Monitor 2.0	PCR	600–700,000
Cobas Amplicor HCV Monitor 2.0	PCR	600–700,000
Versant HCV RNA 3.0	bDNA	615–7,700,000
LCx HCV-RNA	PCR	25–2,630,000
SuperQuant	PCR	30–1,500,000

treatment schedules, being 800,000 IU/ml the decision threshold for extending the duration of combination therapy in patients infected by HCV genotypes 1, 4 and 5 (Pawlotsky et al., 2000). In addition, these tests indicate during treatment whether antiviral therapy is effective or not by measuring decreases in viral load (Davis et al., 2003). However, as quantitative HCV-RNA detection methods are commonly less sensitive than the qualitative ones (Table 2), they cannot be used to determine complete viral clearance from circulation during or after treatment.

Recently, "real-time" PCR techniques have been developed. These methods are based on target amplification and the amplified DNA can be detected during the PCR process, in real-time rather than at the end of the process. Their dynamic range of quantification is consistently wider (up to 10^8 IU/ml) and more sensitive (5–20 IU/ml) (Forman and Valsamakis, 2004; Konnick et al., 2005). For these reasons, "real-time" PCR will replace in the future the other assays for HCV-RNA detection and quantification.

HCV-RNA detection in liver and peripheral blood mononuclear cells

No commercial kits are available for detection of HCV-RNA in liver or in other tissues or cells, such as PBMC, because it has been considered that these assays do not have any clinical relevance for diagnosis of HCV infection or for assessing antiviral responses. However, recent reports have demonstrated that testing for HCV-RNA in liver or in PBMC is crucial to identify the existence of an HCV infection in patients with abnormal values of liver enzymes in the absence of anti-HCV and of serum HCV-RNA (Castillo et al., 2004) and to assess the persistence of HCV infection in patients who cleared serum HCV-RNA and normalized ALT levels years after a successful antiviral treatment as well as in healthy anti-HCV subjects without detectable viremia (Pham et al., 2004; Carreño et al., 2005; López-Alcorocho et al., 2005; Radkowski et al., 2005a, b). This form of HCV infection is known as "occult HCV infection".

These reports have detected HCV-RNA in liver and in PBMC by in-house RT-PCR or "real-time" PCR. The critical step for an accurate viral RNA detection in liver is preservation of HCV-RNA integrity and so, the liver biopsy must be immediately frozen in liquid nitrogen or embedded in a chemical agent that inhibits RNases to preserve the integrity of RNA. In this sense, it has been proven that the time-elapsed between obtaining the liver biopsy and its freezing (to inhibit intracellular RNases) must not be exceed 3 min in order to prevent RNA degradation and assure detection of both HCV-RNA-positive- and negative-strands (Madejon et al., 2000).

Another technique for detecting HCV-RNA in liver or in PBMC is *in situ* hybridization, based on the hybridization of the viral RNA present in cells with a labeled-probe (Gosálvez et al., 1998, 2003). This technique is more tedious than PCR methods but have the advantage that it can be applied to archived liver samples (routinely obtained for histological diagnosis), cross-contamination among samples does not occur and allows identification of the HCV-infected cell type. In addition, a recent paper has demonstrated that the percentage of HCV-infected hepatocytes is a better predictor factor of response to antiviral treatment than serum viremia levels (Rodriguez-Iñigo et al., 2005).

HCV genotyping

There are molecular and serological commercially available tests to determine HCV genotypes. Based on the nucleotide differences in the 5'UTR among genotypes, molecular methods are PCR-techniques that detect these genotypes by direct sequencing or by hybridization with specific-probes of amplicons. The serological assay identifies HCV genotypes by testing for type-specific antibodies against epitopes in the NS4 or core region. This assay is easier to perform than the other ones but has a lower sensitivity and specificity,

References

Agnello V, Abel G, Elfahal M, Knight GB, Zhang QX. Hepatitis C virus and other flaviviridae viruses enter cells via low density lipoprotein receptor. Proc Natl Acad Sci USA 1999; 96: 12766.

Alberti A, Morsica G, Chemello L, Cavalletto D, Noventa F, Pontisso P, Ruol A. Hepatitis C viraemia and liver disease in symptom-free individuals with anti-HCV. Lancet 1992; 340: 697.

Alter HJ. New kit on the block: evaluation of second-generation assays for detection of antibody to the hepatitis C virus. Hepatology 1992; 15: 350.

Alter HJ, Purcell RH, Shih JW, Melpolder JC, Houghton M, Choo QL, Kuo G. Detection of antibody to hepatitis C virus in prospectively followed transfusion recipients with acute and chronic non-A, non-B hepatitis. N Engl J Med 1989; 321: 1494.

Arrieta JJ, Rodriguez-Inigo E, Casqueiro M, Bartolome J, Manzarbeitia F, Herrero M, Pardo M, Carreño V. Detection of hepatitis C virus replication by *In situ* hybridization in epithelial cells of anti-hepatitis C virus-positive patients with and without oral lichen planus. Hepatology 2000; 32: 97.

Arrieta JJ, Rodriguez-Iñigo E, Ortiz-Movilla N, Bartolomé J, Pardo M, Manzarbeitia F, Oliva H, Macias DM, Carreño V. *In situ* detection of hepatitis C virus RNA in salivary glands. Am J Pathol 2001; 158: 259.

Bartosch B, Dubuisson J, Cosset FL. Infectious hepatitis C virus pseudo-particles containing functional E1–E2 envelope protein complexes. J Exp Med 2003a; 197: 633.

Bartosch B, Verney G, Dreux M, Donot P, Morice Y, Penin F, Pawlotsky JM, Lavillette D, Cosset FL. An interplay between hypervariable region 1 of the hepatitis C virus E2 glycoprotein, the scavenger receptor BI, and high-density lipoprotein promotes both enhancement of infection and protection against neutralizing antibodies. J Virol 2005; 79: 8217.

Bartosch B, Vitelli A, Granier C, Goujon C, Dubuisson J, Pascale S, Scarselli E, Cortese R, Nicosia A, Cosset FL. Cell entry of hepatitis C virus requires a set of co-receptors that include the CD81 tetraspanin and the SR-B1 scavenger receptor. J Biol Chem 2003b; 278: 41624.

Bavand M, Feitelson MA, Laub O. The hepatitis B virus-associated reverse transcriptase is encoded by the viral pol gene. J Virol 1989; 63: 1019.

Behrens SE, Tomei L, De Francesco R. Identification and properties of the RNA-dependent RNA polymerase of hepatitis C virus. EMBO J 1996; 15: 12.

Berninger M, Hammer M, Hoyer B, Gerin JL. An assay for the detection of the DNA genome of hepatitis B virus in serum. J Med Virol 1982; 9: 57.

Blight KJ, Kolykhavov AA, Rice CM. Efficient initiation of HCV-RNA replication in cell culture. Science 2000; 290: 1972.

Bonchard MJ, Schneider RJ. The enzymatic X gene of hepatitis B Virus. J Virol 2004; 78: 12725.

Bouvier-Alias M, Patel K, Dahari H, Beaucourt S, Larderie P, Blatt L, Hezode C, Picchio G, Dhumeaux D, Neumann AU, McHutchison JG, Pawlotsky JM. Clinical utility of total HCV core antigen quantification: a new indirect marker of HCV replication. Hepatology 2002; 36: 211.

Brechot C. Hepatitis C virus 1b, cirrhosis and hepatocellular carcinoma. Hepatology 1997; 25: 772.

Brillanti S, Masci C, Miglioli M, Barbara L. Serum IgM antibodies to hepatitis C virus in acute and chronic hepatitis C. Arch Virol 1993; Suppl 8: 213.

Brown EA, Zhang H, Ping LH, Lemon SM. Secondary structure of the 5′ nontranslated regions of the hepatitis C virus and pestivirus genomic RNAs. Nucleic Acid Res 1992; 20: 5041.

Brunetto MR, Cerenzia MT, Oliveri F, Piantino P, Randone A, Calvo PL, Manzini P, Rocca G, Galli C, Bonino F. Monitoring the natural course and response to therapy of chronic hepatitis B with an automated semi-quantitative assay for IgM anti-HBc. J Hepatol 1993; 19: 431.

Bukh J, Miller RH, Purcell RH. Genetic heterogeneity of hepatitis C virus: quasispecies and genotypes. Semin Liver Dis 1995; 15: 41.

Bukh J, Pietschmann T, Lohmann V, Krieger N, Faulk K, Engle RE, Govindarajan S, Shapiro M, St Claire M, Bartenschlager R. Mutations that permit efficient replication of hepatitis C virus RNA in Huh-7 cells prevent productive replication in chimpanzees. Proc Natl Acad Sci USA 2002; 99: 14416.

Cabrerizo M, Bartolomé J, de Sequera P, Caramelo C, Carreño V. Hepatitis B virus DNA in serum and blood cells of hepatitis B surface antigen-negative hemodialysis patients and staff. J Am Soc Nephrol 1997; 8: 1443.

Carman WF, Jacyna MR, Hadziyannis S, Karayiannis P, McGarvey MJ, Makris A, Thomas HC. Mutation preventing formation of hepatitis B e antigen in patients with chronic hepatitis B infection. Lancet 1989; 2: 588.

Carreño V, Castillo I, Bartolomé J, Rodriguez-Iñigo E, Ortiz-Movilla N, de Lucas S, Pardo M. Comparison of hepatitis C virus RNA detection in plasma, whole blood and peripheral blood mononuclear cells of patients with occult hepatitis C virus infection. J Clin Virol 2004; 31: 312.

Carreño V, Castillo I, Rodríguez-Iñigo E, López-Alcorocho JM, Bartolomé J, Quiroga JA, Pardo M. Hepatitis C virus persists and replicates in the liver of the majority of sustained responder patients to antiviral treatment. Hepatology 2005; 42(Suppl 1): 284A.

Castillo I, Pardo M, Bartolomé J, Ortiz-Movilla N, Rodríguez-Iñigo E, Lucas S, Salas C, Jiménez-Hefferman JA, Pérez-Mota A, Graus J, López-Alcorocho JM, Carreño V. Occult hepatitis C virus infection in patients in whom the etiology of persistently abnormal results of liver-function tests is unknown. J Infect Dis 2004; 189: 7.

Castillo I, Rodriguez-Iñigo E, Bartolomé J, de Lucas S, Ortiz-Movilla N, Lopez-Alcorocho JM, Pardo M, Carreño V. Hepatitis C virus replicates in peripheral blood mononuclear cells of patients with occult hepatitis C virus infection. Gut 2005; 54: 682.

Chambers TJ, Hahn CS, Galler R, Rice CM. Flavivirus genome organization, expression and replication. Annu Rev Microbiol 1990; 44: 649.

Chang C, Zhou S, Ganem D, Standring DN. Phenotypic mixing between different hepadnavirus nucleocapsid proteins reveals C protein dimerization to be cis preferential. J Virol 1994; 68: 5225.

Chen PJ, Lin MH, Tai KF, Liu PC, Lin CJ, Chen DS. The Taiwanese hepatitis C virus genome. Virology 1992; 188: 102.

Choo QL, Kuo G, Weiner A, Overby LR, Bradley DW, Hougthon M. Isolation of a cDNA clone derived from a blood-borne non-A, non-B viral hepatitis genome. Science 1989; 244: 359.

Cramp ME, Carucci P, Rossol S, Chokshi S, Maertens G, Williams R, Naoumov NV. Hepatitis C virus (HCV) specific immune responses in anti-HCV positive patients without hepatitis C viremia. Gut 1999; 44: 424.

Dane DS, Cameron CH, Briggs M. Virus-like particles in serum of patients with Australia-antigen-associated hepatitis. Lancet 1970; 2: 695.

Davis GL, Wong JB, McHutchison JG, Manns MP, Harvey J, Albrecht J. Early virologic response to treatment with PEG-interferon alfa-2b plus ribavirin in patients with chronic hepatitis C. Hepatology 2003; 38: 645.

De Lamballerie X, Gallian P, De Micco PH. Evaluation of a chemiluminiscent molecular hybridization assay for the detection and quantitation of hepatitis B virus-DNA in serum. New Microbiol 1995; 18: 207.

De Lucas S, Bartolomé J, Carreño V. Hepatitis C virus core protein down-regulates transcription of interferon-induced antiviral genes. J Infect Dis 2005; 191: 93.

Duckworth GJ, Heptonstall J, Aitken C. Transmission of hepatitis C virus from a surgeon to a patient. The incident control team. Commun. Dis. Public. Health. 1999; 2: 188.

Egger D, Wolk B, Gosert R, Bianchi L, Blum HE, Moradpour D, Bienz K. Expression of hepatitis C virus proteins induces distinct membrane alterations including a candidate viral replication complex. J Virol 2002; 76: 5974.

Enomoto N, Sakuma I, Asahina Y, Kurosaki M, Murakami T, Yamamoto C, Izumi N, Marumo F, Sato C. Comparison of full-length sequences of interferon-sensitive and resistant hepatitis C virus 1b. Sensitivity to interferon is conferred by amino acid substitutions in the NS5A region. J Clin Invest 1995; 96: 224.

Enomoto N, Sakuma I, Asahina Y, Kurosaki M, Murakami T, Yamamoto C, Ogura Y, Izumi N, Marumo F, Sato C. Mutations in the nonstructural protein 5A gene and response to interferon in patients with chronic hepatitis C virus 1b infection. N Engl J Med 1996; 334: 77.

Everhart JE, DiBisceglie AM, Murray LM, Alter HJ, Melpolder JJ, Kuo G, Hoofnagle JH. Risk for non-A, non-B (type C) hepatitis through sexual or household contact with chronic carriers. Ann Intern Med 1990; 112: 544.

Eyster ME, Alter HJ, Aledort LM, Quan S, Hatzakis A, Goedert J. Heterosexual co-transmission of hepatitis C virus (HCV) and human immunodeficiency virus (HIV). Ann Intern Med 1991; 115: 764.

Farci P, Alter HJ, Wong D, Miller RH, Shi JW, Jett B, Purcell RH. A long-term study of hepatitis C virus replication in non-A, non-B hepatitis. N Engl J Med 1991; 325: 98.

Farci P, Shimoda A, Wong D, Cabezon T, De Gioannis D, Strazzera A, Shimizu Y, Shapiro M, Alter HJ, Purcell RH. Prevention of hepatitis C virus infection in chimpanzees by hyperimmune serum against the hypervariable region 1 of the envelope 2 protein. Proc Natl Acad Sci USA 1996; 93: 15394.

Fong TL, Shindo M, Feinstone SM, Hoofnagle JH, Di Bisceglie AM. Detection of replicative intermediates of hepatitis C viral RNA in liver and serum of patients with chronic hepatitis C. J Clin Invest 1991; 88: 1058.

Forman MS, Valsamakis A. Verification of an assay for quantification of hepatitis C virus RNA by use of an analyte-specific reagent and two different extraction methods. J Clin Microbiol 2004; 42: 3581.

Franco A, Paroli M, Testa U, Benvenuto R, Peschle C, Balsano F, Barnaba V. Transferrin receptor mediated uptake and presentation of hepatitis B envelope antigen by T lymphocytes. J Exp Med 1992; 175: 1195.

Gale MJ, Korth MJ, Katze MG. Repression of the PKR protein kinase by the hepatitis C virus NS5A protein: a potential mechanism of interferon resistance. Clin Diagn Virol 1998; 10: 157.

Galibert F, Mandart E, Fitonssi F, Tiollais P, Charnay P. Nucleotide sequence of the hepatitis B virus genome (subtype ayw) cloned in *E. coli.* Nature 1979; 281: 646.

Gallinari P, Brennan D, Nardi C, Brunetti M, Tomei L, Steinkuhler C, De Francesco R. Multiple enzymatic activities associated with recombinant NS3 protein of hepatitis C virus. J Virol 1998; 72: 6758.

Gerken G, Gomes J, Lampertico P, Colombo M, Rothaar T, Trippler M, Colucci G. Clinical evaluation and applications of the Amplicor HBV Monitor tests, a quantitative HBV-DNA PCR assay. J Virol Methods 1998; 74: 155.

Gerlich WH, Robinson WS. Hepatitis B virus contains protein attached to the 5′ terminus of its complete DNA strand. Cell 1980; 21: 801.

Gordillo RM, Gutierrez J, Casal M. Evaluation of the COBAS Taqman 48 real-time PCR system for quantitation of hepatitis B virus DNA. J Clin Microbiol 2005; 43: 3504.

Gosálvez J, Ortiz-Movilla N, Gosálbez A, Rodríguez-Iñigo E, Bartolomé J, Carreño V. Improved sensitivity for cell mapping of hepatitis C virus RNA sequences and cellular surface antigens in blood cells. Lab Invest 2003; 83: 1089.

Gosálvez J, Rodriguez-Iñigo E, Ramiro-Diaz JL, Bartolomé J, Tomas JF, Oliva H, Carreño V. Relative quantification and mapping of hepatitis C virus by *in situ* hybridization and digital image analysis. Hepatology 1998; 27: 1428.

Gosert R, Egger D, Lohmann V, Bartenschlager R, Blum HE, Bienz K, Moradpour D. Identification of the hepatitis C virus RNA replication complex in Huh-7 cells harboring subgenomic replicons. J Virol 2003; 77: 5487.

Gretch DR. Diagnostic tests for hepatitis C. Hepatology 1997; 26(Suppl 3): 43S.

Griffin SD, Beales LP, Clarke DS, Worsfold O, Evans SD, Jaeger J, Harris MP, Rowlands DJ. The p7 protein of hepatitis C virus forms an ion channel that is blocked by the antiviral drug amantadine. FEBS Lett 2003; 535: 34.

Guidotti LG, Matzke B, Pasquinelli C, Shoenberger JM, Rogler C, Chisari FV. The hepatitis B virus (HBV) precore protein inhibits HBV replication in transgenic mice. J Virol 1996; 70: 7056.

Hadziyannis S, Gerber MA, Vissonlis C, Popper H. Cytoplasmic hepatitis B antigen in "ground-glass" hepatocytes of carriers. Arch Pathol 1973; 96: 327.

Hadziyannis SJ. The spectrum of extrahepatic manifestations in hepatitis C virus infection. J Viral Hepat 1997; 4: 9.

Han JH, Shyamala V, Richman KH, Brauer MJ, Irvine B, Urdea MS, Tekamp-Olson P, Kuo G, Choo QL, Houghton M. Characterization of the terminal regions of hepatitis C viral RNA: identification of conserved sequences in the 5' untranslated region and poly(A) tails at the 3' end. Proc Natl Acad Sci USA 1991; 88: 1711.

Heerman KH, Kruse F, Seifer M, Gerlich WH. Immunogenicity of the gene S and Pre-S domains in hepatitis B virions and HBsAg filaments. Intervirology 1987; 28: 14.

Hellen CUT, Pestova TV. Translation of hepatitis C virus RNA. J Viral Hepat 1999; 6: 79.

Heller T, Saito S, Auerbach J, Williams T, Moreen TR, Jazwinski A, Cruz B, Jeurkar N, Sapp R, Luo G, Liang TJ. An in vitro model of hepatitis C virion production. Proc Natl Acad Sci USA 2005; 102: 2579.

Hertogs K, Leenders WPJ, Depla E, DeBruin WCC, Mehens L, Raymackers J, Moshage H, Yap SH. Endonexin II, present in human liver plasma membranes, is a specific binding protein of small hepatitis B virus envelope protein. Virology 1993; 197: 549.

Hijikata M, Shimizu YK, Kato H, Iwamoto A, Shih JW, Alter HJ, Purcell RH, Yoshikura H. Equilibrium centrifugation studies of hepatitis C virus: evidence for circulating immune complexes. J Virol 1993; 67: 1953.

Hino K, Sainokami S, Shimoda K, Niwa H, Iino S. Clinical course of acute hepatitis C and changes in HCV markers. Dig Dis Sci 1994; 39: 19.

Honda M, Kaneko S, Matsushita E, Kobayashi K, Abell GA, Lemon SM. Cell cycle regulation of hepatitis C virus internal ribosomal entry site-directed translation. Gastroenterology 2000; 118: 152.

Hoofnagle JH. Serologic markers of hepatitis B virus infection. Ann Rev Med 1981; 32: 1.

Houghton M, Weiner A, Han J, Kuo G, Choo Q. Molecular biology of the hepatitis C viruses: implications for diagnosis, development and control of viral disease. Hepatology 1991; 14: 381.

Hsu YS, Chien RN, Yeh CT, Sheen IS, Chiou HY, Chu CM, Liaw YF. Long-term outcome after spontaneous HBeAg seroconversion in patients with chronic hepatitis B. Hepatology 2002; 35: 1522.

Ito T, Tahara SM, Lai MM. The 3'-untranslated region of hepatitis C virus RNA enhances translation from an internal ribosomal entry site. J Virol 1998; 72: 8789.

Jamal MM, Soni A, Quinn PG, Wheeler DE, Arora S, Johnston DE. Clinical features of hepatitis C-infected patients with persistently normal alanine transaminase levels in the Southwestern United States. Hepatology 1999; 30: 1307.

Kaito M, Watanabe S, Tsukiyama-Kohara K, Yamaguchi K, Kobayashi Y, Konishi M, Yokoi M, Ishida S, Suzuki SS, Kohara M. Hepatitis C virus particle detected by immunoelectron microscopic study. J Gen Virol 1994; 75: 1755.

Kamer G, Argos P. Primary structural comparison of RNA-dependent polymerases from plant, animal and bacterial viruses. Nucleic Acids Res 1984; 12: 7269.

Kanto T, Hayashi N, Takehara T, Hagiwara H, Mita E, Naito M, Kasahara A, Fusamoto H, Kamada T. Buoyant density of hepatitis C virus recovered from infected hosts: two different features in sucrose equilibrium density-gradient centrifugation related to degree of liver inflammation. Hepatology 1994; 19: 296.

Kao JH, Lai MY, Hwang YT, Yang PM, Chen PJ, Shen JC, Wang TH, Hsu HC, Chen DS. Chronic hepatitis C without anti-hepatitis C antibodies by second-generation assay: a clinico pathologic study and demonstration of the usefulness of a third-generation assay. Dig Dis Sci 1996; 41: 161.

Kato N, Hijikata M, Ootsuyama Y, Nakagawa M, Ohkoshi S, Sugimura T, Shimotono K. Molecular cloning of the human hepatitis C virus genome from Japanese patients with non A, non B hepatitis. Proc Natl Acad Sci USA 1990; 87: 9524.

Khorsi H, Castelain S, Wyseur A, Izopet J, Canva V, Rombout A, Capron D, Capron JP, Lunel F, Stuyver L, Duverlie G. Mutations of hepatitis C virus 1b NS5A 2209–2248 amino acid sequence do not predict the response to recombinant interferon-alfa therapy in French patients. J Hepatol 1997; 27: 72.

Kokubo S, Horii T, Yonekawa O, Ozawa M, Mukaide M. A phylogenetic-tree analysis elucidating nosocomial transmission of hepatitis C virus in a hemodialysis unit. J Viral Hepat 2002; 9: 450.

Kolykhalov AA, Feinstone SM, Rice CM. Identification of a highly conserved sequence element at the 3′ terminus of hepatitis C virus genome RNA. J Virol 1996; 70: 3363.

Kolykhalov AA, Mihalik K, Feinstone SM, Rice CM. Hepatitis C virus-encoded enzymatic activities and conserved RNA elements in the 3′ nontranslated region are essential for virus replication *in vivo*. J Virol 2000; 74: 2046.

Konnick EQ, Williams SM, Ashwood ER, Hillyard DR. Evaluation of the COBAS Hepatitis C Virus (HCV) TaqMan Analyte-Specific Reagent Assay and Comparison to the COBAS Amplicor HCV Monitor V2.0 and Versant HCV bDNA 3.0 Assays. J Clin Microbiol 2005; 43: 2133.

Kumar U, Monjardino J, Thomas HC. Hypervariable region of hepatitis C virus envelope glycoprotein (E2/NS1) in an agammaglobulinemic patient. Gastroenterology 1994; 106: 1072.

Kuo G, Choo QL, Alter HJ, Gitnik GL, Redeker AG, Purcell RH, Dienstag JL, Alter MJ, Stevens CE, Tegtmeier GE, Bonino F, Colombo M, Lee WS, Kuo C, Berger K, Shuster JR, Overby LR, Bradley DW, Houghton M. An assay for circulating antibodies to a major etiologic virus of human non-A, non-B hepatitis. Science 1989; 244: 362.

Lamberts C, Nassal M, Velhagen I, Zentgraf H, Schroder CH. Pre-core-mediated inhibition of hepatitis B virus progeny DNA synthesis. J Virol 1993; 67: 3756.

Landford RE, Chavez D, Brasky KM, Borns RB, Rico-Hesse R. Isolation of a hepadnavirus from the wooly monkey, a New World primate. Proc Natl Acad Sci USA 1998; 95: 5757.

Landford RE, Kim YH, Lee H, Notwall L, Beames B. Mapping of the HBV reverse transcriptase TP and RT domains by transcomplementation for nucleotide priming and by protein-protein interaction. J Virol 1999; 73: 1885.

Large M, Kittleson D, Hahn Y. Suppression of host immune response by the core protein of hepatitis C virus: implications for hepatitis C virus persistence. J Immunol 1999; 168: 931.

Laskus T, Radkowski M, Wang LF, Vargas H, Rakela J. Search for hepatitis C virus extrahepatic replication sites in patients with acquired immunodeficiency syndrome: specific detection of negative-strand viral RNA in various tissues. Hepatology 1998; 28: 1398.

Lauer GM, Walker BD. Hepatitis C virus infection. N Engl J Med 2001; 345: 41.

Lazaro P, Olalquiaga J, Bartolomé J, Ortiz-Movilla N, Rodriguez-Iñigo E, Pardo M, Lecona M, Pico M, Longo I, Garcia-Morras P, Carreño V. Detection of hepatitis C virus RNA and core protein in keratinocytes from patients with cutaneous lichen planus and chronic hepatitis C. J Invest Dermatol 2002; 119: 798.

Lee WM, Polson JE, Carney DS, Sahin B, Gale M. Reemergence of hepatitis C virus after 8.5 years in a patient with hypogammaglobulinemia: evidence for an occult viral reservoir. J Infect Dis 2005; 192: 1088.

Lindenbach BD, Evans MJ, Syder AJ, Wolk B, Tellinghuisen TL, Liu CC, Maruyama T, Hynes RO, Burton DR, McKeating JA, Rice CM. Complete replication of hepatitis C virus in cell culture. Science 2005; 309: 623.

Lohmann V, Korner F, Herian U, Bartenschlager R. Biochemical properties of hepatitis C virus NS5B RNA-dependent RNA polymerase and identification of amino acid sequence motifs essential for enzymatic activity. J Virol 1997; 71: 8416.

Lok ASF, McMahon BJ. Chronic hepatitis B. Hepatology 2001; 34: 1225.

Lopez VA, Bourne EJ, Lutz MW, Condreay LD. Assessment of the COBAS Amplicor HCV Monitor test for quantitation of serum hepatitis B virus DNA levels. J Clin Microbiol 2002; 40: 1972.

López-Alcorocho JM, Rodríguez-Iñigo E, Pardo M, Castillo I, Quiroga JA, Carreño V. Persistence of HCV infection in apparently healthy anti-HCV positive patients with constantly serum HCV-RNA negative and normal ALT levels. Hepatology 2005; 42(Suppl 1): 433A.

Loriot MA, Marcellin P, Bismuth E, Martinot- Peignoux M, Boyer N, Degott C, Erlinger S, Benhamou JP. Demonstration of hepatitis B virus DNA by polymerase chain reaction in the serum and the liver after spontaneous or therapeutically induced HBeAg to anti-HBe or HBsAg to anti-HBs seroconversion in patients with chronic hepatitis B. Hepatology 1992; 15: 32.

Luo G. Cellular proteins bind to the poly(U) tract of the 3′ untranslated region of hepatitis C virus RNA genome. Virology 1999; 256: 105.

Machida A, Kishimoto S, Ohnuma H, Miyamoto H, Baba K, Oda K, Nakamura T, Miyakawa Y, Mayumi M. A hepatitis B surface antigen polypeptide (P31) with the receptor for polymerized human as well as chimpanzee albumins. Gastroenterology 1983; 85: 268.

Madejon A, Manzano ML, Arocena C, Castillo I, Carreño V. Effects of delayed freezing of liver biopsies on the detection of hepatitis C virus RNA strands. J Hepatol 2000; 32: 1019.

Magnius LO, Espmark JA. New specificities in Australia antigen positive sera distinct from LeBourier determinants. J Immunol 1972; 109: 1017.

Magnius LO, Lindholm A, Lundin P, Iwarson S. Clinical significance of a new antigen-antibody system in long-term carriers of hepatitis B surface antigen. J Am Med Assoc 1975; 231: 356.

Maillard P, Krawczynski K, Nitkiewicz J, Bronnert C, Sidorkiewicz M, Gounon P, Dubuisson J, Faure G, Crainic R, Budkowska A. Nonenveloped nucleocapsids of hepatitis C virus in the serum of infected patients. J Virol 2001; 75: 8240.

Marion PL, Oshiro LS, Regnery DC, Scullard GH, Robinson WS. A virus in Beechey ground squirrels that is related to hepatitis B virus in humans. Proc Natl Acad Sci USA 1980; 77: 2941.

Martell M, Esteban JI, Quer J, Genescá J, Weiner A, Esteban R, Guardia J, Gómez J. Hepatitis C virus (HCV) circulates as a population of different but closely related genomes: quasispecies nature of HCV genome distribution. J Virol 1992; 66: 3225.

Mason WS, Seal G, Summers J. Virus of Pekin ducks with structural and biochemical relatedness to human hepatitis B virus. J Virol 1980; 36: 829.

Mathurin P, Moussalli J, Cadranel JF, Thibault V, Charlotte F, Dumouchel P, Cazier A, Huraux JM, Devergie B, Vidaud M, Opolon P, Poynard T. Slow progression rate of fibrosis in hepatitis C virus patients with persistently normal alanine transaminase activity. Hepatology 1998; 27: 868.

Matsumori A, Yutani C, Ikeda Y, Kawai S, Sasayama S. Hepatitis C virus from the hearts of patients with myocarditis and cardiomyopathy. Lab Invest 2000; 80: 1137.

McGwire GB, Tan F, Michel B, Rehli M, Skidgel RA. Identification of a membrane-bound carboxypeptidase as the mammalian homolog of duck gp180, a hepatitis B virus-binding protein. Life Sci 1997; 60: 715.

McMahon BJ, Alward WL, Hall DB, Heyward WL, Bender TR, Francis DP, Maynard JE. Acute hepatitis B virus infection: relation of age to the clinical expression of disease and subsequent development of the carrier state. J Infect Dis 1985; 151: 599.

Mehdi H, Kaplan MK, Anlar FY, Yang X, Bayer R, Sutherland K, Peeples ME. Hepatitis B virus surface antigen binds to a polyprotein H. J Virol 1994; 68: 2415.

Michalak TI, Pasquinelli C, Guilhot S, Chisari FV. Hepatitis B virus persistence after recovery from acute viral hepatitis. J Clin Invest 1994; 93: 230.

Milich DR, Chen MK, Hughes JL, Jones JE. The secreted hepatitis B precore antigen can modulate the immune response to the nucleocapsid: a mechanism for persistence. J Immunol 1998; 160: 2013.

Milich DR, Jones JE, Hughes JL, Price J, Raney AK, McLachan A. Is a function of the secreted hepatitis B e antigen to induce immunologic tolerance in utero? Proc Natl Acad Sci USA 1990; 87: 6599.

Miller RH, Kaneko S, Chung CT, Girones R, Purcell RH. Compact organization of the hepatitis B virus genome. Hepatology 1989; 9: 322.

Naito M, Hayashi N, Hagiwara H, Hiramatsu N, Kasahara A, Fusamoto H, Kamada T. Serum hepatitis C virus RNA quantity and histological features of hepatitis C virus carriers with persistently normal ALT levels. Hepatology 1994; 19: 871.

Navas S, Castillo I, Bartolomé J, Marriott E, Herrero M, Carreño V. Positive and negative hepatitis C virus RNA strands in serum, liver and peripheral blood mononuclear cells in anti-HCV patients: relation with the liver lesion. J Hepatol 1994; 21: 182.

Neville JA, Prescott LE, Bhattacherjee V, Adams N, Pike L, Rodgers B, El-Zayadi A, Hamid S, Dusheiko GM, Saeed AA, Haydon GH, Simmonds P. Antigenic variation of core, NS3 and NS5 proteins among genotypes of hepatitis C virus. J Clin Microbiol 1997; 35: 3062.

Norder H, Courouce A-M, Cousaget P, Echevarria JM, Lee S-D, Mushahwar IK, Robertson RH, Locarnini S, Magnius LO. Genetic diversity of hepatitis B virus strains derived worldwide: genotypes, subgenotypes, and HBsAg subtypes. Intervirology 2004; 47: 289.

Ogata N, Alter HJ, Miller RH, Purcell RH. Nucleotide sequence and mutation rate of the H strain of hepatitis C virus. Proc Natl Acad Sci USA 1991; 88: 3392.

Ohba K, Mizokami M, Lau JYN, Orito E, Ikeo K, Gojobori T. Evolutionary relationship of hepatitis C, pesti-flavi-planviruses and newly discovered GB hepatitis agents. FEBS Lett 1996; 378: 232.

Okamoto H, Imai M, Tsuda F, Tanaka T, Miyakawa Y, mayumi M. Point mutation in the S gene of hepatitis B virus for a d/y or w/r subtypic changes in two blood donors carrying a surface antigen of compound subtype adyr or adwr. J Virol 1987; 61: 3030.

Okamoto H, Tsuda F, Akahane Y, Sugai Y, Yoshiba M, Moriyama K, Tanaka T, Miyakawa Y, Mayumi M. Hepatitis B virus with mutations in the core promoter for an e antigen-negative phenotype in carriers with antibody to e antigen. J Virol 1994; 68: 8102.

Ortiz-Movilla N, Lazaro P, Rodriguez-Iñigo E, Bartolomé J, Longo I, Lecona M, Pardo M, Carreño V. Hepatitis C virus replicates in sweat glands and is released into sweat in patients with chronic hepatitis C. J Med Virol 2002; 68: 529.

Ou JH, Laub O, Rutter WJ. Hepatitis B virus gene function: the precore region targets the core antigen to cellular membranes and causes the secretion of the e antigen. Proc Natl Acad Sci USA 1986; 83: 1578.

Pan CQ, Zhang JX. Natural history and clinical consequences of hepatitis B virus infection. Int J Med Sci 2005; 2: 36.

Paterson M, Laxton CD, Thomas HC, Ackrill AM, Foster GR. Hepatitis C virus NS5A protein inhibits interferon antiviral activity, but the effects do not correlate with clinical response. Gastroenterology 1999; 117: 1187.

Pawlotsky JM. Diagnostics tests for hepatitis C. J Hepatol 1999; 34(Suppl 1): S71–S79.

Pawlotsky JM, Bouvier-Alias M, Hezode C, Darthuy F, Remire J, Dhumeaux D. Standardization of hepatitis C virus RNA quantification. Hepatology 2000; 32: 654.

Pestova TV, Shatsky IN, Fletcher SP, Jackson RJ, Hellen CUT. A prokaryotic-like mode of cytoplasmic eukaryotic ribosome binding to the initiation codon during internal translation initiation of hepatitis C and classical swine fever virus RNAs. Genes Dev 1998; 12: 67.

Pham TNQ, MacParland SA, Mulrooney PM, Cooksley H, Naumov NV, Michalak TI. Hepatitis C virus persistence after spontaneous or treatment-induced resolution of hepatitis C. J Virol 2004; 78: 5867.

Pieroni L, Santolini E, Fipaldini C, Pacini L, Migliaccio G, La Monica N. In vitro study of the NS2-3 protease of hepatitis C virus. J Virol 1997; 71: 6373.

Pietschmann T, Bartenschlager R. The hepatitis C virus replicon system and its application to molecular studies. Curr Opin Drug Dis Dev 2001; 4: 657.

Pietschmann T, Lohmann V, Rutter G, Kurpanek K, Bartenschlager R. Characterization of cell lines carrying self-replicating hepatitis C virus RNAs. J Virol 2001; 75: 1252.

Pileri P, Uematsu Y, Campagnoli S, Galli G, Falugi F, Petracca R, Weiner AJ, Houghton M, Rosa D, Grandi G, Abrignani S. Binding of hepatitis C virus to CD81. Science 1998; 282: 938.

Pöhlmann S, Zhang J, Baribaud F, Chen Z, Leslie GJ, Lin G, Granelli-Piperno A, Doms RW, Rice CM, McKeating JA. Hepatitis C virus glycoproteins interact with DC-SIGN and DC-SIGNR. J Virol 2003; 77: 4070.

Pollack JR, Ganem D. An RNA stem-loop structure directs hepatitis B virus genomic RNA encapsidation. J Virol 1993; 67: 3254.

Pollack JR, Ganem D. Site-specific RNA binding by a hepatitis B virus reverse transcriptase initiates two distinct reactions: RNA packaging and DNA synthesis. J Virol 1994; 68: 5579.

Pult I, Netter HJ, Bruns M, Prassolov A, Sirma H, Hohemberg H, Chang SF, Frolich K, Krone O, Kaleta EF, Will H. Identification and analysis of a new hepadnavirus in white storks. Virology 2001; 289: 114.

Puoti M, Zonaro A, Ravaggi A, Marin MG, Castelnuovo F, Cariani E. Hepatitis C virus RNA and antibody response in the clinical course of acute hepatitis C virus infection. Hepatology 1992; 16: 877.

Quiroga JA, Campillo ML, Castillo I, Bartolomé J, Porres JC, Carreño V. IgM antibody to hepatitis C virus in acute and chronic hepatitis C. Hepatology 1991; 14: 38.

Radkowski M, Gallegos-Orozco JF, Jablonska J, Colby TV, Walewska-Zelecka B, Kubicka J, Wilkinson J, Adair D, Rakela J, Laskus T. Persistence of hepatitis C virus in patients successfully treated for chronic hepatitis C. Hepatology 2005a; 4: 106.

Radkowski M, Horban A, Gallegos-Orozco JF, Pawelczyk A, Jablonska J, Wilkinson J, Adair D, Laskus T. Evidence for viral persistence in patients who test positive for anti-hepatitis C virus antibodies and have normal alanine aminotransferase levels. J Infect Dis 2005b; 191: 1730.

Radkowski M, Wilkinson J, Nowicki M, Adair D, Vargas H, Ingui C, Rakela J, Laskus T. Search for hepatitis C virus negative-strand RNA sequences and analysis of viral sequences in the central nervous system: evidence of replication. J Virol 2002; 76: 600.

Radziwill G, Tucker W, Schaller H. Mutational analysis of the hepatitis B virus P gene product: domain structure and RNase H activity. J Virol 1990; 64: 613.

Ray RB, Lagging LM, Meyer K, Steele R, Ray R. Transcriptional regulation of cellular and viral promoters by the hepatitis C virus core protein. Virus Res 1995; 37: 209.

Roccasecca R, Ansuini H, Vitelli A, Meola A, Scarselli E, Acali S, Pezzanera M, Ercole BB, McKeating J, Yagnik A, Lahm A, Tramontano A, Cortese R, Nicosia A. Binding of the hepatitis C virus E2 glycoprotein to CD81 is strain specific and is modulated by a complex interplay between hypervariable regions 1 and 2. J Virol 2003; 77: 1856.

Rodriguez-Iñigo E, Casqueiro M, Bartolomé J, Barat A, Caramelo C, Ortiz A, Albalate M, Oliva H, Manzano ML, Carreño V. Hepatitis C virus RNA in kidney biopsies from infected patients with renal diseases. J Viral Hepat 2000; 7: 23.

Rodriguez-Iñigo E, López-Alcorocho JM, Bartolomé J, Ortiz-Movilla N, Pardo M, Carreño V. Percentage of hepatitis C virus-infected hepatocytes is a better predictor of response than serum viremia levels. J Mol Diagn 2005; 7: 535.

Roudot-Thoraval F, Pawlotsky JM, Thier V, Deforges L, Girollet PP, Guillot F, Huraux C, Aumont P, Brechot C, Dhumeaux D. Lack of mother-to-infant transmission of hepatitis C virus in human immunodeficiency virus-seronegative women: a prospective study with hepatitis C virus RNA testing. Hepatology 1993; 17: 772.

Sakai A, Claire MS, Faulk K, Govindarajan S, Emerson SU, Purcell RH, Bukh J. The p7 polypeptide of hepatitis C virus is critical for infectivity and contains functionally important genotype-specific sequences. Proc Natl Acad Sci USA 2003; 100: 11646.

Saldanha J, Gerlich W, Lelie N, Dawson P, Heerman K, Heath A. An international collaborative study to establish a World Health Organization international standard for hepatitis B virus DNA nucleic acid amplification techniques. Vox Sang 2001; 80: 63.

Saldanha J, Lelie N, Heath A. Establishment of the first international standard for nucleic acid amplification technology (NAT) assays for HCV RNA. WHO Collaborative Study Group. Vox Sang 1999; 76: 149.

Sali DL, Ingram R, Wendel M, Gupta D, McNemar C, Tsarbopoulos A, Chen JW, Hong Z, Chase R, Risano C, Zhang R, Yao N, Kwong AD, Ramanathan L, Le HV, Weber PC. Serine protease of hepatitis C virus expressed in insect cells as the NS3/4A complex. Biochemistry 1998; 37: 3392.

Santolini E, Migliaccio G, La Monica N. Biosynthesis and biochemical properties of the hepatitis C virus core protein. J Virol 1994; 68: 3631.

Sattler F, Robinson WS. Hepatitis B viral DNA molecules have cohesive ends. J Virol 1979; 32: 226.

Scarselli E, Ansuini H, Cerino R, Roccasecca RM, Acali S, Filocamo G, Traboni C, Nicosia A, Cortese R, Vitelli A. The human scavenger receptor class B type I is a novel candidate receptor for the hepatitis C virus. EMBO J 2002; 21: 5017.

Seeff LB, Hollinger FB, Alter HJ, Wright EC, Cain CM, Buskell ZJ, Ishak KG, Iber FL, Toro D, Samanta A, Koretz RL, Perrillo RP, Goodman ZD, Knodell RG, Gitnick G, Morgan TR, Schiff ER, Lasky S, Stevens C, Vlahcevic RZ, Weinshel E, Tanwandee T, Lin HJ, Barbosa L. Long-term mortality and morbidity of transfusion-associated non-A, non-B, and type C hepatitis: A National Heart, Lung, and Blood Institute collaborative study. Hepatology 2001; 33: 455.

Shimizu YK, Feinstone SM, Kohara M, Purcell RH, Yoshikura H. Hepatitis C virus: detection of intracellular virus particles by electron microscopy. Hepatology 1996; 23: 205.

Shindo M, Arai K, Sokawa Y, Okuno T. The virological and histological states of anti-hepatitis C virus-positive subjects with normal liver biochemical values. Hepatology 1995; 22: 418.

Shrivastava A, Manna SK, Ray RB, Aggarwal BB. Ectopic expression of hepatitis C virus core protein differentially regulates nuclear transcription factors. J Virol 1998; 72: 9722.

Sprengel R, Kaleta EF, Will H. Isolation and characterization of a hepatitis B virus endemic in herons. J Virol 1988; 62: 3832.

Stelzl E, Muller Z, Marth E, Kessler HH. Rapid quantitation of hepatitis B virus DNA by automated sample preparation and real-time PCR. J Clin Microbiol 2004; 42: 2445.

Summers J, Mason WS. Replication of the genome of a hepatitis B-like virus by reverse transcription of an RNA intermediate. Cell 1982; 29: 403.

Summers J, Smolec JM, Snyder R. A virus similar to human hepatitis B virus associated with hepatitis and hepatoma in woodchucks. Proc Natl Acad Sci USA 1978; 75: 4533.

Tai CL, Chi WK, Chen DS, Hwang LH. The helicase activity associated with hepatitis C virus nonstructural protein 3 (NS3). J Virol 1996; 70: 8477.

Takaki A, Wiese M, Maertens G, Depla E, Seifert U, Liebetrau A, Miller JL, Manns MP, Rehermann B. Cellular immune responses persist and humoral responses decrease two decades after recovery from a single-source outbreak of hepatitis C. Nat Med 2000; 6: 578.

Takamizawa A, Mori C, Fuke I, Manabe S, Murakami S, Fujita J, Onishi E, Andoh T, Yoshida I, Okayama H. Structure and organization of the hepatitis C virus genome isolated from human carriers. J Virol 1991; 65: 1105.

Tallis GF, Ryan GM, Lambert SB, Bowden DS, McCaw R, Birch CJ, Moloney M, Carnie JA, Locarnini SA, Rouch GJ, Catton MG. Evidence of patient-to-patient transmission of hepatitis C virus through contaminated intravenous anaesthetic ampoules. J Viral Hepat 2003; 10: 234.

Tanaka T, Kato N, Cho MJ, Sugiyama K, Shimotono K. Structure of the 3' terminus of the hepatitis C virus genome. J Virol 1996; 70: 3307.

Tanaka Y, Esumi M, Shikata T. Persistence of hepatitis B virus DNA after serological clearance of hepatitis B virus. Liver 1990; 10: 6.

Taylor DR, Shi ST, Romano PR, Barber GN, Lai MM. Inhibition of the interferon-inducible protein kinase PKR by HCV E2 protein. Science 1999; 285: 107.

Terrault NA. Hepatitis C virus and liver transplantation. Semin Gastrointest. Dis 2000; 11: 96.

Testut P, Renard CA, Terradillos O, Vitviski-Trepo L, Tekaia F, Degott C, Blake J, Boyer B, Buendia MA. A new hepadnavirus endemic in Artic ground squirrels in Alaska. J Virol 1996; 70: 4210.

Thomssen R, Bonk S, Propfe C, Heermann KH, Kochel HG, Uy A. Association of hepatitis C virus in human sera with beta-lipoprotein. Med Microbiol Immunol 1992; 181: 293.

Thomssen R, Bonk S, Thiele A. Density heterogeneities of hepatitis C virus in human sera due to the binding of beta-lipoproteins and immunoglobulins. Med Microbiol Immunol 1993; 182: 329.

Tong S, Li J, Wands JR. Carboxypeptidase D is an avian hepatitis B virus receptor. J Virol 1999; 73: 8696.

Valentine-Thon E, Steinmann J, Arnold W. Detection of hepatitis B virus DNA in serum with nucleic acid probes labelled with ^{32}P, biotin, alkaline phosphatase or sulphone. Mol Cell Probes 1991; 5: 299.

Wang GH, Zoulim F, Leber EH, Kitson J, Seeger C. Role of RNA in enzymatic activity of the reverse transcriptase of hepatitis B virus. J Virol 1994; 68: 8437.

Wang J, Wang T, Sheu J, Lin S, Lin J, Chen D. Effects of anticoagulants and storage of blood samples on efficacy of the polymerase chain reaction assay for hepatitis C virus. J Clin Microbiol 1992; 30: 750.

Weiner AJ, Brauer MJ, Rosenblatt J, Richman KH, Tung J, Crawford K, Bonino F, Saracco G, Choo QL, Houhgton M, Han JH. Variable and hypervariable domains are found in the regions of HCV corresponding to the flavivirus envelope and NS1 proteins and the pestivirus envelope glycoproteins. Virology 1991; 180: 842.

Whalley A, Murray JM, Brocon D, Webster GJM, Emery VC, Dusheisko GM, Perelson AS. Kinetics of acute hepatitis B virus infection in humans. J Exp Med 2001; 193: 847.

Yan FM, Chen AS, Hao F, Zhao XP, Gu CH, Zhao LB, Yang DL, Hao LJ. Hepatitis C virus may infect extrahepatic tissues in patients with hepatitis C. World J Gastroenterol 2000; 6: 805.

Yanagi M, St Claire M, Emerson SU, Purcell RH, Bukh J. In vitro analysis of the 3' untranslated region of the hepatitis C virus after in vitro mutagenesis of an infectious cDNA clone. Proc Natl Acad Sci 1999; 96: 2291.

Yao JL, Beld MG, Oon LLE, Sherlock CH, Germer J, Menting S, Thoe SYS, Merrick L, Ziermann R, Surtihadi J, Hnatyszyn HJ. Multicenter evaluation of the Versant hepatitis B virus DNA 3.0 assay. J Clin Microbiol 2004; 42: 800.

You LR, Chen CM, Lee YH. Hepatitis C virus core protein enhances NF-KB signal pathway triggering by lymphotoxin-β receptor ligand and tumor necrosis factor alpha. J Virol 1999; 73: 1672.

Yotsuyanagi H, Yasuda K, Iino S, Moriya K, Shintani Y, Fujie H, Tsutsumi T, Kimura S, Koike K. Persistent viremia after recovery from self-limited acute hepatitis B. Hepatology 1998; 27: 1377.

Zanetti AR, Tanzi E, Paccagnini S, Principi N, Pizzocolo G, Caccamo ML, D'Amico E, Cambie G, Vecchi L. Mother-to-infant transmission of hepatitis C virus. Lombarda study group on vertical HCV transmisión.. Lancet 1995; 345: 289.

Zeuzem S, Lee JH, Roth WK. Mutations in the nonstructural 5A gene of European hepatitis C virus isolates and response to interferon alfa. Hepatology 1997; 25: 740.

Zignego AL, Macchia D, Monti M, Thiers V, Mazzetti M, Foschi M, Maggi E, Romagnani S, Gentilini P, Brechot C. Infection of peripheral mononuclear blood cells by hepatitis C virus. J Hepatol 1992; 15: 382.

Zoulim F, Saputelli J, Seeger C. Woodchuck hepatitis virus X protein is required for viral infection *in vivo*. J Virol 1994; 68: 2026.

Zoulim F, Seeger C. Reverse transcription in hepatitis B viruses is primed by tyrosine residue of the polymerase. J Virol 1994; 68: 6.

Congenital and Other Related Infectious
Diseases of the Newborn
Isa K. Mushahwar (Editor)
© 2007 Elsevier B.V. All rights reserved
DOI 10.1016/S0168-7069(06)13008-6

Perinatal Hepatitis B Virus Infection in Japan

Tomiko Koyama[a], Hidetoshi Mito[b], Kazuaki Takahashi[c],
Junko Tanaka[d], Isa K. Mushahwar[e], Hiroshi Yoshizawa[d]

[a]*Health Service Association, Iwate, Japan*
[b]*Health Service Association, Shizuoka, Japan*
[c]*Department of Medical Sciences, Toshiba General Hospital, Tokyo, Japan*
[d]*Department of Epidemiology, Infectious Disease Control and Prevention, Graduate
School of Biomedical Sciences, Hiroshima University, Hiroshima, Japan*
[e]*Abbott Japan, Tokyo, Japan*

Introduction

In areas where infection by hepatitis B virus (HBV) is prevalent and persistent,
perinatal transmission from HBV-infected mothers is an essential route for establishing a persistent carrier state.

These babies carrying HBV can transmit it via a secondary horizontal route to
infants of the same generation, who frequently acquire persistent HBV infections.
Approximately 30% of the infants exposed to HBV when under 3 years of age
become HBV carriers. Together, they serve as a reservoir of HBV throughout their
lives in the community, and may therefore cause, or contribute to, a continuous
spread of the infection.

Perinatal HBV infections resulting in the persistent carrier state occur in approximately 90% of babies born to mothers who are positive for hepatitis B surface
antigen (HBsAg) as well as hepatitis B e antigen (HBeAg) in the serum (Okada
et al., 1976; Stevens et al., 1979). Persistent infections rarely occur in babies born to
mothers who carry HBsAg, but are negative for HBeAg or are positive for the
antibody to HBeAg (anti-HBe). Only around 10–15% of babies contract transient
HBV infections (Shiraki et al., 1980).

In countries where the prevalence of HBsAg is less than 0.2–1.0% in children,
the perinatal HBV transmission is the major route where the HBV carrier state is
established. In these countries, a selective vaccination program, i.e., combined
passive–active immunoprophylaxis of babies born to mothers with HBsAg and
HBeAg by anti-HBs hyper-immune globulin (HBIG) and hepatitis B vaccine (HB
vaccine), is a rational approach to the control of HBV infection.

In contrast, in countries where the prevalence of HBsAg exceeds 8%, perinatal transmission accounts for only 10–20% of infants who are persistently infected with HBV (Yao, 1996; Lee, 1997). Since horizontal transmission to children younger than 5 years old is the major route by which the HBV carrier state becomes established in these hyperendemic countries, universal vaccination of babies is recommended.

It is important to realize that universal vaccination prevents mainly horizontal HBV transmission, but not perinatal HBV infection. In addition, the fact that universal vaccination has the potential for inducing HBV mutants remains a serious problem of this particular approach (Zanetti et al., 1988; Brunetto et al., 1999).

In two model areas in Japan, Shizuoka and Iwate prefectures, the immunoprophylaxis of babies born to HBV carrier mothers with HBeAg, by means of combined hepatitis B HBIG and HB vaccine, was started as a clinical trial in the early 1980s and became a national project in 1986. This chapter presents an account of the experience gained in the prevention of perinatal HBV transmission from the 1980s into the 1990s in Shizuoka and Iwate prefectures.

Carrier rates of hepatitis B virus in Japan

To understand the sero-epidemiological background of HBV infection in Japan, the age-specific HBV carrier rates were estimated on a national basis (Tanaka et al., 2004). To avoid selection bias, only the data of first-time blood donors aged 16–64 years in the Japanese Red Cross Blood Center were collected and analyzed.

During the 6 years from January 1995 to December 2000, 3,485,648 individuals visited their local Japanese Red Cross Blood Centers for the first time to donate blood. The proportion of HBsAg-positive subjects, determined by reversed-passive hemagglutination (R-PHA) reagents made in-house by the Japanese Red Cross Blood Center, was calculated. To ascertain the influence of age on the proportion of HBsAg-positives, the ages of all first-time blood donors were adjusted, taking the year 2000 as the current year. The sex- and age-specific HBsAg-positive rates are shown in Table 1. Overall, HBsAg was detected in 22,018 (0.63%) of 3,485,648 blood donors. The prevalence of HBsAg was significantly higher in men (0.73%) than in women (0.53%, $p < 0.001$), and increased in both with time until the age of 60 years. The HBsAg-positive rates were lowest in the age group under 20: 0.26 and 0.20% in men and women, respectively.

These data suggest that the improvement of sanitary conditions in Japan has helped to decrease the horizontal transmission of HBV and the HBV carrier state in the age groups born before the prevention of perinatal HBV transmission was started in the 1980s.

Prevention of perinatal transmission of hepatitis B virus in Japan

The prevention of perinatal HBV infections has been followed up in two model areas of Japan, namely, Shizuoka and Iwate prefectures.

Table 1

Age-specific HBsAg positive rates in first-time male and female blood donors in Japanese Red Cross Blood Center from 1995 to 2000

Age groups in 2000 (year of birth)	Total number of first-time donors	HBsAg positives (%)	Men		Women	
			Number	HBsAg positives (%)	Number	HBsAg positives (%)
16–19 (1981–1984)	582,415	1327 (0.23)	273,842	709 (0.26)	308,573	618 (0.20)
20–29 (1971–1980)	1,929,147	10,054 (0.52)	1,004,986	5955 (0.59)	924,161	4099 (0.44)
30–39 (1961–1970)	472,447	3988 (0.84)	277,627	2828 (1.02)	194,820	1160 (0.60)
40–49 (1951–1960)	247,020	2950 (1.19)	120,576	1796 (1.49)	126,444	1154 (0.91)
50–59 (1941–1950)	198,477	2984 (1.50)	80,336	1388 (1.73)	118,141	1596 (1.35)
60–69 (1931–1940)	56,142	715 (1.27)	22,782	314 (1.38)	33,360	401 (1.20)
Total	3,485,648	22,018 (0.63)	1,780,149	12,990 (0.73)	1,705,499	9028 (0.53)

In Shizuoka prefecture, immunoprophylaxis of perinatal HBV infection was initiated in 1980 as a clinical trial and became a national project in April 1986 (Noto et al., 2003). In a similar way in Iwate prefecture, following the clinical trial that began in 1981, prophylaxis of perinatal HBV infection in all babies was started in 1986 (Koyama et al., 2003).

The same protocol was used in both prefectures, and was executed as follows: babies born to HBV carrier mothers who were HBeAg reactive (high-risk babies) received HBIG at birth (within a maximum of 48 h after delivery) and the second injection was given 2 months thereafter. The babies were inoculated with HB vaccine 2, 3 and 5 months after birth and were followed until the baby reached 12 months of age (arrows, Fig. 1). In cases in which the antibody titer fell to less than 22–23 PHA, inoculation was repeated as necessary at months 9 and 12 (arrows in parentheses).

Immunoprophylaxis of perinatal HBV transmission in Shizuoka prefecture and its effectiveness in decreasing the transmission of the HBV carrier state

Shizuoka prefecture is located near the center of the main island of Japan, at the foot of Mt. Fuji, and has 3.6 million residents. In this prefecture, the first clinical trial was started in 1980 (Tanaka et al., 2004).

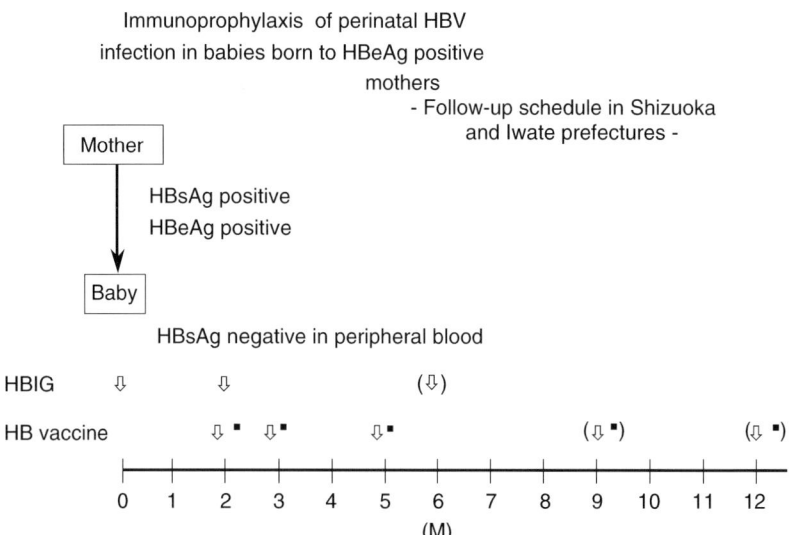

Fig. 1 Prevention of perinatal transmission of HBV: follow-up schedule in Shizuoka and Iwate pre-fectures. Babies born to HBsAg and HBeAg-positive mothers received two injections of HBIG ⇩ and three inoculations of HB vaccines ↓ at indicated time points. Serological tests for HBsAg and anti-HBs were performed monthly. During the follow-up period, anti-HBs titer was maintained at more than 2^3 PHA titer (equivalent to 200 mIU/ml) with appropriate use of HBIG or HB vaccine, or both, (⇩), and (↓), until 12 months after birth. During the follow-up period, when HBsAg became positive, all the prevention programs were stopped.

During the 5 years from 1980 to 1985, a total of 172 high-risk babies received immunophylaxis in a clinical trial. Of them, 166 (96.5%) were protected success-fully so that they did not become HBV carriers, but this outcome could not be prevented in the remaining 6 babies (3.5%).

In 1985, the year of transition of the clinical trial to a national program status, out of 94 high-risk babies receiving immunoprophylaxis, 85 (90.4%) were pro-tected, while the treatment failed in 9 (9.6%). During the first 9 years of the national project from 1986 to 1994, 764 high-risk babies received immunoproph-ylaxis. A total of 729 (95.4%) were protected, but the HBV carrier state developed in the remaining 35 (4.6%).

Overall, passive–active immunoprophylaxis following the protocol shown in Fig. 1 was effective in preventing persistent HBV infection in 980 (95.1%) of the 1030 babies born to HBeAg-positive HBV carrier mothers, but the HBV carrier state developed in the remaining 50 babies (4.9%) (Noto et al., 2003).

To estimate the efficacy of immunoprophylaxis of HBV infection, changes in the prevalence of HBsAg and anti-HBs in elementary school children (7–12 years of age) were compared in groups divided according to their birth year (Table 2). The children in group I were born before 1980 the year when the immunoprophylaxis of HBV was initiated. Those in group III were born after 1985, when the national

Table 2

Prevalence of HBsAg and anti-HBs among elementary school children in Shizuoka prefecture, divided into 3 groups according to birth year

Group	Number tested	HBsAg positives (%)	Anti-HBs positives (%)
I. Born before 1980	3446	7 (0.20)	33 (0.96)
II. Born in 1980–1985	46,993	77 (0.16)	260 (0.55)
III. Born after 1985	23,792	2 (0.01)	51 (0.21)
Total	74,231	86 (0.21)	344 (0.46)

program to prevent perinatal HBV infection commenced. The group II children were born in the period sandwiched between the clinical trial and the national program.

The prevalence of HBsAg gradually decreased from group I (0.20%), to group II (0.16%) to group III (0.01%). Likewise, the prevalence of anti-HBs decreased in a similar manner from group I (0.96%), to group II (0.55%) and group III (0.21%).

These results indicate that, in Japan, preventive measures taken against perinatal HBV infection were largely effective in decreasing the transmission of the HBV carrier state including that due to horizontal infection.

Prevention of perinatal HBV transmission in Iwate from 1981–1992 and sero-epidemiological evidence for its effectiveness

In Iwate prefecture, which has a population of 1.4 million, the clinical trial of prevention of perinatal HBV transmission was started in 1981. In 1985, the year of transition from clinical trial to national program, almost all babies born to HBeAg-positive HBV carrier mothers were given immunoprophylactic treatment (Koyama et al., 2003).

During that year, 39 (86.7%) of 45 babies who received immunoprophylaxis were protected against HBV. During the 7 years from 1986 to 1992, 100,286 (96.0%) of 104,493 pregnant women received tests for HBsAg, and it was detected in 1242 (1.2%) of them. Of those HBsAg-positives, 257 (20.7%) were positive also for HBeAg and all of their babies received immunoprophylaxis (Table 3).

The effectiveness of the immunoprophylaxis of perinatal HBV infection was clearly reflected in the changes in prevalence of HBsAg among elementary school children aged 7–12 years (Table 4). They were divided into three groups according to their birth year. In the group born between 1978 and 1980, before the start of the clinical trial of immunoprophylaxis, the prevalence of HBsAg was 0.75% (78/10,437). The prevalence of HBsAg was already decreasing among those who were born from 1981 to 1985, during the period of the clinical trial on prevention. In this group of subjects, the prevalence of HBsAg was 0.22% (46/20,812). The decrease was more prominent in children born after 1985, since the national program of

Table 3

Babies who were treated to prevent perinatal HBV transmission from 1981 to 1992 in Iwate, Japan

Year	Number of deliveries	HBsAg tested (% of deliveries)	HBsAg (+) (% of tested)	HBeAg (+) (% in HBsAg)	Prevention (% of HBeAg (+))
Before national program (1981–1985)					
1981	18,600	ND	ND	ND	1
1982	18,581	ND	ND	ND	12
1983	19,582	ND	ND	ND	18
1984	18,043	ND	ND	ND	29
1985	17,232	10,628 (61.7)	ND	45	39 (86.7%)
After start of national program (1986–1992)					
1986	16,536	15,872 (96.0)	244 (1.4)	47 (19.3)	47 (100.0)
1987	15,567	15,205 (97.7)	241 (1.6)	60 (24.9)	60 (100.0)
1988	15,410	14,282 (92.7)	166 (1.2)	40 (24.1)	40 (100.0)
1989	14,548	14,541 (99.9)	179 (1.2)	25 (14.0)	25 (100.0)
1990	14,254	13,997 (98.2)	161 (1.2)	42 (26.1)	42 (100.0)
1991	14,270	13,245 (92.8)	136 (1.0)	21 (15.4)	21 (100.0)
1992	13,908	13,144 (94.5)	115 (0.9)	22 (19.1)	22 (100.0)
Total	104,493	100,286 (96.0)	1242 (1.2)	257 (20.7)	257 (100.0)

Note: ND, no data available.

immunoprophylaxis was set in motion. HBsAg was detected in only 12 (0.04%) of 32,049 children born between 1986 and 1990 ($p < 0.001$ against the prevalence in t he children born between 1981 and 1985). Likewise, the prevalence of anti-HBs decreased from 1.52% (159/10,437) in those born from 1978 to 1980, to 0.79% (165/20,812) in those born from 1981 to 1985, and 0.85% (274/32,049) in the children born between 1986 and 1990 ($p < 0.001$).

The rate of anti-HBc-positives among the children with anti-HBs decreased from 81.9% (127/155) among those who were born in the years 1978–1980 to 43.3% (68/157) in those born in 1981–1985, and finally to 11.0% (59/536) in those born in 1986–1994 (Table 5). These results indicate that preventive measures against perinatal HBV infection could eventually result in the prevention of horizontal transmission among children in the same age groups.

Prevalence of surface antigen mutants

Serum HBV DNA from 15 infants and 11 mothers with chronic hepatitis acquired by either intra-uterine infection or post-vaccination prophylaxis were cloned then followed by direct sequencing of the HBV genome encoding the major antigenic

Table 4

Changes in prevalence of HBsAg and anti-HBs in 3 groups of elementary school children devided according to birth year

Year of birth	Number tested	HBsAg positives (%)	Anti-HBs positives (%)
Before immunoprophylaxis (1978–1980)			
1978	2666	26 (0.94)	52 (1.95)
1979	4212	27 (0.64)	72 (1.71)
1980	3559	25 (0.70)	35 (0.98)
Subtotal	10,437	78 (0.75)	159 (1.52)
During clinical trials of immunoprophylaxis (1981–1985)			
1981	2541	12 (0.47)	30 (1.18)
1982	1594	4 (0.25)	12 (0.75)
1983	3847	6 (0.16)	17 (0.44)
1984	6206	11 (0.18)	58 (0.93)
1985	6624	13 (0.20)	48 (0.72)
Subtotal	20,812	46 (0.22)	165 (0.79)
After start of national immunoprophylaxis program (1986–1990)			
1986	6775	3 (0.04)	41 (0.61)
1987	6505	4 (0.06)	62 (0.95)
1988	6310	2 (0.03)	58 (0.92)
1989	6436	2 (0.03)	64 (0.71)
1990	6023	1 (0.02)	67 (1.11)
Subtotal	32,049	12 (0.04)	292 (0.91)

epitopes of HBsAg (amino acids 100–200). The results of this analysis are listed in Table 6, and the following observations are listed as noted below:

1. Three novel HBV variants were detected in babies and their mothers, namely, I126T and S114T (Cases 1/I and 5/I) that were acquired by intrauterine infection. Also variant P127T in both mother and baby (Case 5/L) indicating vertical transmission. To our knowledge, these variants have not been reported previously.
2. Another novel variant, namely, G145A (Case 4/L) was detected in the baby but not his mother. This variant has been reported to occur naturally in sera of HBV chronic carriers in Korea (Song et al., 2005).
3. Analysis of all other remaining cases revealed that mixed populations of wild type and mutant viruses are found in all the tested infants and their mothers.
4. Many of the surface antigen mutants that were identified in the babies were not found in their mothers. This finding is similar to previously reported work (Nainan et al., 2002).
5. A surprising finding was the absence of supposedly the most predominant HBsAg variant, namely, G145R from the sera of the babies and their mothers.

Table 5

Prevalence of anti-HBc among elementary school children positive for anti-HBs, divided by birth year

Year of birth	Anti-HBs positive children	Anti-HBc positives (%)
Before immunoprophylaxis (1978–1980)		
1978	49	40 (81.6)
1979	72	64 (88.9)
1980	34	23 (76.7)
Subtotal	155	127 (81.9)
During clinical trials of immunoprophylaxis (1981–1985)		
1981	30	23 (76.7)
1982	12	9 (75.0)
1983	14	6 (42.9)
1984	58	18 (31.0)
1985	43	12 (27.9)
Subtotal	157	68 (43.3)
After start of national immunoprophylaxis program (1986–1994)		
1986	41	10 (24.4)
1987	61	11 (18.0)
1988	58	9 (15.5)
1989	46	6 (13.0)
1990	67	6 (9.0)
1991	62	7 (11.3)
1992	72	2 (2.8)
1993	63	5 (7.9)
1994	66	3 (4.6)
Subtotal	536	59 (11.0)

Instead, variant G145A was idetified (Cases 5/I, 2/L and 4/L). This variant has already been reported to occur naturally in sera of HBV chronic carriers in Korea (Song et al., 2005).

6. Another novel HBV variant, namely, K141E was found in a baby (Case 4/I). This is the second report of such a finding. Originally, this unique variant was identified in the sera of two Gambian children (Karthigesu et al., 1994).

7. Of interest is the presence of the novel mutant T118K (Case 2/L). This mutant has been reported once in the literature (Kfoury et al., 2001), and it is found outside the HBsAg "a" determinatnt region (amino acids 124–147) just as the case with mutant S114T (Cases 1/I and 5/I). HBsAg mutations outside the "a" determinant have been reported to damage the immunodominant region structure and thus alter the group specific dominant antigenicity (Kfoury et al., 2001). Hence, the reason we are reporting in Table 6 a variety of HBsAg mutants outside the "a" determinant itself. Current studies show that the HBsAg loop extends much further than initially believed, because other

Table 6

Mutation in the S gene of HBV DNA clones from 15 HBV positive babies and some of their mothers

Babies			Mothers		
Case/group	Clones tested	Variant[a]	Case/group	Clones tested	Variant[a]
1/I	21	I126T[b]	1/I	23	I126T[b]
2/I	22	Q101R, Q129R, W156R, W172R	2/I	23	P105L, T116I, K122E, C137R, L162P
3/I	6	M133T, S174G	3/I	20	A157T, L162P
4/I	12	P135S, K141E, F158S, F161S, L176P	4/I	17	Y100H, S132P, S154P, F158S, F161S
5/I	14	S114T[b], G145A[b]	5/I	16	S114T[b], G145A[b]
6/I	24	L109P, S136P, S155Y	6/I	23	T113A, G119R, S136P, T148A
7/I	22	S113A, S117C, T118P, C139Y N146D, L176P	7/I	24	G112E, S117N, Q129H, S132L, C149Y, R160G, F170L
8/I	23	P142L	8/I	23	L109P, S114P, C124R, T131A, C138R, S171F, W172C, W172R
9/I	24	G130E, T148A, C149R, S171F	9/I	24	S117R, C121G, Q129P, M133I, P135L, S171P
10/I	17	C121S, T115A	10/I	0	NT
1/L	10	T116A[b]	1/L	0	NT
2/L	10	T118K, G145A	2/L	0	NT
3/L	10	I126T, T131A	3/L	0	NT
4/L	16	G145A[b]	4/L	14	C124R, C137R
5/L	19	P127T[b]	5/L	20	P127T[b]

Note: I, intrauterine infection; L, late-phase infection; NT, Not Tested.
[a]Amino acid substitution in "a" determinant (124–147) and outside "a" determinant (100–123 and 148–176).
[b]Novel variants, no wild-type virus present.

conserved epitopes have been found also between amino acids 100 and 200 (Kfoury et al., 2001; Gerlich, 2004).

The data shown in Table 6 illustrate that changes in either the major hydrophilic loop of HBsAg or outside it are common and do play an important role in transfusion safety, HBV vaccine efficacy and diagnostic accuracy and reliability.

Acknowledgments

This work was executed under the guidance of the Special Committee for Preventing Hepatitis B both in Iwate and Shizuoka, supported by the Department of Public Health of Iwate and Shizuoka Prefecture Government, respectively. We are very appreciative of all medical and co-medical staff members in departments of obstetrics and pediatrics in Iwate and Shizuoka who participated actively and practically in this project.

References

Brunetto MR, Rodriguez UA, Bonio F. Hepatitis B virus mutants. Intervirology 1999; 42: 69–80.

Gerlich WH. Diagnostic problems caused by HBsAg mutants. Intervirology 2004; 47: 310–313.

Karthigesu VD, Allison LM, Fortuin M, Mendy M, Whittle HC, Howard CR. A novel hepatitis B virus variant in the sera of immunized children. J Gen Virol 1994; 75: 443–448.

Kfoury Baz EM, Zheng J, Mazuruk K, Van Le A, Peterson DL. Characterization of a novel hepatitis B virus mutant: demonstration of mutation-induced hepatitis B virus surface antigen group specific "a" determinant conformation change and its application in diagnostic assays. Transfus Med 2001; 5(3): 55–362.

Koyama T, Matsuda I, Sato S, Yoshizawa H. Prevention of perinatal hepatitis B virus transmission by combined passive-active immuno-prophylaxis in Iwate, Japan (1991–1992) and epidemiological evidence for its efficacy. Hepatol Res 2003; 26: 287–292.

Lee WN. Hepatitis virus infection. N Engl J Med 1997; 337: 1733–1744.

Nainan OV, Khristova ML, Byun K, Xia G, Taylor PE, Stephens CE, Margolis HS. Genetic variation of hepatitis B surface antigen coding region among infants with chronic hepatitis B virus infection. J Med Virol 2002; 68: 319–327.

Noto H, Terao T, Ryou S, Hirose Y, Yoshida T, Ookubo H, Mito H, Yoshizawa H. Combined passive and active immunoprophylaxis for preventing perinatal transmission of the hepatitis B virus carrier state in Shizuoka, Japan during 1980–1994. J Gastroenterol Hepatol 2003; 18: 943–949.

Okada K, Kamiyama I, Inomata M, Imai M, Miyakawa Y, Mayumi M. e antigen and anti-e in the serum of asymptomatic carrier mothers as indicators of positive and negative transmission of hepatitis B virus to their infants. N Engl J Med 1976; 294: 746–749.

Shiraki K, Yoshihara N, Sakurai M, Eto T, Kawana T. Acute hepatitis B in infants born to carrier mothers with the antibody to hepatitis B e antigen. J Pediatr 1980; 97: 768–770.

Song BC, Kim S-H, Kim H, Ying Y-H, Kim H-J, Kim Y-J, Yoon J-H, Lee H-S, Cha CY, Kook Y-H, Kim B-J. Prevalence of naturally occurring surface antigen variants of hepatitis B virus in Korean patients infected chronically. J Med Virol 2005; 74: 194–202.

Stevens CE, Neurath RA, Beasleg RP, Szmuness W. HBeAg and anti-HBe detection by radioimmunoassay in correlation with vertical transmission of hepatitis B virus in Taiwan. J Med Virol 1979; 3: 337–341.

Tanaka J, Kumagai J, Katayama K, Komiya Y, Mizui M, Yamanaka R, Suzuki K, Yoshizawa H. Sex- and age-specific carriers of hepatitis B and C viruses in Japan estimated by
the prevalence in the 3,485,648 first-time blood donors during 1995–2000. Intervirology
2004; 47: 32–40.

Yao GB. Importance of perinatal virus horizontal transmission of hepatitis B virus infection
in China. Gut 1996; 38: S39–S42.

Zanetti AR, Tanzi E, Manzillo G, Maio G, Sbreglia C, Caporaso N, Thomas H, Zuckerman
AJ. Hepatitis B variant in Europe. Lancet 1998; 2(8620): 1132–1133.

Congenital and Other Related Infectious
Diseases of the Newborn
Isa K. Mushahwar (Editor)
DOI 10.1016/S0168-7069(06)13009-8

Hepatitis C in Pregnancy and Mother-to-Infant Transmission of HCV

Alessandro R. Zanetti[a], Elisabetta Tanzi[a], Augusto E. Semprini[b]

[a]*Department of Public Health-Microbiology-Virology, University of Milan, Via Pascal 36/38, 20133 Milan, Italy*
[b]*Department of Obstetrics and Gynaecology, University of Milan, Hospital L. Sacco, Via G.B. Grassi, 20157 Milan, Italy*

Abstract

Pregnancy is not contraindicated to women infected with HCV and HCV infection does not adversely affect pregnancy. The risk of mother-to-infant transmission of HCV is approximately 5%, but may be higher in children born to mothers with HCV/HIV co-infection. Transmission of infection is usually restricted to mothers who are HCV-RNA positive. Higher HCV-RNA levels seem to be associated with a greater risk, but a specific cut-off value predicting transmission cannot be defined. Interferon and ribavirin are contraindicated during pregnancy. There is no evidence that Caesarean delivery may reduce risk of vertical infection compared to vaginal delivery. Caution should be recommended in using invasive procedures (amniocentesis, villocentesis, and funicolocentesis), which may potentially expose the foetus or the neonate to the infected maternal blood. Avoiding foetal scalp monitoring and prolonged labour after rupture of membranes may reduce the risk of vertical transmission of HCV. Breastfeeding appears to be safe and is not contraindicated. Infected children usually progress to chronic disease with a benign course, at least initially. Longitudinal studies are needed to determine the long-term natural history of vertical HCV infections. Interferon plus ribavirin combination has been shown to be safe and effective in treating hepatitis C during childhood. Vaccinations against both hepatitis A and hepatitis B are highly recommended to children infected with HCV.

Introduction

Viral Hepatitis type C is a major worldwide public health problem, being a leading cause of acute and chronic liver disease including cirrhosis and primary hepato-cellular carcinoma. Hepatitis C virus (HCV), first identified in 1989, is a single-stranded RNA virus belonging to the *Hepacivirus* genus within the *Flaviviridae* family, which also includes GB virus C, yellow fever, West Nile and dengue viruses, and the animal pestiviruses (Choo et al., 1989; Kuo et al., 1989; Robertson et al., 1998; Lauer and Walker, 2001). Viral replication occurs through an RNA-de-pendent RNA polymerase devoid of 3'-exonuclease proofreading activity. This lack provides the biochemical basis for the rapid evolution of diverse but related qua-sispecies co-existing within an infected individual. A lengthy evolutionary process gave origin to six different genotypes (from 1 to 6), each with several subtypes (Simmonds, 1999). These genotypes/subtypes have different worldwide geograph-ical distribution patterns (Hoofnagle, 2002). Current evidence indicates that the different genotypes do not seem to differ for what concerns the natural course of infection nor the ability of person-to-person transmission. On the contrary, the response to therapy with interferon and ribavirin appears different for certain genotypes/subtypes, with genotype 2 and 3 responding better than genotype 1 and 4 (Manns et al., 2001; Fried et al., 2002; Hadziyannis et al., 2004).

Estimate indicates that at least 170 million people in the world (or approx-imately 3% of the global population) are infected with the HCV, a part of whom are at risk of developing life-threatening diseases, resulting in nearly half a million deaths per year. In industrialized countries, the incidence of acute hepatitis C is currently around 1–3 cases per 100,000 persons annually (EASL International Consensus Conference on Hepatitis C, 1999). However, since most HCV infections are asymptomatic and remain unnoticed to the surveillance systems, the number of those infected per year is estimated to be at least 10 times than reported. Progres-sion to chronic disease occurs in the majority of HCV-infected persons with a variable outcome over time (Hoofnagle, 2002; Seeff, 2002). Different outcomes seem to be linked to the route of transmission, age at infection, and, possibly, to gender (Roudot-Thoraval et al., 1997; Gordon et al., 1998; Bellentani et al., 1999; Kenny-Walsh et al., 1999; Rodger et al., 2000; Wiese et al., 2000; Barrett et al., 2001; Poynard et al., 2001; Hoofnagle, 2002). Infections encountered in adulthood carry a significantly higher probability of advancing to cirrhosis within 20 years in comparison to those acquired during infancy (Bortolotti et al., 1994; Matsuoka et al., 1994; Dike et al., 1998; Garcia-Monzon et al., 1998; O'Riordan et al., 1998; Vogt et al., 1999; Seeff et al., 2000, 2001; Poynard et al., 2001; Harris et al., 2002; Seeff, 2002). In industrialized countries, HCV accounts for approximately 20% of cases of acute hepatitis, 70% of cases of chronic hepatitis, 40% of cases of end-stage cirrhosis, and 30% of liver transplant (EASL International Consensus Con-ference on Hepatitis C, 1999). Co-infections and co-morbid conditions, which usually increase with age, may also be important contributors to the progression of hepatitis C infection (Zarski et al., 1998; Benhamou et al., 1999; Harris et al., 2001;

Monto et al., 2002). Although, the burden of hepatitis C is still high, the rate of new infections has dramatically declined in recent years as a result of the general improvements in standard of living and hygiene and the introduction of several public health measures including use of disposable syringes and needles, implementation of universal precautions in medical settings, and refinement of blood screening.

HCV is efficiently transmitted parenterally, and the main route of transmission in adults is through needle sharing during intravenous drug injections. Prior to the discovery of HCV and the introduction of anti-HCV antibody screening of blood donors in 1991, transfusion of HCV-infected blood or blood products was the predominant route of infection during childhood. Following the substantial increase in safety of the blood supply achieved in the last years, vertical/perinatal transmission has become the major route of HCV infection in children. The incidence of new vertical/perinatal infections in children depends on the prevalence of HCV infections among women of childbearing age and on the risk of viral transmission during pregnancy.

This chapter focuses on the prevalence of HCV infection in pregnant women in different populations, reproductive counselling, and management of HCV-infected pregnant women, factors that may influence the risk of vertical transmission, and the outcome of HCV infection in children.

Prevalence of HCV infection among women of childbearing age

Antenatal HCV prevalence ranges from less than 1–2.5% in Western Europe, the United States, Japan, and Australia but is higher in eastern Europe, Middle East, and Africa, particularly in some sub-Saharan populations where the prevalence of infection may exceed 10% (Roudot-Thoraval et al., 1993; Boxall et al., 1994; Louis et al., 1994; El-Gohary et al., 1995; Floreani et al., 1996; Pipan et al., 1996; Conte et al., 2000; Okamoto et al., 2000; Goldberg et al., 2001). Very high prevalence has been reported in Egypt (up to 40% in some parts of the country), resulting from the widespread use of contaminated needles and syringes during the mass campaigns to treat schistosomiasis infections, conducted in the Nile Delta region between the 1960s and the early 1980s (Rao et al, 2002). In industrialized countries, high prevalence of infection has been reported in certain groups, such as intravenous drug users and those infected with HIV (Pembrey et al., 2003). Other risk factors which may increase the probability for a pregnant woman of being infected with HCV include blood transfusions received prior to the introduction of donors screening, and parenteral exposure to the virus through surgery, dental care or following piercing and tattooing. However, a substantial proportion (up to 50%) of women with HCV has no evidence of exposure to known risk factors in their history (Zanetti et al., 1999).

At present, routine HCV screening is not recommended to all pregnant women since no effective interventions are available to control and prevent the mother-to-infant transmission of the infection (American Academy of Pediatrics, 1998; Zanetti et al., 1999; Pembrey et al., 2005). In some settings, women are tested if considered at high risk of being infected with HCV (i.e. women with history of intravenous drug use or those infected with HIV) in order to identify babies at risk of vertical transmission and to offer post-pregnancy therapeutic options to the infected women. Selective screening policies targeting women at increased risk seem to be somewhat more cost-effective than universal testing, but such approach would exclude from detection a consistent number of infected women without any known risk factors.

Infected pregnant women are usually identified by the detection of anti-HCV antibodies by enzyme immunoassays (EIA). These assays are reliable in immuno-competent individuals but less sensitive in patients with renal failure and in those with immune deficiency. In low-risk populations, such as childbearing women in industrialized countries, systematic testing may result in a number of false-positive detections. Therefore, an initially positive or indeterminate test should be confirmed by a second EIA or by a confirmatory recombinant immunoblot assay (RIBA) performed on the same sample. Detection of HCV-RNA by nucleic acid tests (NAT) is usually performed on anti-HCV positive samples to identify the presence of viraemia. Approximately 50–85% of women with anti-HCV antibody have detectable HCV-RNA in their blood, as a marker of ongoing infection (Zanetti et al., 1999; Conte et al., 2000; Yeung et al., 2001; Resti et al., 2003). Diversities in the prevalence of viraemia, found in different studies, likely reflect differences in the characteristics of the samples of women examined [i.e. study populations with or without women with HIV, those with abnormal alanine aminotransferase (ALT), those with risk factors such as injecting drug, etc.] or due to differences in the sensitivity of the assays and procedures utilized in the laboratories for HCV-RNA detection (i.e. qualitative/quantitative assays, in-house versus commercially available assays). Last-generation NAT are of greatly higher sensitivity compared to first-generation assays, with lower detection threshold limits of fewer than 100 copies of HCV-RNA per ml.

Reproductive counselling

Pregnancy is not contraindicated in women infected with HCV, but reproductive counselling and assistance allow to provide specific obstetrical care. Women infected with HCV planning for a child may worry whether pregnancy could adversely influence the course of HCV hepatic disease, and on the other hand, whether HCV infection might alter the course of pregnancy. Another issue of primary importance regards the risk of vertical transmission and the possibility that the child might acquire the infection should be discussed. Although such risk is low, the ensuing infection can become chronic with the inherent potential risk of progression, later in life, to cirrhosis or even to hepatocellular carcinoma. Women should also be informed that up-to-date no measures (i.e. type of feeding and mode of delivery) were proven effective in reducing the risk of vertical transmission, and that treatment of paediatric HCV infection is still not optimal.

Women infected with HCV should be counselled regarding prevention of viral transmission to others and advised to test for co-infection with HBV or HIV, which share similar risk factors and modes of transmission. The possibility that infection could be due to intravenous drug use should be investigated, and women who are active drug users should be informed about the negative consequences of drug use during pregnancy. Pregnant women with HCV infection should also be advised to avoid hepatotoxic medications and alcohol.

Sexual transmission during unprotected intercourses is unlikely in heterosexual monogamous couples (Terrault, 2002; Vandelli et al., 2004). An HCV-infected woman planning to conceive should notify her HCV status to the partner, who should be reassured that the risk of sexual transmission is so low that the use of barrier precautions (i.e. latex condom) is not deemed necessary for individuals in monogamous partnership with an HCV-infected partner (Strader et al., 2004).

Infection with HCV is not associated with decreased fertility, even in the presence of advanced liver disease. Infected women, who fail to conceive in the expected conception delay and require reproductive assistance, can assume fertility drugs and tolerate the increased levels of estrogens induced by these drugs. However, careful considerations should be given to the additional metabolic burden of these therapies in women with substantial liver damage.

Due to their associated toxic effect, both interferon alpha and ribavirin are contraindicated during pregnancy. However, women who come for consultation ahead of pregnancy should be advised to undergo a course of treatment with the combination therapy prior to conception in order to decrease or to eliminate active viral replication and, consequently, to reduce the risk of vertical transmission. In this case, women should be advised to postpone pregnancy for at least 6 months after cessation of ribavirin treatment, because of its potential toxicity to germ cells (Chutaputti, 2000). Deferral of conception should also be recommended to couples in which the male partner is infected with HCV and undergoing ribavirin treatment.

Hepatitis C and pregnancy

There is no evidence that pregnancy could accelerate the progression of HCV-induced liver damage. During pregnancy, ALT levels usually decrease or even normalize in the second and third trimesters, despite possible increase in HCV viral load (Floreani et al., 1996; Conte et al., 2000; Gervais et al., 2000). The modifications return to pre-pregnancy levels within 3–6 months after delivery.

In pregnant women, albumin concentrations decrease possibly due to haemodilution, while alkaline phosphatase levels rise, due to the production by the placenta. Estrogen levels increase several fold in comparison to pre-pregnancy values, and this positively influences the hepatic synthesis of several proteins, including the alpha-1, alpha-2, and beta fractions, coagulation factors, and fibrinogen. Worsening of HCV infection during pregnancy is uncommon, but cholestasis might complicate gestation as of the first trimester and can be severe enough to warrant treatment to control itching and monitor foetal wellbeing (Riely, 1994; Nicastri et al., 1998). This alteration usually disappears shortly after delivery.

In the presence of significant liver fibrosis, return of portal blood flow through the hepatic sinusoid system can be impaired with ensuing portal hypertension and increased risk of bleeding from oesofageal varicosities. Bleeding can be customarily treated, but delivery of the child should be considered if the pregnancy is close to term, to reduce volaemia and facilitate diagnostic and therapeutic procedures. In the presence of severe portal hypertension before pregnancy, women should be informed about the increased risk of gastrointestinal bleeding during pregnancy.

The management of pregnancy is particularly delicate in women with cirrhosis, especially when uncompensated (Krol-Van Straaten and De Maat, 1984). Normal pregnancies and deliveries have been reported in women who underwent liver transplant, and there is no evidence that pregnancy can negatively influence the tolerance of the grafted liver or the transplant's long-term outcome (Radomski et al., 1995; Jain et al., 1997; Wu et al., 1998).

Overall, pregnancy does not induce a deterioration of HCV-associated liver disease and, conversely HCV does not seem to increase the risk of congenital anomalies and obstetrical complications (Floreani et al., 1996; Paternoster et al., 2002).

Rates and risk factors for vertical transmission of HCV

Women infected with HCV can transmit the virus to their children, and most cases of paediatric HCV infections are due to vertical transmission. The rate of mother-to-child transmission is currently estimated to be 5%, ranging from 3% to 10% (Zanetti et al., 1995, 1998; Thomas et al., 1998; Conte et al., 2000; Gibb et al., 2000; Resti et al., 2002, 2003; European Paediatric Hepatitis C Virus Network, 2005a; Mast et al., 2005; Pembrey et al., 2005). Transmission is strongly associated with the detection of HCV-RNA in maternal blood. Women with high viral load during pregnancy or at delivery are those at increased risk of transmitting HCV to their children, although a threshold value above which transmission can be predicted or below which can be excluded is not available (Giacchino et al., 1998; Thomas et al., 1998; Zanetti et al., 1998; Okamoto et al., 2000; Dal Molin et al., 2002; Steininger et al., 2003; Pembrey et al., 2005). Rarely, infection has been reported in children born to mothers with undetectable HCV-RNA (Pembrey et al., 2005). Fluctuations in viral load during pregnancy, with viraemia levels above and below the sensitivity limit of the NAT used for nucleic acid detection, might provide an at least partial explanation to such finding.

There is no evidence that the rate of transmission is influenced by HCV genotypes (Zanetti et al., 1999; Dal Molin et al., 2002; Resti et al., 2003) The quasispecies nature of HCV and maternal antibody titres could also influence the rate of transmission, but this association should be further explored (Kudo et al., 1997; Manzin et al., 2000).

Maternal history of chronic hepatitis and elevated serum ALT levels at delivery do not seem to increase the likelihood of HCV transmission infection to their children (Zanetti et al., 1999; Mast et al., 2005).

HCV/HIV co-infected mothers are at increased risk of transmitting HCV vertically in comparison to women infected by HCV alone, probably due to higher circulating HCV viral loads associated with HIV-induced immunosuppression (Zanetti et al., 1995, 1998; European Paediatric Hepatitis C Virus Network, 1999, 2001; Yeung et al., 2001; Mast et al., 2005).

However, the risk seems to be substantially attenuated with the increasing use of highly active antiretroviral therapy (HAART) for the suppression of HIV replication in pregnancy. The improvement of the HIV-induced immunosuppression may indirectly limit HCV replication (European Paediatric Hepatitis C Virus Network, 2005a).

Data concerning the influence of maternal injecting drug use as a potential risk factor for mother-to-child transmission of HCV is conflicting.

In a large multicentre study carried out in Italy on 1372 mothers–infants pairs (Resti et al., 2002), history of maternal drug use was linked to an increased risk of transmission, while such association was not observed by others (European Paediatric Hepatitis C Virus Network, 2005a).

A recent study (European Paediatric Hepatitis C Virus Network, 2005a) indicates that female gender of children born to HCV-positive mothers significantly increased the risk of acquiring infection, compared to male gender. This finding needs to be further confirmed, but it is intriguing to know that a similar gender effect was also observed in mother-to-child transmission of HIV (European Collaborative Study, 2004).

There is no evidence to suggest that gestational age may influence the rate of mother-to-infant transmission of HCV and no difference in frequency of infection has been observed between term (>36 months) and premature (<36 months) infants (European Paediatric Hepatitis C Virus Network, 2005a).

In the same way, maternal age at delivery as well as weight at birth of the infant do not seem to influence the rate of vertical transmission of HCV (European Paediatric Hepatitis C Virus Network, 2005a).

Mode of delivery and timing of mother-to-infant transmission of HCV

The timing and mechanisms of mother-to-infant transmission of HCV remain largely unknown. Transfer of the virus can occur during pregnancy, through placental breaks during labour or, in the birth canal through exposure of the infant to the maternal blood and cervical secretions. In some studies, HCV-RNA has been found immediately after birth suggesting *in utero* infection. In other studies, infected children were HCV-RNA negative at birth and became positive weeks later suggesting peripartum transmission. Mok et al. (2005) suggested that one-third to a half of HCV-infected children acquire infection during the intrauterine period, in line with what reported by Resti et al. (1998), who found that at least 46% (95%

CI: 19% to 75%) of transmission occurred *in utero*, as six of the 13 infected children had HCV-RNA detectable immediately after birth.

Elective Caesarean section has been suggested as a possible measure to prevent intrapartum transmission of the virus. A protective effect has been suggested (Paccagnini et al., 1995; Gibb et al., 2000), but most studies agree that the rate of mother-to-infant transmission does not differ significantly between infants delivered by Caesarean section compared to those delivered vaginally (Zanetti et al., 1999; Conte et al., 2000; Fiore et al., 2001; Resti et al., 2002). In a large study conducted by the European Paediatric Hepatitis C Virus Network (2001) on a total of 1.474 HCV-infected women, multivariate analysis did not show a significant protective effect of mode of delivery among mothers with HCV infection alone. Vice versa, mothers co-infected with HIV delivered by Caesarean section had 60% lesser likelihood to transmit the infection in comparison to co-infected mothers who delivered vaginally. A more recent European study carried out on 1787 mother–child pairs further confirms such findings (European Paediatric Hepatitis C Virus Network, 2005a). Failure to prove a beneficial effect of Caesarean delivery is consistent with the large proportion of intrauterine transmission of HCV. Thus, at present, there is no indication to recommend elective Caesarean section to pregnant women with HCV alone, while it is highly recommended for those co-infected with HIV/HCV, in accordance with the current HIV guidelines (Newell, 2002).

Other obstetric factors

Pre-natal sampling of amniotic fluid (amniocentesis), placental tissue (villocentesis), or foetal blood (funicolocentesis) are all procedures that might facilitate passage of HCV into the foetal compartment as samples are obtained with a needle inserted through the maternal abdomen. The reported rate of infection with HCV following accidental needle-stick from HCV positive sources has been estimated at around 0.3% and increases to 0.7% in cases of large sizes inocula (hollow needle containing blood) (De Carli et al., 2003) However, needles used in pre-natal diagnosis are mandrinated and, therefore, the risk of transferring infected blood through this procedure could be lower.

There are very few reports of vertical transmission of HCV in women who underwent invasive pre-natal procedures. Hence, the role of these procedures in transmitting the virus to the child is difficult to assess. In a study carried out by Delamare et al. (1999), HCV-RNA was detected in one of the 16 amniotic fluid samples collected during the fourth month of pregnancy from viraemic women. The child born to the woman whose amniotic fluid was HCV-RNA positive was not viraemic upon examination performed shortly after birth.

There has been no viral detection in amniotic fluid samples collected at mid-gestation or at term from 17 HCV viraemic women (personal data).

Amniocentesis was considered a possible explanation for a case of diamniotic twins discordant for HCV, where the needle punctured the amniotic sac of only the infected child (Minola et al., 2001). According to Davies et al. (2003) there is no evidence that amniocentesis may increase the risk of vertical infection. However, HCV-infected pregnant women should be counselled since the current limited evidence on this issue does not allow for definitive conclusions.

No association between the length of ruptured membranes and HCV transmission was found in a study carried out in the USA (Thomas et al., 1998), while duration of membranes rupture was found to be significantly longer in transmitting than in non-transmitting mothers in other studies (Spencer et al., 1997; European Paediatric Hepatitis C Virus Network, 2005a; Mast et al., 2005).

During labour, the use of internal scalp electrodes to monitor foetal heart should be avoided, as these may damage the infant's scalp and facilitate contamination with the infected maternal blood (Mast et al., 2005).

In some women, operative delivery may be required. However, the procedure employs devices, such as vacuum cups or forceps which might lacerate foetal scalp, and are usually associated with significant maternal bleeding due to perineal incision or vaginal laceration, all of which may increase risk of viral transmission (Steininger et al., 2003). In a French case–control study, the use of forceps in vaginal delivery was associated with a significant (3-fold) risk of vertical transmission (Poiraud et al., 2001).

In HCV-viraemic women, if operative delivery is required, the potential risk for foetal infection associated with this procedure, should be balanced against the alternative of Caesarean delivery.

Breastfeeding

Current evidence does not suggest that breastfeeding can increase the risk of mother-to-infant transmission of HCV (Resti et al., 1998, 2003; European Paediatric Hepatitis C Virus Network, 2005a; Mast et al., 2005; Pembrey et al., 2005). However, the impact of factors such as duration of breastfeeding, levels of HCV-RNA and anti-HCV antibodies in colostrum and milk, and exposure to maternal-infected blood through chapped nipples in influencing HCV transmission through breastfeeding has not been sufficiently investigated. HCV-RNA has been found in colostrum and milk in some studies (Lin et al., 1995; Kumar and Shahul, 1998; Thomas et al., 1998; Ruiz-Extremera et al., 2000; Mast et al., 2005). Two studies suggest that HCV-RNA detection in breast milk may be associated with higher risk of transmission (Lin et al., 1995; Ruiz-Extremera et al., 2000), but other studies fail to demonstrate any association between type of infant feeding and risk of vertical transmission. In a large multi-centre Italian study conducted by Resti et al. (2002), the adjusted odds ratio for breastfeeding was 0.95 (95% CI: 0.58–1.40, $p = 0.74$). Multivariate analyses did not show a significant effect of breastfeeding in 916 women with HCV infection alone. However, HIV/HCV co-infected women who breastfed were more likely to infect their children than those who did not (OR = 6.41, $p = 0.03$) (European Paediatric Hepatitis C Virus Network, 2001). More recently, the European Paediatric Hepatitis C Virus Network Group further confirmed in a multicentre international study on 1787 mother–child pairs enrolled at 33 different centres, that breastfeeding does not increase the risk of viral trans-mission (adjusted OR, 0.88 (95% CI: 0.48–1.61), $p = 0.68$) (European Paediatric Hepatitis C Virus Network, 2005a).

Diagnosis and outcome of HCV vertical infection

Due to the passive transfer of maternal antibody, the diagnosis of HCV infection in exposed children cannot be based solely on anti-HCV testing at birth or during the first months of life. Maternal antibody can be detected in most infants born to HCV-infected mothers for several months and usually disappears within the first year of life, although in some cases may persist longer (up to 18 months) (Resti et al., 2003; Pembrey et al., 2005). ALT is not a useful marker for diagnosis since levels may be normal in most HCV infected children, and transiently elevated in some uninfected children. Approximately 70% of infected children become HCV-RNA positive by 1 month and 90% by 3 months of age, and viraemia is usually accompanied by a subsequent active production of anti-HCV antibody. Thus, an early diagnosis of infant infection should be based on the detection of HCV-RNA at the first well-child visit or preferably between 3 and 6 months of life, confirmed by anti-HCV serological status at 18 months.

It is advisable that the diagnosis of infection be confirmed by at least two positive HCV-RNA detections performed on separate samples.

Viral hepatitis C has a high probability of evolving towards chronicity with a variable outcome over time. Infected babies tend to progress to chronic infection with benign course, at least in the short medium term, and extrahepatic manifes-tations are rare (European Paediatric Hepatitis C Virus Network, 2000, 2005b; Pembrey et al., 2005; Tovo et al., 2005). Histological findings usually show features of minimal to mild hepatitis, but in few cases, liver damage may be severe (Bortol-otti et al., 1997; Jonas, 2002; El-Raziky et al., 2004). Periportal fibrosis is relatively common and appears to progress with age and duration of infection (Badizadegan et al., 1998; Guido et al., 1998; Jara et al., 2003; Strader et al., 2004).

A prospective study carried out on 266 children with vertically acquired HCV infection who were prospectively followed up from birth till 16 years of age (median 4.2 years) in 30 European health care centres showed low prevalence of HCV-related symptoms and signs in the first 10–15 years of life (European Paediatric Hepatitis C Virus Network, 2005b). Approximately 20% of infected children had spontaneous clearance of HCV-RNA, 50% had evidence of chronic asymptomatic infection characterized by normal ALT levels and intermittent viraemia, and 30% had evidence of chronic, active infection characterized by persistent viraemia, ab-normal ALT levels, and, in some cases, hepatomegaly.

Most of the children who loose HCV-RNA maintain antibody in absence of detectable viraemia for long periods of time, though few may serorevert to anti-HCV negativity (European Paediatric Hepatitis C Virus Network, 2005b).

Information about the long-term consequences of vertically acquired HCV beyond 2 decades is scarce. There is evidence that patients infected at young age are at lower risk of progressive liver disease than those infected at older age (Kenny-Walsh et al., 1999; Vogt et al., 1999; Wiese et al., 2000). Over half of 67 children who acquired HCV during cardiac surgery before the implementation of blood donor screening were still HCV-RNA positive after 20 years of infection, but only a minority had histological signs of progressive liver damage, despite infection with the most aggressive genotype 1 (Vogt et al., 1999). A similar slow rate of progression was observed in a group of 35-year-old individuals who were infected by HCV of genotype 1b through mini transfusions of blood given at birth. 90% of such persons were still viraemic after more than 3 decades from primary infection, but the majority showed no sign of fibrosis (Casiraghi et al., 2004). A study conducted in seven European centres on 224 HCV-infected children supports the view that hepatitis C is generally mild in children, but that may slowly progress over the time since the mean fibrosis score was found to be higher among older children (> 15 years) than younger children (Jara et al., 2003). This finding is in line with what has been reported by Guido et al. (1998) about the histological features of hepatitis C in liver samples obtained from 80 children.

Therefore, since the rate of progression of HCV infection is slow, usually over decades, and the development of severe disease as cirrhosis and hepatocellular carcinoma commonly exceed 20–25 years of established chronic hepatitis C, it is possible that vertically infected children may not manifest severe symptoms until adulthood.

Because of the paucity of information regarding the long-term natural history of vertically acquired infections, further studies are needed to clarify this issue.

According to the American Association for the Study of the Liver Diseases practice guidelines (Strader et al., 2004), treatment is contraindicated in children below the age of 3 years. Vice versa, children aged from 3 to 17 years old, who are considered appropriate candidates for therapy, may receive interferon alpha-2b and ribavirin. The combination has been shown to be effective and reasonably safe for the treatment of childhood chronic hepatitis C (Gonzales-Peralta et al., 2005).

Finally, as a super infection with HAV or with HBV may worsen the prognosis of the underlying HCV infection (Akriviadis and Redeker, 1989; Tsai et al., 1996; Vento et al., 1998; ACIP, 1999), vaccination against both hepatitis A and B should be recommended to HCV infected children.

Conclusion

Based on the current evidence, HCV prevalence is around 1–2.5% among unselected childbearing women from Europe and the USA, but is higher in developing countries. History of drug use, blood transfusion performed prior to 1991 or of other modes of parenteral exposure is associated with HCV infection in pregnant women. However, up to 50% of infected women may have no known risk factors, and would be missed in selective antenatal screening.

Pregnancy is not contraindicated in women with HCV, and HCV infection does not appear to adversely affect pregnancy, delivery, or the perinatal health of mother and newborn. The risk of mother-to-infant transmission is estimated at approximately 5% and higher for babies born to HIV co-infected women, although HAART treatment during pregnancy seems to decrease such effect. Vertical transmission is usually restricted to infants whose mothers are viraemic and rates of transmission increase with increasing maternal viral load, but a specific cut-off value which predicts transmission cannot be defined. Transmission is not related to specific HCV genotypes. Available drugs cannot be used in pregnancy due to their teratogenic (ribavirin) or to possible adverse effects on foetal growth (interferon). At present there is no evidence that Caesarean delivery can reduce the risk of HCV transmission compared to vaginal delivery. The role of obstetric variables such as type of vaginal delivery (spontaneous, induced, or operative) and timing of Caesarean section (before and during labour) remains largely unknown. Caution should be recommended in using any invasive procedures (i.e. chorionic villous sampling, amniocentesis, and cord blood sampling) that may expose the foetus or the neonate to infected maternal blood. Avoiding foetal scalp monitoring and prolonged labour after rupture of membranes may reduce the risk of viral transmission to the infant.

Breastfeeding is safe and not contraindicated, but factors that may influence the risk of transmission through this route (i.e. duration of lactation, levels of HCV-RNA in colostrums and milk, exposure to chapped nipples) require further study.

Testing babies born to HCV infected mothers for anti-HCV should be performed at 18 months or late, but if an earlier diagnosis is desired, HCV-RNA detection is suggested at the first well-child visit or at 3–6 months. Infected babies usually progress to chronic disease with a benign course, at least initially. Longitudinal studies are needed to determine the long-term outcome of hepatitis C in vertically infected children. Interferon alpha-2b in combination with ribavirin can be of benefit for the treatment of chronic hepatitis C in children. Vaccination against hepatitis A and B is highly recommended in children with HCV infection.

References

ACIP. Prevention of hepatitis A through active or passive immunization: recommendations of the Advisory Committee on Immunization Practices (ACIP). MMWR 1999; 48(RR-12): 1–37.

Akriviadis EA, Redeker AG. Fulminant hepatitis A in intravenous drug users with chronic liver disease. Ann Intern Med 1989; 118: 838–839.

American Academy of Pediatrics (Committee on Infectious Diseases). Hepatitis C virus infection. Pediatrics 1998; 101: 481–485.

Badizadegan K, Jonas MM, Ott MJ, Nelson SP, Perez-Atayde AR. Histopathology of the liver in children with chronic hepatitis C viral infection. Hepatology 1998; 28: 1416–1423.

Barrett S, Goh J, Coughlan B, Ryan E, Stewart S, Cockram A, O'Keane JC, Crowe J. The natural course of hepatitis C virus infection after 22 years in a unique homogenous cohort: spontaneous viral clearance and chronic HCV infection. Gut 2001; 49: 423–430.

Bellentani S, Pozzato G, Saccoccio G, Crovatto M, Crocè LS, Mazzoran L, Masutti F, Cristianini G, Tiribelli C. Clinical course and risk factors of hepatitis C virus related liver disease in the general population: report from the Dionysis Study. Gut 1999; 44: 874–880.

Benhamou Y, Bochet M, Di Martino V, Charlotte F, Azria F, Coutellier A, Vidaud M, Bricaire F, Opolon P, Katlama C, Poynard T. Liver fibrosis progression in human immunodeficiency virus and hepatitis C virus coinfected patients. The Multivirc Group. Hepatology 1999; 30: 1054–1058.

Bortolotti F, Jara P, Diaz C, Vajro P, Hierro L, Giacchino R, de la Vega A, Crivellaro C, Camarena C, Barbera C, Nebbia G, Cancan L, de Moliner L. Posttransfusion and community-acquired hepatitis C in childhood. J Pediatr Gastroenterol Nutr 1994; 18: 279–283.

Bortolotti F, Resti M, Giacchino R, Azzari C, Gussetti N, Crivellaro C, Barbera C, Mannelli F, Zancan L, Bertolini A. Hepatitis C virus infection and related liver disease in children of mothers with antibodies to the virus. J Pediatr 1997; 130: 990–993.

Boxall E, Skidmore S, Evans C, Nightingale S. The prevalence of hepatitis B and C in an antenatal population of various ethnic origin. Epidemiol Infect 1994; 113: 523–528.

Casiraghi MA, De Paschale M, Romanò L, Biffi R, Assi A, Binelli G, Zanetti AR. Long-term outcome (35 years) of hepatitis C after acquisition of infection through mini transfusions of blood given at birth. Hepatology 2004; 39: 90–96.

Choo QL, Kuo G, Weiner AJ, Overby LR, Bradley DW. Isolation of a cDNA clone derived from a blood-borne non-A, non-B viral hepatitis genome. Science 1989; 244: 359–362.

Chutaputti A. Adverse effects and other safety aspects of the hepatitis C antivirals. J Gastroenterol Hepatol 2000; 15: E156–E163.

Conte D, Frenguelli M, Prati D, Colucci A, Minola E. Prevalence and clinical course of chronic hepatitis C virus (HCV) infection: rate of HCV vertical transmission in a cohort of 15250 pregnant women. Hepatology 2000; 31: 751–755.

Dal Molin G, D'Agaro P, Ansaldi F, Ciana G, Fertz C, Alberico S, Campello C. Mother to infant transmission of hepatitis C virus: rate of infection and assessment of viral load and IgM anti-HCV as risk factors. J Med Virol 2002; 67: 137–142.

Davies G, Wilson RD, Desilets V, Reid GJ, Shaw D, Summers A, Wyatt P, Young D. Amniocentesis and women with hepatitis B, hepatitis C, or human immunodeficiency virus. J Obstet Gynaecol Can 2003; 25: 145–152.

De Carli G, Puro V, Ippolito G, Studio Italiano Rischio Occupazionale da HIV Group. Risk of hepatitis C virus transmission following percutaneous exposure in healthcare workers. Infection 2003; 31(Suppl 2): 22–27.

Delamare C, Carbonne B, Heim N, Berkane N, Petit JC, Uzan S, Grangé J-D. Detection of hepatitis C virus RNA (HCV RNA) in amniotic fluid. A Prospective Study. J Hepatol 1999; 31: 416–420.

Dike AE, Christie JML, Kurtz JB, Teo C-G. Hepatitis C in blood transfusion recipients identified at the Oxford blood centre in the national HCV look-back programme. Transfus Med 1998; 8: 87–95.

EASL International Consensus Conference on Hepatitis C. Paris, 26–28 February, 1999. Consensus Statement. J. Hepatol 1999; 30: 956–961.

El-Gohary A, Hassan A, Nooman Z, Lavanchy D, Mayerat C, El-Ayat A, Fawaz N, Gobran F, Ahmed M, Kawano F, Kiyokawa T, Yamaguchi K. High prevalence of hepatitis C virus among urban and rural population groups in Egypt. Acta Trop 1995; 59: 155–161.

El-Raziky MS, El-Hawary M, El-Koofy N, Okasha S, Kotb M, Salama K, Esmat G, El-Raziky M, Abouzied AM, El-Karaksy H. Hepatitis C virus infection in Egyptian children: single centre experience. J Viral Hep 2004; 11: 471–476.

European Collaborative Study. Are girls more at risk of intra-uterine-acquired HIV infection than boys? AIDS 2004; 18: 344–347.

European Paediatric Hepatitis C Virus Network. Antenatal hepatitis C virus screening and management of infected women and their children: policies in Europe. Eur J Pediatr 1999; 158: 842–846.

European Paediatric Hepatitis C Virus Network. Persistence rate and progression of vertically acquired hepatitis C infection. J Infect Dis 2000; 181: 419–424.

European Paediatric Hepatitis C Virus Network. Effects of mode of delivery and infant feeding on the risk of mother-to-child transmission of hepattis C virus. Br J Obstet Gynaecol 2001; 108: 371–377.

European Paediatric Hepatitis C Virus Network. A significant sex—but not elective caesarean section—effect on mother-to-child transmission of hepatitis C virus infection. J Infect Dis 2005a; 192: 1872–1879.

European Paediatric Hepatitis C Virus Network. Three broad modalities in the natural history of vertically acquired hepatitis C virus infection. Clin Infect Dis 2005b; 41: 45–51.

Fiore S, Newell M-L, Zanetti AR, Coll O. Mother-to-child HCV transmission. Lancet 2001; 357: 141–142.

Floreani A, Paternoster D, Zappalà F, Cucinato R, Bombi G, Grella P, Chiaramonte M. Hepatitis C virus infection in pregnancy. Br J Obstet Gynaecol 1996; 103: 325–329.

Fried MW, Shiffman ML, Reddy KR, Smith C, Marinos G, Goncales Jr. FL, Haussinger D, Diago M, Carosi G, Dhumeaux D, Craxi A, Lin A, Hoffman J, Yu J. Peginterferon alfa-2a plus ribavirin for chronic hepatitis C virus infection. N Engl J Med 2002; 347: 975–982.

Garcia-Monzon C, Jara P, Fernandez-Bermejo M, Hierro L, Frauca E, Camarena C, Diaz C, de la Vega A, Larrauri J, Garcia-Iglesias C, Borque MJ, Sanz P, Garcia-Buey L, Moreno-Monteagudo JA, Moreno-Otero R. Chronic hepatitis C in children: a clinical and immunohistochemical comparative study with adult patients. Hepatology 1998; 28: 1696–1701.

Gervais A, Bacq Y, Bernuau J, Martinot M, Auperin A, Boyer N, Kilani A, Erlimger S, Valla D, Marcellin P. Decrease in serum ALT and increase in serum HCV RNA during pregnancy in women with chronic hepatitis C. J Hepatol 2000; 32: 293–299.

Giacchino R, Tasso L, Timitilli A, Castagnola E, Cristina E, Sinelli N, Gotta C, Giambartolomei G, Moscatelli P, Picciotto A. Vertical transmission of hepatitis C virus infection: usefulness of viremia detection in HIV-seronegative hepatitis C virus-seropositive mothers. J Pediatr 1998; 132: 167–169.

Gibb DM, Goodall RL, Dunn DT, Healy M, Neave P, Cafferkey M, Butler K. Mother-to-child transmission of hepatitis C virus: evidence for preventable peripartum transmission. Lancet 2000; 356: 904–907.

Goldberg D, McIntyre PG, Smith R, Appleyard K, Dunlop J, Taylor A, Hutchinson S. Hepatitis C virus among high and low risk pregnant women in Dundee: unliked anonymous testing. Br J Obstet Gynaecol 2001; 108: 365–370.

Gonzalez-Peralta RP, Kelly DA, Haber B, Molleston J, Murray KF, Jonas MM, Shelton M, Mieli-Vergani G, Lurie Y, Martin S, Lang T, Baczkowski A, Geffner M, Gupta S, Laughlin M (for the International Pediatric Hepatitis C Therapy Group). Interferon alfa-2b in combination with ribavirin for the treatment of chronic hepatitis C in children: efficacy, safety, and pharmacokinetics. Hepatology 2005; 42: 1010–1018.

Gordon SC, Bayati N, Silverman AL. Clinical outcome of hepatitis C as a function of mode of transmission. Hepatology 1998; 28: 562–567.

Guido M, Rugger M, Jara P, Hierro L, Giacchino R, Larrauri J, Zancan L, Leandro G, Marino CE, Balli F, Bagni A, Timitilli A, Bortolotti F. Chronic hepatitis C in children: the pathological and clinical spectrum. Gastroenterology 1998; 115: 1525–1529.

Hadziyannis SJ, Sette H, Morgan TR, Balan V, Diago M, Marcellin P, Ramadori G, Bodenheimer Jr. H, Bernstein D, Rizzetto M, Zeuzem S, Pockros PJ, Lin A, Ackrill AM. Peginterferon alfa-2a (40 kilodaltons) and ribavirin combination therapy in chronic hepatitis C: randomized study of the effect of treatment duration and ribavirin dose. Ann Intern Med 2004; 140: 346–355.

Harris DR, Gonin R, Alter HJ, Wright EC, Buskell ZJ, Hollinger FB, Seeff LB (for the National Heart, Lung and Blood Institute Study Group). The relationship of acute transfusion-associated hepatitis to the development of cirrhosis in the presence of alcohol abuse. Ann Intern Med 2001; 134: 120–124.

Harris HE, Ramsay ME, Andrews N, Eldridge KP (on behalf of the HCV National Register Steering Group). Clinical course of hepatitis C virus during the first decade of infection: cohort study. BMJ 2002; 324: 1–6.

Hoofnagle JH. Course and outcome of hepatitis C. Hepatology 2002; 36(Suppl 1): S21–S29.

Kenny-Walsh E. (for the Irish Hepatology Research Group) Clinical outcomes after hepatitis C infection from contaminated anti-D immune globulin. N Engl J Med 1999; 340: 1228–1233.

Krol-Van Straaten J, De Maat CE. Successful pregnancies in cirrhosis of the liver before and after portocaval anastomosis. Neth J Med 1984; 27: 14–15.

Kudo T, Yanase Y, Ohshiro M, Yamamoto M, Morita M, Shibata M, Morishima T. Analysis of mother-to-infant transmission of hepatitis C virus: quasispecies nature and buoyant densities of maternal virus populations. J Med Virol 1997; 51: 225–230.

Kumar RM, Shahul S. Role of breast-feeding in transmission of hepatitis C virus to infants of HCV-infected mothers. J Hepatol 1998; 29: 191–197.

Kuo G, Choo QL, Alter HJ, Gitnick GL, Redeker AG, Purcell RH, Miyamura T, Dienstag JL, Alter MJ, Stevens CE. An assay for circulating antibodies to a major etiologic virus of human non-A, non-B hepatitis. Science 1989; 244: 362–364.

Jain A, Venkataramanan R, Fung JJ, Gartner JC, Lever J, Balan V, Warty V, Starzl TE. Pregnancy after liver transplantation under tacrolimus. Transplantation 1997; 64: 559–565.

Jara P, Resti M, Hierro L, Giacchino R, Barbera C, Zancan L, Crivellaro C, Sokal E, Azzari C, Guido M, Bortolotti F. Chronic hepatitis C virus infection in childhood: clinical patterns and evolution in 224 white children. Clin Infect Dis 2003; 36: 275–280.

Jonas MM. Children with hepatitis C. Hepatology 2002; 36(Suppl 1): S173–S178.

Lauer GM, Walker BD. Hepatitis C virus infection. N Engl J Med 2001; 345: 41–52.

Lin H-H, Kao J-H, Hsu H-Y, Ni Y-H, Chang M-H, Huang S-C, Hwang L-H, Chen P-J, Chen D-S. Absence of infection in breast-fed infants born to hepatitis C virus-infected mothers. J Pediatr 1995; 126: 589–591.

Louis FJ, Maubert B, Le Hesran J-Y, Kemmegne J, Delaporte E, Louis J-P. High prevalence of anti-hepatitis C virus antibodies in Cameroon rural forest area. Trans R Soc Trop Med Hyg 1994; 88: 53–54.

Manns MP, McHutchinson JG, Gordon SC, Rustgi VK, Shiffman M, Reindollar R, Goodman ZD, Kouri K, Ling MH, Albrecht JK and the International Hepatitis

Interventional Therapy Group. Peginterferon alfa-2b plus ribavirin compared with inter-
    feron alfa-2b plus ribavirin for initial treatment of chronic hepatitis C: a randomized trial.
    Lancet 2001; 358: 958–965.

Manzin A, Solforosi L, Debiaggi M, Zara F, Tanzi E, Romanò L, Zanetti AR, Clementi M.
    Dominant role of host selective pressure in driving hepatitis C virus evolution in perinatal
    infection. J Virol 2000; 74: 4327–4334.

Mast EE, Hwang L-Y, Seto DSY, Nolte FS, Nainan OV, Wurtzel H, Alter MJ. Risk factors
    for perinatal transmission of hepatitis C virus (HCV) and the natural history of HCV
    infection acquired in infancy. J Infect Dis 2005; 192: 1880–1889.

Matsuoka S, Tatara K, Hayabuchi Y, Taguchi Y, Mori K, Honda H, Itou S, Yuasa Y,
    Kuroda Y. Serologic, virologic, and histologic characteristics of chronic phase hepatitis C
    virus disease in children infected by transfusion. Pediatrics 1994; 94: 919–922.

Minola E, Maccabruni A, Pacati I, Martinetti M. Amniocentesis as a possible risk factor for
    mother-to-infant transmission of hepatitis C virus. Hepatology 2001; 33: 1341–1342.

Mok J, Pembrey L, Tovo P-A, Newell ML (for the European Paediatric Hepatitis C Virus
    Network). When does mother to child transmission of hepatitis C virus occur? Arch Dis
    Child Fetal Neonatal Ed 2005; 90: F156–F160.

Monto A, Alonzo J, Watson JJ, Grunfeld C, Wright TL. Steatosis in chronic hepatitis C:
    relative contributions of obesity, diabetes mellitus, and alcohol. Hepatology 2002; 36:
    729–736.

Newell M-L (editor). Pregnancy and HIV infection: a European consensus on management.
    Executive summary. AIDS 2002; 16(Suppl 2): S1–S18.

Nicastri PL, Diaferia A, Tartagni M, Loizzi P, Fanelli M. A randomised placebo-controlled
    trial of ursodeoxycolic acid and S-adenosylmethionine in the treatment of intrahepatic
    cholestasis of pregnancy. Br Obstet Gynaecol 1998; 105: 1205–1207.

Okamoto M, Nagata I, Murakami J, Kaji S, Iitsuka T, Hoshika T, Matsuda R, Tazawa Y,
    Shiraki K, Hino S. Prospective reevaluation of risk factors in mother-to-child transmis-
    sion of hepatitis C virus: high virus load, vaginal delivery, and negative anti-NS4 anti-
    body. J Infect Dis 2000; 182: 1511–1514.

O'Riordan JM, Conroy A, Nourse C, Yap PL, McDonald GSA, Kaminski G, Leong K,
    Lawlor E, Davoren A, Strong K, Davidson F, Lloyd A, Power J. Risk of hepatitis C
    infection in neonates transfused with blood from donors infected with hepatitis C.
    Transfus Med 1998; 8: 303–308.

Paccagnini S, Principi N, Massironi E, Tanzi E, Romano L, Muggiasca ML, Ragni MC,
    Salvaggio L. Perinatal transmission and manifestation of hepatitis C virus infection in a
    high risk population. Pediatr Infect Dis J 1995; 14: 195–199.

Paternoster DM, Fabris F, Palù G, Santarossa C, Bracciante R, Snijders D, Floreani A.
    Intra-hepatic cholestasis of pregnancy in hepatitis C virus infection. Acta Obstet Gynecol
    Scand 2002; 81: 99–103.

Pembrey L, Newell M-L, Peckham C. Is there a case for hepatitis C infection screening in the
    antenatal period? J Med Screen 2003; 10: 161–168.

Pembrey L, Newell M-L, Tovo P-A, the EPHN Collaborators. The management of HCV
    infected pregnant women and their children. European Paediatric HCV Network. J He-
    patol 2005; 43: 515–525.

Pipan C, Amici S, Aston G, Ceci GP, Botta GA. Vertical transmission of hepatitis C virus in
    low risk pregnant women. Eur J Clin Microbiol Infect Dis 1996; 15: 116–120.

Poiraud S, Cohen J, Amiot X, Berkane N, Flahault A, Dussaix E Mother-to-child transmission of hepatitis C virus: a case-control study of risk factors. The American Gastroenterological Association and Digestive Disease Week. Atlanta, GA, 2001; Abstract no.1879, A366.

Poynard T, Ratziu V, Charlotte F, Goodman Z, McHutchison J, Albrecht J. Rates and risk factors of liver fibrosis progression in patients with chronic hepatitis C. J Hepatol 2001; 34: 730–739.

Radomski JS, Moritz MJ, Munoz SJ, Cater JR, Jarrell BE, Armenti VT. National transplantation pregnancy registry: analysis of pregnancy outcomes in female liver transplant recipients. Liver Transplant Surg 1995; 1: 281–284.

Rao MR, Naficy AB, Darwish MA, Darwish NM, Schisterman E, Clemens JD, Edelman R. Further evidence for association of hepatitis C infection with parenteral schistosomiasis treatment in Egypt. BMC Infect Dis 2002; 2: 30–33.

Resti M, Azzari C, Galli L, Zuin G, Giacchino R, Bortolotti F, Marcellini M, Moriondo M, de Martino M, Vierucci A for the Italian study group on mother-to-infant hepatitis C virus transmission. Maternal drug use is a pre-eminent risk factor for mother-to-child hepatitis C virus transmission: results from a multicenter study of 1372 mother–infant pairs. J Infect Dis 2002; 185: 567–572.

Resti M, Azzari C, Mannelli F, Moriondo M, Novembre E, de Martino M, Vierucci A, and Tuscany study group on hepatitis C virus infection in children. Mother to child transmission of hepatitis C virus: prospective study of risk factors and timing of infection in children born to women seronegative for HIV-1. BMJ 1998; 317: 437–441.

Resti M, Bortolotti F, Vajro P, Maggiore G on behalf of the Committee of hepatology of the Italian Society of Pediatric Gastroenterology and Hepatology Guidelines for the screening and follow-up of infants born to anti-HCV positive mothers. Digest Liver Dis 2003; 35: 453–457.

Riely CA. Hepatic disease in pregnancy. Am J Med 1994; 96(1A): 18S–22S.

Robertson B, Myers G, Howard C, Brettin T, Bukh J, Gaschen B, Gojobori T, Maertens G, Mizokami M, Nainan O, Netesov S, Nishioka K, Shin-I T, Simmonds P, Smith D, Stuyver L, Weiner A. Classification, nomenclature, and database development for hepatitis C virus (HCV) and related viruses: proposals for standardization. Arch Virol 1998; 143: 2493–2503.

Rodger AJ, Roberts S, Lanigan A, Bowden S, Brown T, Crofts N. Assessment of long-term outcomes of community-acquired hepatitis C infection in a cohort with sera stored from 1971 to 1975. Hepatology 2000; 32: 582–587.

Roudot-Thoraval F, Bastie A, Pawlotsky J-M, Dhumeaux D and the Study Group for the prevalence and the epidemiology of hepatitis C virus. Epidemiological factors affecting the severity of hepatitis C virus-related liver disease: a French survey of 6,664 patients. Hepatology 1997; 26: 485–490.

Roudot-Thoraval F, Pawlotsky JM, Deforges L, Girollet PP, Dhumeaux D. Anti-HCV seroprevalence in pregnant women in France. Gut 1993; 34(2 Suppl): S55–S56.

Ruiz-Extremera A, Salmeron J, Torres C, Munoz de Rueda P, Gimenez F, Robles C, Miranda MT. Follow-up of transmission of hepatitis C to babies of human immunodeficiency virus-negative women: the role of breast-feeding in transmission. Pediatr Infect Dis J 2000; 19: 511–516.

Seeff LB. Natural history of chronic hepatitis C. Hepatology 2002; 36(Suppl 1): S35–S46.

Seeff LB, Hollinger FB, Alter HJ, Wright EC, Cain CMB, Buskell ZJ, Ishak KG, Iber FL, Toro D, Samanta A, Koretz RL, Perrillo RP, Goodman ZD, Knodell RG, Gitnick G, Morgan TR, Schiff ER, Lasky S, Stevens C, Vlahcevic RZ, Weinshel E, Tanwandee T, Lin HJ, Barbosa L. Long-term mortality and morbidity of transfusion-associated non-A, non-B, and type C hepatitis: A National Heart, Lung, and Blood Institute Collaborative Study. Hepatology 2001; 33: 455–463.

Seeff LB, Miller RN, Rabkin CS, Buskell-Bales Z, Straley-Eason KD, Smoak BL, Johnson LD, Lee SR, Kaplan EL. 45-year follow-up of hepatitis C virus infection in healthy young adults. Ann Intern Med 2000; 132: 105–111.

Simmonds P. Viral heterogeneity of the hepatitis C virus. J Hepatol 1999; 31(Suppl 1): 54–60.

Spencer JD, Latt N, Beeby PJ, Collins E, Saunders JB, McCaughan GW, Cossart YE. Transmission of hepatitis C virus to infants of human immunodeficiency virus-negative intravenous drug-using mothers: rate of infection and assessment of risk factors for transmission. J Viral Hep 1997; 4: 395–409.

Steininger C, Kundi M, Jatzko G, Kiss H, Lischka A, Holzmann H. Increased risk of mother-to-infant transmission of hepatitis C virus by intrapartum infantile exposure to maternal blood. J Infect Dis 2003; 187: 345–351.

Strader DB, Wright T, Thomas DL, Seeff LB. AASLD guideline. Diagnosis, management, and treatment of hepatitis C. Hepatology 2004; 39: 1147–1171.

Terrault NA. Sexual activity as a risk factor for hepatitis C. Hepatology 2002; 36(Suppl 1): S99–S105.

Thomas DL, Villano SA, Riester K, Hershow R, Mofenson LM, Landesman SH, Hollinger FB, Davenny K, Riley L, Diaz C, Tang HB, Quinn TC, for the Women and Infants Transmission Study Perinatal transmission of hepatitis C virus from human immunodeficiency virus type 1-infected mothers. J Infect Dis 1998; 177: 1480–1488.

Thomas SL, Newell M-L, Peckham CS, Ades AE, Hall AJ. A review of hepatitis C virus (HCV) vertical transmission to infants born to mothers with and without HCV viraemia or human immunodeficiency virus infection. Int J Epidemiol 1998; 27: 108–117.

Tovo P-A, Lazier L, Versace A. Hepatitis B virus and hepatitis C virus infections in children. Curr Opin Infect Dis 2005; 18: 261–266.

Tsai JF, Jeng JE, Ho MS, Chang WY, Lin ZY, Tsai JH. Independent and additive effect modification of hepatitis B and C virus infection on the development of chronic hepatitis. J Hepatol 1996; 24: 271–276.

Vandelli C, Renzo F, Romanò L, Tisminetzky S, De Palma M, Stroffolini T, Ventura E, Zanetti A. Lack of evidence of sexual transmission of hepatitis C among monogamous couples: results of a 10-year prospective follow-up study. Am J Gastroenterol 2004; 99: 855–859.

Vento S, Garofano T, Renzini C, Cairelli F, Casali F, Ghironzi G, Ferraro T, Concia E. Fulminant hepatitis associated with hepatitis A virus superinfection in patients with chronic hepatitis C. N Engl J Med 1998; 338: 286–290.

Vogt M, Lang T, Frosner G, Klingler C, Sendl AF, Zeller A, Wiebecke B, Langer B, Meisner H, Hess J. Prevalence and clinical outcome of hepatitis C infection in children who underwent cardiac surgery before the implementation of blood-donor screening. N Engl J Med 1999; 341: 866–870.

Wiese M, Berr F, Lafrenz M, Porst H, Oesen U for the East German Hepatitis C Study Group Low frequency of cirrhosis in a hepatitis C (genotype 1b) single-source outbreak in Germany: a 20-year multicenter study. Hepatology 2000; 32: 91–96.

Wu A, Nashan B, Messner U, Schmidt HH, Guenther HH, Niesert S, Pichmayr R. Outcome of 22 successful pregnancies after liver transplantation. Clin Transplant 1998; 12: 454–464.

Yeung LTF, King SM, Roberts EA. Mother-to-infant transmission of hepatitis C virus. Hepatology 2001; 34: 223–229.

Zanetti AR, Tanzi E, Newell M-L. Mother-to-infant transmission of hepatitis C virus. J Hepatol 1999; 31(Suppl 1): 96–100.

Zanetti AR, Tanzi E, Paccagnini S, Principi N, Pizzocolo G, Caccamo ML, D'Amico E, Cambiè G, Vecchi L and The Lombardy Study Group on Vertical HCV Transmission Mother-to-infant transmission of hepatitis C virus. Lancet 1995; 345: 289–291.

Zanetti AR, Tanzi E, Romanò L, Zuin G, Minola E, Vecchi L, Principi N. A prospective study on mother to infant transmission of hepatitis C virus. Intervirology 1998; 41: 208–212.

Zarski JP, Bohn B, Bastie A, Pawlotsky JM, Baud M, Bost-Bezeaux F, Tran van Nhieu J, Seigneurin JM, Buffett C, Dhumeaux D. Characteristics of patients with dual infection by hepatitis B and C viruses. J Hepatol 1998; 28: 27–33.

Congenital and Other Related Infectious
Diseases of the Newborn
Isa K. Mushahwar (Editor)
© 2007 Elsevier B.V. All rights reserved
DOI 10.1016/S0168-7069(06)13010-4

Human Parvovirus B19: Molecular Virology, Clinical Features, Prevalence, Diagnosis and Control [☆]

Amanda Corcoran[a], Sean Doyle[b]

[a]*Biotrin International, The Rise, Mount Merrion Co. Dublin, Ireland*
[b]*National Institute for Cellular Biotechnology, Department of Biology, National University of Ireland Maynooth, Maynooth, Co. Kildare, Ireland*

Parvovirus B19-introduction

Parvovirus B19 (B19) is an erythrovirus and recent studies have classified B19 as a genotype 1 erythrovirus with genotypes 2 (erythrovirus K71 or A6) and 3 (erythrovirus V9) also present in the human population. B19 is a significant human pathogen which can cause foetal hydrops and foetal death if maternal infection, followed by transplacental foetal infection, occurs during pregnancy. The virus is also transmitted by inter-personal contact and potentially via blood product administration. Symptoms of B19 infection include malaise, rash and anthralgia. Significantly, maternal B19 infection during pregnancy can be asymptomatic and so careful monitoring of at-risk pregnancies is recommended. Both antibody- and cell-mediated immunity play an important role in the anti-viral response and effective diagnostic test systems, for both B19 antibody and DNA detection, are now available. B19-induced foetal hydrops can be effectively treated by intrauterine blood transfusion; however, no vaccine is available to prevent infection at present.

Molecular virology

Human parvovirus B19 (B19) was first identified in 1975 by Yvonne Cossart (Cossart et al., 1975). The virus was first associated with disease in 1981 when it was

---

[☆] This chapter is dedicated to Ben.

linked to an aplastic crisis in a patient with sickle-cell disease. Subsequently, B19 has since been shown to be the causative agent of erythema infectiosum (EI) (Fifth disease of childhood), spontaneous abortion and some forms of acute arthritis (Anderson et al., 1983; Kinney et al., 1988; Woolf and Cohen, 1995). B19 is approximately 20 nm in diameter, has a genome of 5.6 kb (Clewley, 1984; Cotmore and Tattersall, 1984) and is a small, non-enveloped, single-stranded DNA virus. Like all parvoviruses, the constituent capsid proteins (VP1 and VP2) are arranged with icosahedral symmetry. The B19 capsid consists of an 83 kDa low-abundance structural protein, VP1, and a 58 kDa major structural protein, VP2. VP2 makes up about 95% of total capsid structure with VP1 accounting for the remaining 5% (Ozawa et al., 1987). The sequences of the two proteins are co-linear and the entire VP2 sequence is identical to the carboxyl-terminus of VP1. However, VP1 comprises an additional 227 amino acids unique to the amino-terminal, the so-called VP1 unique region (VP1u). To the left of these sequences on the B19 genome is the open-reading frame for a non-structural protein, NS1 which encodes a 77 kDa protein. NS1 is a phosphoprotein with important regulatory functions including transcriptional control (Momoeda et al., 1994a, b), virus replication and also plays a role in host cell death (Ozawa et al., 1988). NS1 also exhibits DNA-binding properties (Raab et al., 2002), and a multitude of enzymatic functions including ATPase, helicase and site-specific endonuclease activity, as well as containing nuclear localisation signals (Li and Rhode, 1990; McCarthy et al., 1992; Jindal et al., 1994; Brown and Young, 1998). It has been demonstrated that B19 NS1 also effects G(1), but not G(2), arrest in erythroid UT7/Epo-S1 cells (Morita et al., 2003).

A single promoter, p6, is employed by B19 which is capable of differentially expressing both structural and non-structural genes (Blundell et al., 1987; Ozawa et al., 1987). The NS1 protein interacts directly with the p6 promoter and with cellular transcription factors Sp1/Sp3 to effect transcriptional regulation (Raab et al., 2002). Two additional smaller polypeptides (p7.5 and p11) have been identified, one encoded by a region near the centre of the B19 genome with a predicted M_r of 7.5 kDa and the other which is encoded at the extreme right-hand end of the genome of predicted $M_r = 11$ kDa (St Amand et al., 1991). Spliced transcripts of both proteins have been detected in infected cells but specific functions have not, as yet, been assigned to either protein (Luo, 1993).

As a result of the increased interest in, and molecular detection of, parvovirus B19 a number of new erythrovirus genotypes have been identified. Servant et al. (2002) has suggested that B19 be classified as a genotype 1 erythrovirus with newly identified strains A6 (Nguyen et al., 2002) and K71 (Hokynar et al., 2002) classified as genotypes 2 and erythrovirus V9 (Nguyen et al., 1998) as the prototype genotype 3. Based on inter-genotype phylogenetic relationships between NS1 and VP1u regions, respectively, erythrovirus genotype 3 (erythrovirus variant V9) has been shown to be the most prevalent erythrovirus in Ghana and appears to divide into two sub-types (Candotti et al., 2004).

B19 has only been shown to infect humans and replicates in human erythroid progenitor cells (late erythroid cell precursors and burst-forming erythroid progenitors (BFU-E)) of the bone marrow and blood, resulting in an inhibition of erythropoiesis (Mortimer et al., 1983). Brown et al. (1993,1994) elegantly demonstrated that the restrictive tropism of productive B19 infection is primarily due to the P blood group antigen, globoside (Gb4). This molecule is a significant cellular receptor for B19 and is most often found on cells of the erythroid lineage but also on platelets and tissues from the heart, kidney, lung, liver, endothelium and on synovia (Cooling et al., 1995; Jordan and DeLoia, 1999). Individuals lacking erythrocyte P antigens are very rare (1 in 200,000) and exhibit much diminished susceptibility to B19 infection (Brown et al., 1994; Chipman et al., 1996). However, the limited tropism of B19 is not fully understood as low-level capsid expression has actually been observed in non-permissive cells; nonetheless, intracellular factors unique to erythroid cells are thought to be essential for optimal transcription and viral replication (Ozawa et al., 1987; Kurpad et al., 1999; Gallinella et al., 2000).

Weigel-Kelley et al. (2001) have demonstrated that the P antigen-expression level on cell surfaces is not directly related to the efficiency of viral binding. In addition, despite P antigen expression and viral adherence to the P antigen, some cell lines could not be transduced with a B19 vector thereby indicating that a co-receptor is likely to be necessary for B19 entry into human cells. Thus, the presence of P antigen alone is not sufficient for B19 to gain entry into cells (Weigel-Kelley et al., 2001) and it has been suggested that multiple β-integrins may additionally function as co-receptors for B19 cellular uptake (Weigel-Kelley et al., 2003).

In vitro studies of B19 infectivity have been greatly hampered by difficulties in propagating the virus *in vitro*. Indeed, no continuous cell line propagating B19 has been established, due to the cytotoxic nature of the non-structural protein, NS1 (Ozawa et al., 1987; Momoeda et al., 1994b). However, recent studies have shown that infection under hypoxic conditions (1%(v/v) O_2) causes an upregulation of B19 expression which is associated with increased viral replication and of infectious virion production (Pillet et al., 2004). It has been demonstrated that hypoxia-inducible factor-1 (HIF-1), a key transcription factor involved in the cellular response to reduced oxygenation, binds an HIF-binding site (HBS) present in the B19 promoter region (Pillet et al., 2004). In a parallel work, Caillet-Fauquet et al. (2004) have shown that human plasma containing known amounts of B19 DNA (virus) could infect the human erythroid cell line KU812F and that under low oxygen pressure, higher yields of infectious B19 progeny virus and increased viral transcription were observed. These authors also demonstrated that anti-B19 IgG reduced B19 infectivity and suggest that system represents a promising model to study B19 infectivity and infectivity control methodologies.

Transmission of B19 infection most often occurs by personal contact via aerosol or respiratory secretions, however contaminated blood products such as clotting factor concentrates are also a source of iatrogenic transmission (Anderson et al., 1985; Lyon et al., 1989; Williams et al., 1990; Santagostino et al., 1994; Erdman et al., 1997). Significantly, B19 can also be transmitted transplacentally from an infected mother to the foetus, on occasion leading to non-immune foetal hydrops (NIHF), spontaneous abortion or intrauterine foetal death (IUFD)

(Clewley et al., 1987; Miller et al., 1998; Skjoldebrand-Sparre et al., 2000). A range of vertical transmission rates for maternal–foetal infection of 7–33% have been reported (Enders and Biber, 1990; Hall et al., 1990; Yaegashi, 2000). The P blood group antigen, which acts as a receptor for B19, has been detected on cells of the villous trophoblast of placental tissues in varying amounts during the course of pregnancy. In the first trimester, P antigen levels are elevated, begin to decline in the second trimester and become undetectable by the mid-stages of trimester 3 (Jordan and DeLoia, 1999). It has been proposed that this high level of globoside receptor on placental cells in early pregnancy may act as a pathway for mater- nal–foetus B19 transmission whereby the virus can then infect erythroid precursor cells for replication. Indeed, Wegner and Jordan (2004) have conclusively shown that I^{125}-labelled B19 VP2 capsids interact with villous cytotrophoblast cells via the P antigen. Moreover, in a detailed review of viral transmission at the uteri- ne–placental interface, Pereira et al. (2005) have shown that cytotrophoblasts in- fected with human cytomegalovirus exhibit altered differentiation patterns and suggest that such abberant behaviour may contribute to foetal growth restriction.

Clinical features and prevalence

B19 has been associated with an ever-expanding range of clinical disorders since the discovery that it is the aetiologic agent of EI, a facial and occasionally body-wide red rash. It is also associated with complications during pregnancy, acute art- hropathy, severe disease in immunocompromised patients and transient aplastic crisis.

General clinical features and chronic infection

Infection with B19 occurs worldwide and cases of infection have been reported in all seasons. Seroprevalence increases with age and by adulthood at least 70% of the adult population are B19 IgG seropositive (Cohen and Buckley, 1988). B19 out- breaks can persist for months in schools as seronegative children represent a sig- nificant reservoir for B19 infection. Recently infected children therefore are the main source of transmission in day-care centres due to the relatively large number of seronegative children and the close contact of children within this environment (Tuckerman et al., 1986; Grilli et al., 1989). The annual seroconversion rate among women of childbearing age has been estimated to be 1.5% during endemic periods and 13% during epidemics (Koch and Adler, 1989; Valeur-Jensen et al., 1999).

B19 infection has also been linked to arthritis and arthralgias, most commonly in adults but also in children (Reid et al., 1985) as has been documented for the rubella virus (Lee, 1962). On average, 50% of adult cases reported with EI have associated joint symptomologies, which may last for up to 1 month (Cassinotti et al., 1995). B19 arthritis is usually symmetrical and affects mainly the small joints of the hands, wrists and knees (Reid et al., 1985). It is more common in females and an estimated 60% of women with symptomatic disease exhibit signs of arthropathy

(White et al., 1985; Woolf et al., 1989). Symptoms generally diminish within 3 weeks without any permanent joint damage (Woolf et al., 1991), however about 20% of affected women suffer a persistent or recurrent arthropathy. About 75% of these patients have an associated rash and less than 20% have the typical 'slapped cheeks' facial exanthem. It has been hypothesised that B19-associated arthritis may be related to certain patient human leucocyte antigen (HLA) haplotypes, with individuals classified as either HLA DR4 or B27 exhibited increased susceptibility (Klouda et al., 1986; Jawad, 1993). At present, it is unclear how B19 produces symptoms associated with arthritis. Like the appearance of exanthema in EI, arthritis usually occurs after the development of B19-specific antibodies which suggests that symptoms may be due to immune-complex formation. Although the P antigen is expressed on synovium, it has been shown that synovial membrane cells are non-permissive to B19 (Miki and Chantler, 1992; Cooling et al., 1995). B19 may gain entry to B19 receptor positive cells, that are not actively dividing, resulting in the production of excessive, cytotoxic NS1 (Ozawa et al., 1988). The presence of the NS1 protein induces the expression of pro-inflammatory cytokines, which could cause the inflammation and cell damage seen in patients with B19-associated arthritis and other inflammatory and autoimmune disorders which have been associated with B19 infection (Moffatt et al., 1996; Mitchell, 2002). The precise significance of antibodies against the non-structural protein is unclear. Antibodies specific for NS1 were found in individuals manifesting persistent B19-associated arthropathy but not in convalescent serum (von Poblotzki et al., 1995a) thus suggesting a differential host response in these cohorts. However, similar NS1 antibody reactivity in patients with either chronic or acute B19-associated arthropathy (Mitchell et al., 2001) and recently infected healthy individuals (Searle et al., 1998; Ennis et al., 2001; Mitchell, et al., 2001; Heegaard et al., 2002b). Von Landenberg et al. (2003) have suggested that B19 may be directly involved in the induction of autoimmune reactions mediated, at least in part, by anti-phospholipid antibodies because of the prevalence of these antibodies in persistently B19-infected individuals.

Chronic infection with B19 may be of significance in pregnancy because, it can be speculated that, the altered maternal immune status may facilitate re-activation of viral infection (Bültmann et al., 2005). However, the clinical significance of chronic B19 infection is often unclear. Chronic infection may be due to the fact that B19 DNA persists in bone marrow, peripheral blood and synovial tissues of patients with chronic B19-associated arthropathy (Foto et al., 1993; Musiani et al., 1995; Toivanen, 1995). However, it has also been shown that although B19 DNA persisted in the synovium tissue of 28% of children presenting with chronic arthritis, an even higher proportion (48%) of seropositive immunocompetent volunteers had B19 DNA in their synovium tissues. These data suggest that B19 DNA in synovial tissue may be indirectly associated with symptoms of chronic arthropathy. None of the individuals tested had evidence of B19 DNA in synovial fluid, bone marrow or blood and all were positive for B19 IgG antibodies (Soderlund et al., 1997). Nonetheless, a recent report further enhances the correlation between B19 infection and rheumatic childhood disease (Lehmann et al., 2003). This work clearly elucidates a significant difference in serum and/or synovial fluid-derived B19 DNA ($P < 0.0001$) between control (9/124; 7%) and patient (26/74; 35%) specimens and concludes that the rate of persistent B19 infection in these patients is significantly higher than in age-matched controls. However, the recent finding of B19 DNA in 64% (14/22) of control skin biopsies compared to 50% (18/36) of chronic urticaria patients confirms that caution should be exercised in drawing conclusions regarding B19 involvement in skin disorders, and possibly in other B19-associated clinical disorders (Vuorinen et al., 2002).

B19 infection and pregnancy

Exposure to, and infection with B19 can lead to serious complications during pregnancy (Fig. 1). Infection during pregnancy may result in foetal anaemia, spontaneous abortion and hydrops foetalis (Brown et al., 1984; Kinney et al., 1988; Heegaard and Hornsleth, 1995). Seroprevalence studies have shown that approximately 30–40% of women are not immune, therefore do not possess B19 antibodies, and are consequently at risk of B19 infection. A vertical transmission rate of 33% has been reported by the United Kingdom Public Health Laboratory Service (PHLS, 1990) and similar rates have been reported in other studies (Brown et al., 1984; Hall et al., 1990), although a recent report has disclosed a transmission rate of 51% (Yaegashi, 2000). On the basis of 4 million births occurring in Europe per annum (Eurostat, 1998), an average B19 seronegativity of 30% among pregnant women and a seroconversion rate for women of child-bearing age of 0.1–1%, it can be estimated, that up to 14,000 women will seroconvert during pregnancy. About 20% of B19 infections in pregnancy are thought to result in foetal loss, thus implying that 2800 incidences of foetal death will occur each year, in Europe, as a consequence of B19 infection (Levy et al., 1997; Miller et al., 1998; Wattre et al., 1998). This figure is based solely on live births and as the number of actual pregnancies is much higher, the above estimate is conservative. Based on overall birth rates, similar incidences of foetal death due to B19 infection can be predicted for the US and Canada.

Pregnant women are most susceptible to B19 infection during epidemics and also when exposed to recently infected children in the home (Valeur-Jensen et al., 1999). During outbreaks, transmission rates of 25% in the school and 50% in the home have been reported (Anderson et al., 1990). It is somewhat unfortunate that most pregnant women acutely infected with B19 remain asymptomatic (Fig. 1), however some do experience symptoms such as exanthema and arthralgia (Komischke et al., 1997; Enders et al., 2004). As these symptoms are commonly associated with pregnancy, acute B19 infection can often be overlooked, however routine analysis of maternal immune status with respect to B19 infection would overcome this problem. Although open to debate, we propose that pregnant women should be carefully monitored during pregnancy for acute B19 infection due to the high level of seroconversion in young women and because infection with

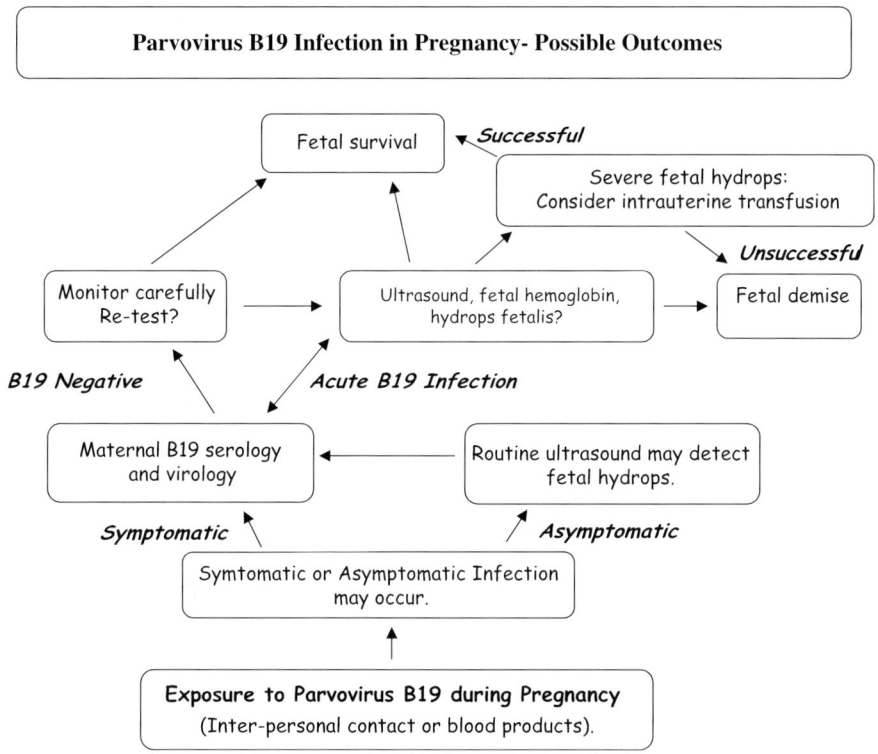

Fig. 1 Parvovirus B19 infection in pregnancy—possible outcomes. Exposure to B19 during pregnancy may result in either symptomatic or asymptomatic infection. Symptomatic infection can generally be identifed by B19 serological or virological analyses. In the case of asymptomatic maternal infection, ultrasound and foetal haemoglobin determination will be required to diagnose foetal hydrops, in addition to B19 DNA detection. Recent evidence indicates that intrauterine foetal transfusion may be an important tool in the successful treatment of severe fetal hydrops (Enders et al., 2004).

B19 during pregnancy can lead to spontaneous abortion or foetal anaemia. Given the availability of standardised and reliable diagnostic test systems, such screening should be relatively straightforward to implement.

Foetal death usually occurs 4–6 weeks postinfection but has been reported up to 12 weeks after B19 symptomatic infection (Hedrick, 1996). A study of 427 pregnant women with B19 infection in the UK found that foetal loss was limited to the first 20 weeks of gestation (Miller et al., 1998). This is supported by figures released in the UK and other studies which reported that foetal loss as a consequence of intrauterine B19 infection is highest in, but not restricted to, the first 20 weeks of gestation (PHLS, 1990; Hall et al., 1990). The outcome of one of the largest prospective studies of foetal complications as a result of serologically confirmed maternal B19 infection ($n = 1018$ individuals) was published in 2004 and provides some of the most important information to those involved in the management of B19-infected maternal infection (Enders et al., 2004). Over a 5-year period (1993–1998), B19 infection was serologically confirmed in 1018 pregnant women, 73% of whom presented without the classical symptoms of B19 infection such as rash and arthropathy. The incidences of hydrops foetalis and foetal death were 3.9% (40/1018) and 6.3% (64/1018), respectively with all foetal deaths occurring prior to 20 weeks gestation (11%; 64/579). The risk of foetal hydrops was highest when infection occurred during gestation weeks 13–20 (7.1%; 23/322). Intrauterine foetal transfusions were administered in 13/23 cases of severe foetal hydrops and a survival rate of 85% (11/13) was observed. Strikingly, no foetal survival was evident in the remaining 10/23 cases of severe foetal hydrops where intrauterine transfusion was not administered. Thus one of the major findings of this study has been that prompt intervention, via intrauterine transfusion following confirmation of severe foetal hydrops, can contribute to a reduction in the rate of foetal death (Fig. 1) (Enders et al., 2004).

Anaemia is, therefore, a key underlying factor in the development of hydrops. Foetal hydrops was initially associated with B19 infection in 1984 (Brown et al., 1984). Since then, 10–20% of cases of NIHF have been reported to be B19 associated (Yaegashi et al., 1994; Jordan, 1996), and in a study of B19 infection in Japanese women during pregnancy, the risk of hydrops was determined to be about 10% (Yaegashi et al., 1999). NIHF usually occurs 2–4 weeks after maternal B19 infection (Komischke et al., 1997). Cases of IUFD associated with foetal hydrops and caused by B19 have been most commonly reported in the second trimester and to a lesser extent in the third trimester of pregnancy (Sanghi et al., 1997). When cases of IUFD occurring during an 18-month period in the UK were examined it was discovered that 11 deaths were caused by B19 in the second trimester, and of these only three were hydropic (Wright et al., 1996). In a separate study over a 16-year period, 10 cases of IUFD were reported which were presented in gestational weeks 15–29. Of those cases, 90% of the fetuses were hydropic, 30–40% had associated heart failure and three of the maternal infections had been asymptomatic (Morey et al., 1992).

The critical time of infection has since been narrowed down to the 16th week of gestation (Yaegashi et al., 1999) with most cases of foetal loss due to B19 infection reported in the second trimester (Enders and Biber, 1990; Torok, 1990; Wattre et al., 1998). This susceptibility can be attributed, at least in part, to the relative immaturity of the foetal immune response at this stage. More importantly though, is the tropism B19 has for erythroid progenitor cells (Yaegashi, 2000) and the fact that in the second trimester of pregnancy the lifespan of foetal red blood cells (RBCs) is shortened and the RBC mass increases 3- to 4-fold during this period of gestation (Rodis et al., 1988). During an infection, B19 replication occurs within these cells which undergo apoptosis resulting in an inhibition of erythropoiesis (Morey et al., 1993). As B19 replicates, cell lysis occurs causing erythroblastopenia and therefore severe foetal anaemia, which may be fatal to the foetus. Indeed, Norbeck et al. (2004) have recently demonstrated that VP2 protein alone, or component peptides, have the potential to inhibit haematopoiesis both in and *ex vivo* and suggest its potential use for the treatment of diseases such as polycytemia vera.

However, direct inhibition of haematopoiesis by B19 VP2 may also be associated with the pathogenicity of B19 infection towards the foetus via disruption of red blood cell maturation.

Third-trimester foetal loss or IUFD caused by an acute B19 infection had not been widely reported until recently. Skjoldebrand-Sparre et al. (2000) reported that of 93 cases of IUFD examined, 7.5% had B19 DNA in the placental tissue in the absence of foetal hydrops. None of the infected pregnant women in this study showed any clinical symptoms of B19, which again reinforces the proposal of routine screening for B19 exposure during pregnancy. Skjoldebrand-Sparre et al. suggested that, in the past, B19-associated IUFD in the final stages of gestation may have been overlooked due to inadequate diagnostic procedures and also the difference in clinical features of third-trimester B19 infection. However, one of the most unusual observations in these cases of IUFD was the lack of foetal hydrops and the fact that many of the cases (5/7) had either delayed or absent B19 IgG responses. Histopathological examination of the foetuses revealed no major abnormalities. Another report of non-hydropic third-trimester IUFD associated with B19 infection has been published (Tolfvenstam et al., 2001a). Here, it was revealed by PCR analysis, of the foetal or placental tissues, that 15% of IUFD was attributable to B19 infection. This study also found delayed B19-specific antibody responses, as the mothers involved had no serological evidence of an acute B19 infection. However, follow-up studies detected B19 antibody seroconversion within 6 months. Tissue samples exhibited no signs of viral inclusions and immunochemical analysis revealed no evidence of B19 proteins (Tolfvenstam et al., 2001a). Although the concept of B19-induced third-trimester foetal loss data has proved somewhat controversial (Crowley et al., 2001; Sebire, 2001), it undoubtedly further illustrates the requirements for awareness of B19 pathogenesis and diagnostic B19 quantitative PCR screening during pregnancy. Furthermore, Nunoue et al. (2002) strongly suggest that prospective studies to evaluate the relationship between time of infection and IUFD, with and without signs of foetal hydrops, are necessary. In fact, B19 PCR may be the most sensitive way of diagnosing intrauterine B19 infection especially since more than 50% of infected foetuses test negative for B19 IgM (Dieck et al., 1999).

Although follow-up of foetal status is generally recommended to take place for up to 3 months following diagnosis of material infection, Nyman et al. (2005) have reported a case of IUFD occurring 5 months after primary diagnosis of infection and associated with prolonged B19 viraemia and the presence of serological markers. These authors have suggested that revision of current follow-up criteria may be necessary if extended viraemia is a more common occurrence than heretofore thought.

Rodriguez et al. (2002, 2005) have undertaken the analysis of NIFH in both stillborn and livebirth autopsy scenarios. Following the evaluation of 840 stillborn autopsies (Rodriguez et al., 2002), 51 cases of NIFH were observed which represented 6.07% of all stillbirths. Congenital infection, caused either by bacterial or viral infection was identified in 17 of the 51 cases of NIFH of which B19 was uniquely identified in four cases (7.8%). In fact, B19 infection was the fifth most prevalent of a total of 23 individually classified NIFH aetiologies by these authors. Subsequently, Rodriguez et al. (2005) have also studied the aetiology of NIFH in liveborn infants ($n = 429$, 14-year period) who died soon after birth. Although a similar incidence of NIFH was observed to the previous study (7.45%; 32/429), the aetiology of B19-associated NIFH, in an individual with systemic infection and myocarditis, was only 3.1% (1/32 cases). Given this lower incidence of livebirth with B19-associated NIFH, these observations support the view that the effects of B19 infection during pregnancy are more likely to result in either *in utero* foetal death or the complete resolution of infection, with, or without, the administration of appropriate therapies.

An unusual case of foetal demise, caused by B19 infection, has been described by Marton et al. (2005). Here, despite the successful administration of multiple foetal blood transfusions to prevent anaemia, foetal hydrops worsened and cardiac enlargement was observed upon foetal echocardiographic analysis which resulted in foetal death after delivery at week 31 of gestation. Subsequent autopsy found evidence of liver fibrosis. In addition, cardiomegaly and cardiac failure was caused by B19 infection and B19-infected cardiac myocytes, as shown immunohistochem-ically, were found to have undergone apoptosis. Thus, therapeutic intervention is not always successful.

Although rare, B19 infection occurs during twin pregnancies and while it ap-pears that both twins are equally susceptible to infection, individual foetus survival does occur (Wolff et al., 2005; Graesslin et al., 2005). Graesslin et al. have reported an occurrence of one foetal death at week 13 with foetal hydrops evident in the second twin. Following confirmation of B19 infection via B19 DNA detection in amniotic fluid and maternal B19 IgG reactivity, *in utero* blood transfusion raised foetal haemoglobin levels from 3.9 to 5.9 g/dl and, apart from transient my-ocarditis, the twin survived and was born normally without any negative outcome.

While much focus has rightly been placed on foetal survival following B19 infection, maternal health may not go unaffected. Bültmann et al. (2005) have recently described how peripartum cardiomyopathy (PPCM), a rare disorder whereby left ventricular dysfunction, develops in late pregnancy or early puerper-ium, may be associated with virus-associated inflammatory responses in myocytes. These authors studied 26 cases of PPCM and analysed endomyocardial biopsies for a range of viral genomes and identified B19 ($n = 4$), HHV6 ($n = 2$), CMV ($n = 1$) and EBV ($n = 1$) DNA in eight patients (30.7%). Borderline myocarditis was evident in all cases and one B19 infected patient also exhibited dilated card-iomyopathy with inflammation. Although a similar occurrence of viral DNA was detected in control patients (30.3%), no inflammatory responses were evident. Consequently, Bültmann et al. (2005) have hypothesised that changes to immune function during pregnancy may facilitate reactivation of latent viral infection, or potentiate the effects of a recent infection, resulting in inflammatory cardiomyopa-thy associated with viral infection. In any case, this study clearly shows the re-quirement for virological assessment of PPCM cases.

To date, there is very little evidence to suggest that maternal B19 infections increase the risk of congenital anomalies and generally B19 is considered to be embryocidal rather than teratogenic. However, there have been case reports of central nervous system, eye and craniofacial anomalies (Markenson and Yancey, 1998; Levy et al., 1997).

Immunity to B19 infection

Antibody-mediated immune response

Upon exposure of immunocompetent individuals to B19, high-titre B19 viraemia usually occurs within 1 week and lasts about 5 days with virus titres peaking on the first 2 days. B19-specific IgM antibodies are detected late in the viraemic stage, on about day 10–12 and can persist for up to 5 months postinfection (Anderson et al., 1985; Schwarz et al., 1988; Yaegashi et al., 1989), but in some patients can last even longer (Musiani et al., 1995). B19-specific IgG antibodies appear about 15 days postinfection, remain elevated for many months and generally persist long term (years). Antibodies against linear epitopes of the B19 VP2 protein and to some extent VP1, disappear abruptly after B19 infection whereas IgG reactivity against conformational epitopes of both VP1 and VP2 persist (Soderlund et al., 1995; Kerr et al., 1999). B19 IgA antibodies are detectable for a short period following the onset of clinical symptoms to B19 (Erdman et al., 1991) but have attracted little attention as diagnostic markers of infection. The development of the B19-specific antibody response corresponds with viral clearance and also, in the vast majority of cases of B19 infection in immunocompetent individuals, protection from subsequent infection (Anderson et al., 1985)—although absolute confirmation of protective and neutralising B19-specific antibodies has yet to be established. However, Serjeant et al. (2001) have shown that in children with sickle cell disease, only one episode of B19-associated transient aplastic crisis (TAC) is ever detected, thereby strongly suggesting an absence of re-infection.

The B19 VP1 protein, and in particular the VP1u, was thought to be the immunodominant antigen. Moreover, its incorporation into serological assays was thought essential (Rayment et al., 1990). However, it is now clear that this observation, which was based on the absence of antibodies to linear epitopes within the VP2 protein, when screened by Western blot, is erroneous. It has now been conclusively established that antibodies against capsid VP2 are maintained even when B19 IgG directed against the VP1u is lost (Kerr et al., 1999; Manaresi et al., 1999; Corcoran et al., 2000). Although, the key role of cellular immunity against B19 infection is emerging (see the section on Cellular immunity), specific anti-viral antibody is considered to represent a significant mechanism of immune protection, based on the circumstantial evidence that high-dose immunoglobulin therapy is sometimes beneficial in infected patients (Kurtzman et al., 1989b; Schwarz et al., 1990). Additionally, persistent infections associated with chronic anaemia have been observed where the immune response to B19 has failed to produce neutralising antibodies or they have been at very low levels (Kurtzman et al., 1987,1988; Coulombel et al., 1989).

Cellular immunity

Cellular immunity to parvovirus B19 has not been studied as comprehensively as the humoral response, predominantly due to the fact that antibodies were thought to be the most important response in combatting B19 infection. Initial attempts to demonstrate specific T-cell proliferative responses to B19 were unsuccessful (Kurtzman et al., 1989a) which for some time supported the prevailing theory that neutralising antibody production alone conferred immunity to B19. *Ex vivo* B19-specific CD4+ T-cells responses were first detected in 1996 against *Escherichia coli*-expressed VP1, VP2 and NS1 antigens (von Poblotzki et al., 1996). T cell responses of 16 individuals were analysed *ex vivo* (10 seropositive and six seronegative blood donors), none of whom had evidence of acute infection. Of the seropositive cohort stimulated with VP2, 90% displayed specific T-cell responses and 80% exhibited VP1-specific responses. There was no significant difference in T-cell proliferation for NS1 between seropositive and seronegative individuals. Upon inclusion of HLA class I and II-specific monoclonal antibodies it was determined that HLA class II-specific antibodies inhibited T-cell proliferation, indicating that the effector T-cell population are CD4+ cells. Subsequent peripheral blood mononuclear cells (PBMC) depletion of either CD4+ or CD8+ T cells and stimulation of the remaining population confirmed this observation.

   Subsequent studies showed significant *ex vivo* T-cell reactivity in PBMC of recently and remotely infected individuals using a B19 candidate vaccine (Franssila et al., 2001) and also B19 recombinant proteins, VP1 and VP2 (Corcoran et al., 2000). Recently infected individuals displayed very strong T-cell stimulation responses to the B19 capsids exhibiting average T-cell stimulation indices (S.I.) of 36 (Franssila et al., 2001). Blood donors with past infections gave comparable rates of T-cell stimulation. Seronegative individuals had S.I. values of about 3.3 and this study also showed that the responding population of T cells were CD4+. Although von Poblotzki et al. (1996) found no difference in T-cell responses to NS1 in seronegative and seropositive individuals, significant responses to this antigen have been reported in both recently infected individuals and patients who developed chronic arthropathy following B19 infection (Mitchell et al., 2001). T-cell responses to NS1 were not seen in the group of healthy individuals with past B19 infection except for two individuals who notably, were also NS1 IgG seropositive.

   The cellular immune response to a 15-mer epitope of NS1 that is specifically recognised by cytotoxic CD8+ T cells was investigated using major histocompatibility complex (MHC) tetrameric complex binding (Tolfvenstam et al., 2001b). The response of 21 individuals to this epitope was examined in healthy volunteers and HIV-1-infected adults and children. Sixteen of the volunteers were HLA matched (HLA B35) and 6 were mismatched; 63% of matched individuals displayed specific CD8+ T-cell responses; 72% of matched individuals in the same cohort exhibited specific T-cell responses causing the production of interferon-γ (IFN-γ). The level of B19-specific CD8 + T-cells was similar among healthy and HIV-infected individuals. The results presented in this report showed the important cellular role of cytotoxic T cells in combating B19 infection (Tolfvenstam et al., 2001b). Moreover, B19-specific T-cell responses may now represent a novel method for confirming past B19 infection.

Using a combination of *ex vivo* analytical approaches (e.g. IFN-γ ELISpot and ^{51}Cr-release assays following T-cell stimulation with peptides essentially representing the entire B19 proteome), Norbeck et al. (2005) have demonstrated that CD8 + T-cell responses are induced, and maintained for up to 2 years, following B19 infection of immunocompetent female individuals ($n = 5$). Moreover, these authors have also identified a number of HLA restricted CD8 + T-cell epitopes, most of which are located within the B19 NS1 protein. These workers further showed that while all individuals exhibited *ex vivo* IFN-γ responses to NS1 peptides, only 2/5 individuals were responsive to VP2-derived peptides and none to VP1u peptides. Norbeck et al. concluded that while CD4 + -mediated immunity is directed towards the B19 structural proteins, it appears that CD8 + cytotoxic immunity is primarily directed against epitopes located within NS1 protein and postulated that B19 may represent a model organism to explore temporally extended viral–host interactions.

The importance of evaluating T-cell responses in understanding the nature of B19 infection was demonstrated recently by Chen et al. (2001). An AIDS patient with persistent B19 infection was identified. An initial remission of B19 infection in the patient was evident despite a lack of a specific antibody response, thus indicating a role for cellular immunity in combatting B19 infection. In addition to this case, NS1-specific lymphocytes have been detected in two B19 seronegative individuals who were exposed to B19, indicating a possible sub-clinical B19 infection or perhaps a loss of antibodies against capsid proteins (Mitchell et al., 2001). Investigations by Tolfvenstam (Tolfvenstam et al., 2001b) identified two healthy immunocompetent adults and two HIV-1-infected patients, seronegative for B19, with specific CD8 + T-cell responses against B19 by either IFN-γ ELISpot or tetramer-binding studies, thus implying the presence of a cellular response in the absence of a humoral response.

The production of a number of specific cytokines has thus far been associated with B19 infection. Significant T-cell transcriptional activation has been reported in a patient with acute B19 infection, causing increased levels of interleukin (IL)-1β, IL-6 and IFN-γ messenger RNA (mRNA) (Wagner et al., 1995). In a study of recently infected children it was shown that although strong T-cell proliferative responses were evident to both capsid proteins, production of the Th1 cytokine, IFN-γ, but not IL-2, was impaired when compared to convalescent adults (Corcoran et al., 2000). Corcoran et al. also demonstrated that *ex vivo* T-cell responses from B19 seropositive compared to seronegative individuals pregnant individuals ($n = 149$) exhibited significantly higher IFN-γ levels for following VP1 ($268 + 36$ versus $103 + 19$ pg/ml; $p = 0.003$) and VP2 ($242 + 42$ versus $91 + 16$ pg/ml; $p = 0.01$) antigen stimulation. Significantly higher levels of IL-2 were also observed in B19 seropositive individuals following both VP1 ($p = 0.0003$) and VP2 ($p = 0.0005$) stimulation (Corcoran et al., 2003). However this *ex vivo* production of IFN-γ and IL-2 observed in B19 seropositive pregnant women was lower than previously observed for healthy non-pregnant individuals suggesting a possible diminution of the maternal anti-viral immune response, which may subsequently increase the risk of foetal B19 infection.

The effect of maternal immune status, during pregnancy, on B19 infection has been further clarified by the work of Franssila et al. (2005) whereby weaker T-cell proliferative responses and also specific cytokine secretions (IFN-γ and IL-10) were detected in recently infected pregnant women ($n = 3$) compared to control and recently infected non-pregnant women. In fact, there was no evidence of IL-10 production in the B19-infected pregnant individuals. Interestingly, one of the patients with no symptoms of infection displayed stronger IFN-γ responses against VP1/2 co-capsids than against VP2 capsids only, when compared to the other two pregnant and B19-infected (symptomatic) individuals. Foetal loss occurred only in the case of asymtomatic B19 infection and it could be hypothesised that the greater reactivity to B19 VP1 epitopes, demonstrated by elevated *ex vivo* production of the Th1 cytokine, IFN-γ, may in some way be associated to this observation. Overall, the relatively weaker T cell responses to B19 antigens during pregnancy, observed by Franssila et al. (2005) is in accordance with the data and proposal of Corcoran et al. (2003) that pregnancy may contribute to the pathogenicity of B19 infection through attenuation of the anti-viral immune response.

Expression of the non-structural protein, NS1, causes the production of increased levels of the inflammatory cytokine IL-6 in a number of cell lines including hematopoietic cell lines and human umbilical vein endothelial cells (Moffatt et al., 1996). IL-6 is known to be involved in synovial cell proliferation and in addition, high levels of IL-6 along with other inflammatory cytokines have been found in inflamed joints of patients with rheumatoid arthritis (RA), which would suggest an association between IL-6 production and the joint manifestations observed with B19 infection (Bataille et al., 1995). In addition to IL-6 production, high levels of IFN-γ, TNFα and IL-8 have been detected in the serum of infants with B19-associated acute myocarditis (Nigro et al., 2000). There has been some evidence to suggest that IL-2 production at the maternal–foetal interface of women who seroconvert during pregnancy will determine the outcome of the gestation. There was a trend towards more CD3+ T cells and IL-2 secretion on the foetal side from pregnancies with poor outcome, whereas IL-2 on the maternal side within the intervillous space was associated with a favourable prognosis (Jordan et al., 2001).

Diagnosis of B19 infection

Extremely accurate laboratory diagnosis of recent B19 infection or past exposure relies on testing (i) serum or plasma specimens for either specific antibody reactivity against viral capsid proteins, VP2 or VP1, expressed in eukaryotic expression systems (e.g. baculovirus-expression system) by ELISA or (ii) for B19 DNA in maternal or foetal tissues (e.g. amniotic fluid or blood) by qualitative or quantitative PCR (Fig. 2). It is important to note that B19-specific immunoassays incorporating *E. coli*-expressed B19 proteins only, which have undergone denaturation as part of a manufacturing process, will produce false-negative results due to the absence of conformational epitopes (Jordan, 2000) and the use of such systems should be avoided in the interests of patient care. A specific advantage of the eukaryotic baculovirus-expression system is its ability to enable the post-translational protein folding necessary for the generation of soluble VP2 capsids (Fig. 3) (Brown et al., 1990; Kerr et al., 1995a). Unlike B19 VP2, VP1 does not appear to form soluble capsid structures, however, VP1 has been produced as a 'conformationally intact' protein which has been shown to retain conformational epitopes present in the native virion (Brown et al., 1990; Kerr et al., 1999). Co-expression of VP1 and VP2 in eukaryotic expression systems has been proposed to result in the formation of empty capsids, which are antigenically indistinguishable from native B19 virions. Furthermore, it has been hypothesised that such co-capsids contain

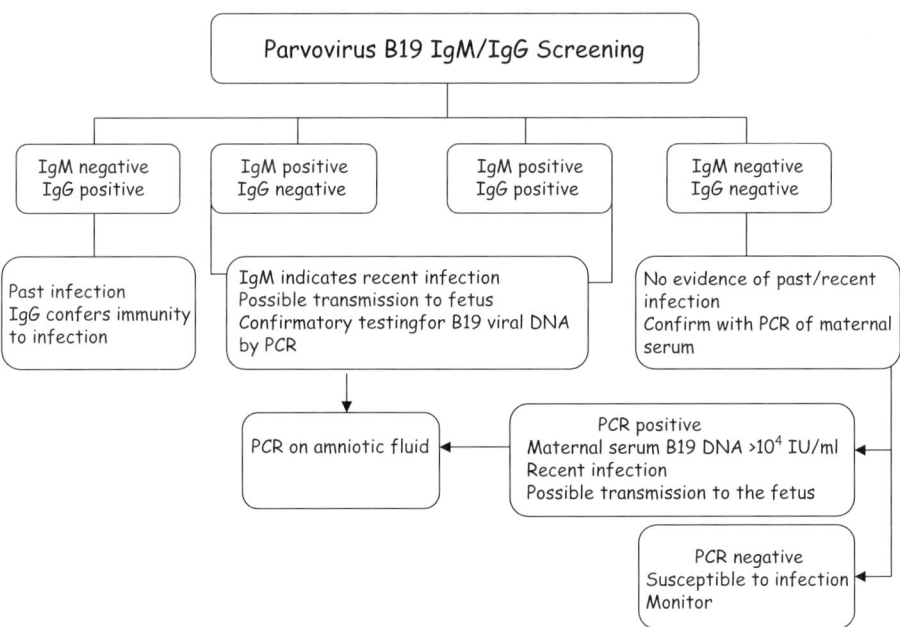

Fig. 2 Detailed serological and virological screening algorithim for the diagnosis of parvovirus B19 infection in pregnancy. Women who are exposed to parvovirus B19 should be assessed to determine if they are susceptible to infection or have an acute infection. If a woman tests negative for parvovirus B19 IgM reactivity and positive for B19 IgG, the woman is immune and can be reassured that she will not develop infection. If the woman is B19 IgG and IgM negative, the woman is not immune and could develop infection. B19 PCR analysis will confirm maternal status. If the woman is positive for B19 IgM and either positive or negative for B19 IgG reactivity, she has been recently infected and there is a risk of a transplacental infection. B19 PCR analysis of the amniotic fluid will confirm transmission to the foetus.

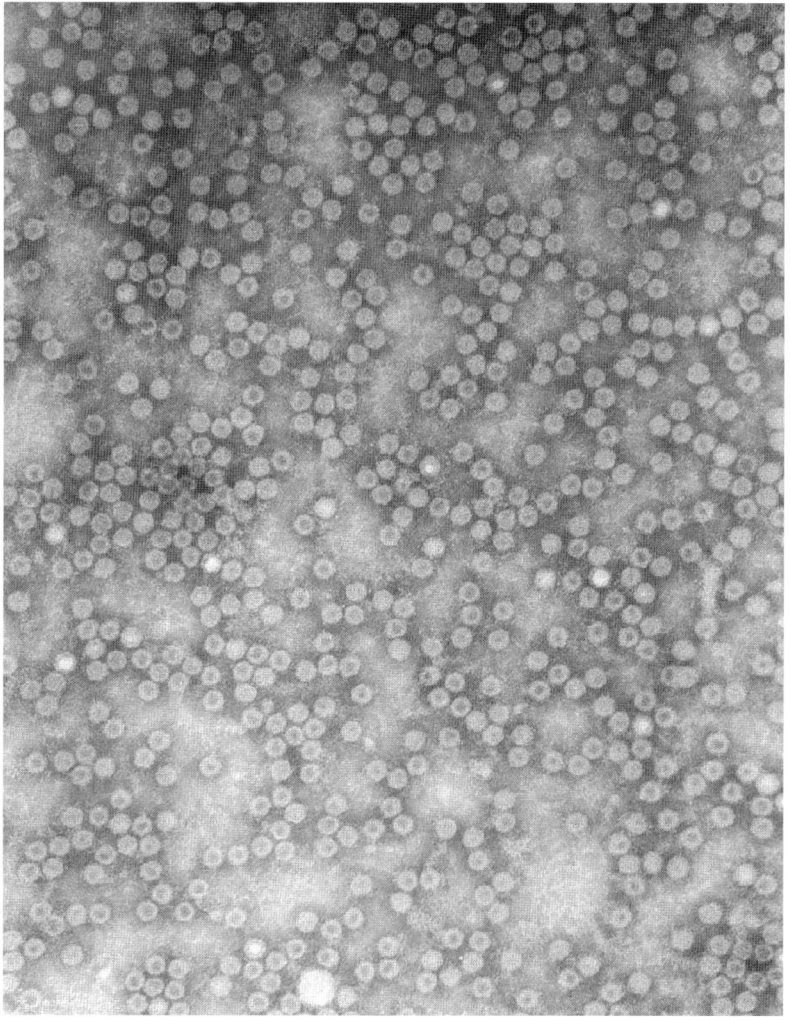

Fig. 3 Parvovirus B19 capsids. Electron microscopic image of B19 capsids, comprising recombinant B19 VP2 only, which are produced using the baculovirus expression system. These capsids are utilised in FDA approved serological assays to detect B19 IgM and IgG. Courtesy of Biotrin Limited, Dublin, Ireland.

conformational epitopes essential for accurate detection of infection (Kajigaya et al., 1989, 1991; Franssila et al., 2001; Ballou et al., 2003).

Evidence has recently emerged that B19 NS1 IgG and IgM detection may also contribute to the diagnosis of acute B19 infection, thereby supplementing the detection of B19-specific antibodies, reactive towards B19 capsid antigens, as diagnostic markers of B19 exposure (Ennis et al., 2001; Heegaard et al., 2002b).

Detection of b19 IgM

Acute B19 infections can be detected and confirmed by the presence of B19-specific IgM reactivity while past infections are detected by IgG reactivity (Anderson et al., 1985) (Fig. 2). Generally, IgM antibodies appear 7–10 days postinfection and are directed against linear and conformational epitopes of VP1 and VP2 (Palmer et al., 1996; Manaresi et al., 2001).

Only one B19 IgM diagnostic test is available that has been approved by the United States Food and Drug Administration (FDA) for the detection of B19-specific IgM as a marker of recent infection in pregnancy. This test system is a μ-capture enzyme immunoassay (EIA) that utilises highly purified recombinant B19 VP2 capsids (Fig. 3) for the detection of B19-specific IgM in either human serum or plasma. The immunoassay has a sensitivity of 89.1% and a specificity of 99.4% (Doyle et al., 2000) and is extensively used for the diagnosis of recent B19 infection (Jordan, 2000; Mitchell et al., 2001; Vuorinen et al., 2002). Validated alteration of the immunoassay cutoff, based on receiver operating charcterisitic (ROC) analysis can accommodate superior immunoassay sensitivity ($>89.1\%$) which may have a utility in the detection of lower levels of B19-specific IgM in pregnancy, immunocompromised individuals and young children (Doyle et al., 2000). Of special significance is the observation that no evidence of cross-reactivity with antibodies specific for other pregnancy-related viral infections (e.g. rubella, mumps, varicella zoster virus, cytomegalovirus and herpes simplex virus-1 (HSV-1)) and HSV-2 is apparent when this immunoassay is used in clinical settings. Although at present there is no international standard preparation for B19 IgM, the widespread utilisation of this immunoassay system means that inter-laboratory results can be compared with confidence. It should be stated that previous studies have reported cross-reactivity with rubella in several commercial B19 IgM assays (Sloots and Devine, 1996; Tolfvenstam et al., 1996) and as the symptoms of rubella infection are similar to those of B19 infection this was a cause for concern, particularly in the diagnosis of infection in pregnant women. A 5% false-positive rate was reported when specimens from healthy volunteers were analysed with a range of commercially available B19 IgM immunoassays, probably due to cross-reactivity and the lack of specificity in these immunoassays (Tolfvenstam et al., 1996). However, as of 2005 many of the systems employed in these studies are no longer available.

Beersma et al. (2005) have shown that B19 DNA levels in sera exhibit significant correlation with the presence of B19 VP2-reactive IgM (Pearson coefficient, $r = 0.44$). Moreover, these authors have demonstrated that in sera with B19 DNA loads greater than 10^6 IU/ml, B19 IgM reactivity (as defined by specimen/assay cutoff ratio) always exceeds 3.0. Thus, it is clear that the presence of B19 VP2 IgM antibodies in sera is predictive for the presence of B19 DNA. Beersma et al. also evaluated differential antibody reactivity between B19 VP1 and VP2 antigens and suggest that because only low levels of B19 DNA were present in the small number of sera (4/212) which were B19 VP1-only IgM reactive that B19 VP2 IgM is sufficient to detect highly B19 viraemic sera. These observations represent extremely useful information in a clinical context as they represent the first data correlating viral load with B19 IgM antibody levels.

Some reports have suggested that IgM directed against conformational epitopes on VP1 and VP2 proteins, and against linear epitopes on VP1, are produced at the same time postinfection and with identical frequencies. However, it has also been suggested that IgM reactivity against the minor capsid protein, VP1, may persist somewhat longer postinfection (Palmer et al., 1996; Manaresi et al., 2001). Thus, should IgM responses against conformational VP1 persist at a time when other B19-specific IgM antibodies are absent, then diagnostic techniques incorporating conformational VP1 may not be the most suitable marker of *acute* B19 infection. However, other work could elucidate no difference in IgM reactivity against conformational epitopes of the capsid proteins in diagnosing B19 infection (Kerr et al., 1999). Furthermore, these authors observed no differences in IgM reactivity against native (conformationally intact) antigens and linearised antigens for either VP1 or VP2.

Although detection of B19 NS1 IgM has received little attention as a marker of recent infection with parvovirus B19, Ennis et al. (2001) observed that 27.5% (11/40) of specimens that were B19 VP2 IgM positive also contained B19 NS1 IgM when tested by ELISA. Interestingly, when these samples were analysed by Western blot there was no evidence of NS1 IgM reactivity which indicates that conformational epitopes of the NS1 protein may be important for detection.

Detection of B19 IgG

After exposure to B19, the appearance of B19 IgG antibodies coincides with diminishing IgM antibody response, and B19 IgG reactivity against conformational epitopes of VP1 and VP2 persists postinfection (Fig. 2). However, for both capsid proteins, reactivity against linear epitopes declines postinfection, abruptly against VP2 but more slowly against VP1 (Soderlund et al., 1995; Kaikkonen et al., 1999; Kerr et al., 1999; Manaresi et al., 1999)—an observation which has significant consequences for diagnosis. Antibody reactivity against linear VP2 epitopes, predominantly directed against a heptapeptide (amino acids 344–350) identified by analysis of acute-phase sera (Kaikkonen et al., 1999), usually disappears within 6 months of B19 infection (Soderlund et al., 1995). Thus detection of B19-specific IgG, directed against linear epitopes of VP2, may assist in timing B19 exposure to within a 6-month period.

Although the antibody response wanes against linear epitopes on B19 capsid proteins it persists against conformational epitopes of both capsid proteins. Only one FDA approved B19 IgG immunoassay is available to detect B19 IgG as a marker of past infection (Corcoran et al., 2000). This microplate immunoassay which utilises capsid VP2 to detect B19 and erythrovirus V9 (genotype 3) IgG (Heegaard et al., 2002a; Candotti et al., 2004; Corcoran et al., 2005b) (Fig. 3). In studies undertaken to fulfill FDA approval criteria, inter-assay reproducibility data for this B19 IgG-specific immunoassay was determined by blinded analysis of a panel of unreactive, weakly reactive and reactive B19 IgG specimens ($n = 16$) across three separate manufactured lots of the immunoassay, at three test sites, over a 3-day period. Consequently, each specimen was assayed three times per day (in duplicate) per lot, on three different days, at each of the three laboratories ($n = 81$ assays per specimen). Total inter-assay reproducibility was excellent, and % coefficient of variation (%CV), ranged from 11.2 to 21.8%CV or 15.6 to 26.8%CV when expressed in terms of either immunoassay index (specimen/cutoff ratio) or OD values, respectively. Linear regression analysis of inter-site data confirmed the high reproducibility and robustness associated with the B19 IgG-specific immunoassay and correlation coefficients of 0.99 were observed for both index and OD values, respectively, for both inter-site (site 1 versus 2, site 2 versus 3 and 1 versus 3) and all inter-lot comparative scenarios. Comparative studies of this baculovirus-based immunoassay to another commercially available *E. coli*-based VP1 immunoassay for the detection of B19 antibodies in pregnant women have been undertaken and confirmed the accuracy of diagnosis, and absence of equivocal results, of the VP2 capsid immunoassay system (Jordan, 2000). The availability of a B19 IgG international standard (2nd International Standard 2003; code 01/602; 77 IU/ampoule) further contributes to the accurate confirmation of past B19 infection by standardising B19 IgG determination from different laboratories using different test systems (Ferguson et al., 1997; Searle et al., 1997).

Candotti et al. (2004) have recently presented controversial data which suggested that enzyme immunoassays utilising B19 VP2 capsids derived from genotype 1 did not detect a subset of erythrovirus genotype 3 (V9)-derived IgG. These findings have been disputed (Corcoran et al., 2005b) and work is currently underway to resolve this significant issue. Initial data (not shown) from analysis of blinded specimens suggest that B19 VP2 capsids can indeed detect all V9-derived IgG, a finding which confirms the diagnostic utility of this validated immunoassay system and that VP1 presence is not necessary to diagnose B19 infection.

The importance of NS1-specific IgG merits consideration with view to improved diagnosis of acute B19 infection. Although the presence of B19 NS1 IgG was originally proposed to be associated with persistent B19 infection (von Poblotzki et al., 1995a, b), it now appears to be the case that no significant difference between the level of NS1 IgG in control patients with past infection and those with chronic B19 infection is evident (Searle et al., 1998; Venturoli et al., 1998; Jones et al., 1999). In addition, Tolfvenstam et al. (2000) have mapped B-cell epitopes on NS1 and identified three antigenic regions (amino acids 191–206, 271–286, 371–386), which exhibited equal reactivity towards antibodies from healthy individuals with past B19 infection and B19-persistently infected patients. Hemauer et al. (2000) showed that NS1 IgG reactivity was most prevalent in serum following recent infection in pregnant women (61%) which, in turn, was supported by the work of Mitchell et al. (2001). Mitchell et al. examined NS1 IgG reactivity in sera from a range of cohorts (i.e. individuals (i) infected with B19, (ii) who had been exposed to B19 but were not infected, (iii) who were suffering from a rash illness, chronic arthropathy or (iv) were healthy controls) and observed that NS1 IgG reactivity was predominant in recently infected specimens. Moreover, when subsequent specimens from these individuals were analysed, the level of NS1-specific IgG reactivity had declined. In addition there was no evidence of a correlation between NS1-specific IgG and the onset or development of arthropathy (Mitchell et al., 2001). Ennis et al. (2001) demonstrated that 69% of children recently infected with B19 were NS1 IgG seropositive and Heegaard et al. (2002b) also observed a seroprevalence of 60% B19 NS1 IgG in recently infected individuals (<6 weeks postinfection) and suggest that NS1 IgG detection may significantly improve immunoassay sensitivity. Thus as the NS1-specific IgG response diminishes, as the virus is cleared, NS1 IgG reactivity may contribute to accurate diagnosis as a marker of recent infection, in parallel with the detection of IgG against linear epitopes on VP2 (Ennis et al., 2001).

In summary, detection of B19-specific IgM indicates recent infection with B19 and B19 IgG detection confirms past exposure. Detection is optimal in immunoassays utilising VP2 capsids for antibody detection. Antibody detection against B19 NS1 protein may contribute to the confirmation of recent B19 infection but only when in association with standardised VP2 capsid-based immunoassays. Genotype 3 (erythrovirus V9) antibody detection is also feasible using immunoassays based on B19 VP2 capsids.

B19 DNA detection by PCR

Without doubt, the most sensitive method of diagnosis of B19 infection in pregnancy is the detection of B19 viral DNA in maternal–foetal blood or tissue by PCR. Many clinical laboratories now provide parallel B19 antibody screening and diagnostic PCR which greatly improves the sensitivity of detection of B19 infection (Skjoldebrand-Sparre et al., 2000; Manaresi et al., 2002). However, caution must be exercised with regard to the deployment of B19 PCR for a number of reasons: (1) the high viral titres associated with B19 infection may cause cross-contamination of samples and hence cause PCR false positivity. This is particularly problematic when nested PCR is used for B19 detection. (2) Low levels of B19 DNA may remain in the host long after infection thus, B19 DNA detection may not always be indicative of an acute infection. B19 viral titres can reach greater than 10^{12} genome equivalents per ml (ge/ml) (Prowse et al., 1997) during the stage of acute infection. In healthy, immunocompetent individuals viral DNA is detectable for at least 1 month postinfection (Erdman et al., 1991) but has also been shown to persist at low levels for long periods (Cassinotti et al., 1993; Kerr et al., 1995b; Musiani et al., 1995; Cassinotti and Siegl, 2000). In cases of chronic B19 infection, viral DNA can persist in the host without the presence of B19-specific IgM or IgG (Kurtzman et al., 1988; Frickhofen et al., 1990). Thus, B19 DNA detected by qualitative PCR analysis is not always indicative of recent infection. In fact, quantitative PCR was used by Cassinotti and Siegl (2000) to determine the amount of B19 viral DNA in an immunocompetent patient from the time of acute B19 infection until convalescence. Over a 1-year period a series of blood samples were taken and analysed using a real-time PCR analysis. The B19 viral titre reached levels of 8.8×10^9 ge/ml of blood during the viremic stage of infection. At this point the patient was positive for B19-specific IgM but had no evidence of IgG reactivity. By week 164 the viral load had declined to 95 ge/ml, IgM reactivity was lost and IgG reactivity against B19 capsid proteins was strong. Subsequent specimens taken had no detectable B19 DNA. Thus, while the actual amount of circulating B19 DNA present following B19 infection diminished dramatically after the first few weeks of infection, it persisted for some time before being cleared from the host despite the development of circulating B19 IgG. This slow rate of B19 DNA clearance from an immunocompetent host could have a negative impact on PCR as a diagnostic tool in differentiating between recent and chronic B19 infection in a situation where a qualitative PCR assay, of unspecified sensitivity of detection is employed. (3) Many PCR assays are developed in-house and employ primer pairs of undefined sensitivity of detection. (4) Many extraction methods are suitable for DNA purification from serum or plasma only and not from solid tissue (e.g. placenta or foetal tissue). (5) Finally , false negativity may be observed with respect to non-B19 strains (e.g. erythrovirus V9, K71 or A6) due to minor sequence differences (Hokynar et al., 2002; Nguyen et al., 2002; [Servant et al., 2002). An in-house nested PCR assay capable of accurately detecting V9 and B19 DNA simultaneously has been developed (Heegaard et al., 2001), which comprises of a primary round of amplification using a pair of consensus primers and a subsequent round of amplification using separate primers for B19 and V9. Using this PCR assay, clinical samples, including 100 B19 IgM-positive specimens and untreated plasma pools representing 100,000 blood donor units from the Danish population, were screened for both V9 and B19 DNA. None of the specimens analysed were positive for V9 DNA, which may be due to the fact that this V9 erythrovirus isolate is an emerging virus and may actually be more divergent than previously thought (Heegaard et al., 2001).

PCR analysis has also revealed another B19 viral genotype, K71, which persists in human skin and has a nucleotide divergence of 10.8% from B19 and 8.6% from V9 (Hokynar et al., 2002). Many of the aforementioned issues associated with 'home-brew' PCR tests to detect the parvovirus B19 in clinical specimens can be overcome with the use of commercially available test systems. Analysis of two commercially available validated quantitative B19 PCR systems, the LightCycler-Parvovirus B19 quantification kit (Roche Diagnostics; http://www.roche-diagnostics.com/) and the RealArt Parvo B19 LC PCR (Artus; http://www.artus-biotech2.com) was performed by Hokynar et al. (2004) to examine their ability to detect, quantify and also differentiate between genotypes. The study revealed that although the Roche system was capable of detecting genotype 1 DNA at high sensitivity, it proved unsuitable for genotype 2, and to some extent, genotype 3 DNA detection. Conversely, the quantitative PCR system manufactured by Artus proved equally efficacious with respect to genotype detection, although again, high-sensitivity genotype 3 DNA detection was somewhat problematic. Schneider et al.

(2004) and Liefeldt et al. (2005) have also recently reported high-sensitivity strategies for quantitative detection and differentiation of all three erythrovirus genotypes.

Notwithstanding these limitations, B19 PCR is an effective technique used to detect B19 infection. In addition, with the introduction of the WHO International Standard for Parvovirus B19 DNA (NIBSC 99/800), PCR assay standardisation has become possible whereby B19 DNA units are quoted in International Units/ml (IU/ml) (Saldanha et al., 2002). Using the WHO standard, a number of compatible B19 PCR assay systems have been established (Daly et al., 2002; Müller et al., 2002; Thomas et al., 2003) and, using real-time PCR technology, a sensitivity of detection of 15.4 IU/ml (10 Baxter-Units/ml) was reached (Aberham et al., 2001).

Alternative detection methods

In cases of foetal infection and also in the immunocompromised host, when no B19-specific antibodies are present, patient histology can be used to assist with the confirmation of B19 infection in foetal tissue, whereby characteristic B19 inclusion bodies can be visualised either by DNA hybridisation or by antigen-detection techniques (van Elsacker-Niele, 1998). However, although these techniques are specific, sensitivity of detection remains problematic (van Elsacker-Niele and Kroes, 1999). Assays based on exploitation of the P antigen receptor of B19, known as receptor-mediated hemagglutination (RHA), have been proposed as a cheap way of screening plasma and apparently detect whole virus, however the assay sensitivity is low when compared to PCR and, more importantly, it has not been assessed in an obstetrics context (Cohen and Bates, 1995; Sato et al., 1995; Wakamatsu et al., 1999). In cases where patients are treated with intravenous immunoglobulin (IVIG) to treat chronic B19 infection, assessment of antigen-specific B cell memory allows one to discriminate IVIG- and individual-derived B19 IgG, which is important in determining the seroconversion status of the individual (Corcoran et al., 2005a).

Elevated maternal serum alpha fetoprotein (MSAFP) levels have been associated with foetal parvovirus B19 infection, probably due to damage to foetal liver cells, thus MSAFP levels could potentially serve as an indirect indicator of foetal infection (Carrington et al., 1987; Bernstein and Capeless, 1989). However, the sensitivity of this test is unknown and as several cases have reported severe foetal infection with normal levels of MSAFP (Saller et al., 1993; Johnson et al., 1994), the association between elevated MSAFP levels and B19 foetal infection is weak and, therefore, cannot be accepted as a reliable marker of infection.

The most reliable way to diagnose acute foetal infection is to detect B19 DNA in amniotic fluid or foetal serum by PCR or viral particles by electron microscopy. Clinical use of these tests however remains to be evaluated. Although B19 infection can be diagnosed through PCR analysis of amniotic fluid obtained by amniocentesis, invasive diagnosis of infection is not required for all suspected/confirmed maternal infections. It must be noted that viral particles are only present at the viremic stage and the method used to detect these, an EIA, is generally insensitive. The presence of B19 IgM in foetal blood cannot be depended on to make a diagnosis of foetal infection as IgM appears in foetal circulation only after 22 gestational weeks (Rodis et al., 1988). Even beyond 22 weeks of foetal development IgM diagnosis can present misleading false-negative results (Pryde et al., 1992).

Blood product safety and pregnancy

Currently, there is no strategy for the best management of foetal hydrops caused by B19 infection during pregnancy but many cases are treated with intravascular transfusion. In a survey of maternal–foetal medicine specialists involving 539 cases of B19-induced hydrops, death occurred after intrauterine transfusion in 6% of cases, and in 30% of cases without intrauterine transfusion (Rodis et al., 1998). Treatment of B19 infection with transfused blood is not always effective and it is imperative that one is cognisant of the potential presence of high titre B19 virus in blood products (Prowse et al., 1997; Santagostino et al., 1997).

Screening of blood donations for the presence of B19 DNA is not routine (Blumel et al., 2002) despite the fact that this virus is highly resilient and can withstand denaturation even at high temperatures (Santagostino et al., 1994). In fact, B19 is thought to withstand processes involving solvent–detergent treatment, lyophilisation and temperatures of $100\,^{\circ}C$ for 30 min, and despite these harsh virucidal processes, still have the capacity to contaminate factor VIII and factor IX concentrates (Santagostino et al., 1997). B19 contamination of such purified blood products is particularly problematic as, in the absence of B19 IgG, the infectious potential of B19 may be enhanced (Blumel et al., 2002). The most-recent determination of B19 prevalence is 1 in 837 blood donations ($n = 5025$, range 7.1×10^4 to 2.1×10^{12} IU B19 DNA/ml) (Henriques et al., 2005) Previously, B19 levels had been estimated to be present in 1:16,000 transfusions based on the average incidence of B19 in a non-epidemic period (320 cases per 100,000 population) and the fact that viraemia lasts about 7 days (Prowse et al., 1997). During epidemics the incidence of viraemia in donations is greatly increased with levels reported as high as 1:167 in Japan (Yoto et al., 1995).

The infectious level of parvovirus B19 in blood products has yet to be established with certainty and is likely to depend on the amount of neutralising B19 IgG co-present in the product, in addition to recipient immune status. As part of a phase IV study, a group of 100 healthy volunteers, seronegative for B19, were given 1 unit of plasma that had been solvent/detergent treated (Davenport et al., 2000). Of the volunteers subsequently screened for incidences of B19 infection, 18% had seroconverted over the subsequent 3 months. Three of the 10 batches of plasma used in the study were retrospectively found to contain high levels of B19 ($> 10^7$ ge/ml) and these batches coincided with the plasma administered to the volunteers who seroconverted. Interestingly, batches with low amounts of B19 ($< 10^4$ ge/ml) did not cause B19 seroconversion. Presently, plasma lots containing high levels of B19 are eliminated from manufacturing batches of plasma. Thus, there is a level of virus, as yet undetermined, that will not cause B19 infection. Notably, Daly et al. (2002) undertook a retrospective study of similar plasma pools ($n = 30$) to those utilised in the study of Davenport et al. (2000) and found B19 IgG levels in the range $64.7 + 17.5\,IU/ml$. Thus it is possible that this level of B19 IgG may be capable of preventing recipient B19 infection when transfused with plasma contaminated with low levels of parvovirus B19 ($<10^4\,ge/ml$). Blumel et al., 2002 however, identified two incidences of B19 transmission by separate lots of clotting factor concentrates, one with $8.6 \times 10^6\,ge/ml$ (volume: 180 ml) and the other shown to have $4 \times 10^3\,ge/ml$ B19 DNA (volume: 966 ml), which were responsible for seroconversion.

Despite the fact that B19 infection can be transmitted via contaminated blood products, regulatory requirements relating to B19 contamination of pooled plasma or blood products prior to product release have only recently been implemented. The European Pharmacopoeia now stipulates that B19 DNA levels must be less than $10^4\,IU/ml$ in plasma pools destined for anti-D IgG manufacture (European Pharmacopoeia, 2004). However, it should be acknowledged that many manufacturers now perform B19 PCR on plasma mini-pools to eliminate high B19 viral load plasma (Aberham et al., 2001) and many blood banks supply this upon request under the designation 'Parvo-safe blood'. PCR screening of blood products has been shown to facilitate removal of 23 B19 PCR-positive donations from a plasma pool of 6000 resulting in a 10–100-fold decrease in viral load (Prowse et al., 1997).

Nonetheless, the issue of whether high-risk populations, such as pregnant women, immunocompromised patients and people with chronic anaemia, should undergo administration of any B19-containing products while the level of infectious B19 DNA is unknown, and minipool screening is not mandatory, must be addressed. The aforementioned availability of an international standard preparation of B19 DNA (Saldanha et al., 2002) in addition to a number of compatible and quantitative B19 PCR detection systems (Aberham et al., 2001; Daly et al., 2002; Knoll et al., 2002; Müller et al., 2002; Thomas et al., 2003), should alleviate problems caused by ambiguity between results from laboratories using various methods of measuring and expressing B19 DNA levels and help determine the infectious dose for parvovirus B19.

Treatment and vaccination

Parvovirus B19 infection is self-limiting in the immunocompetent host and, therefore, no specific therapy is required for such individuals. However, in cases where individuals suffer from arthritic complications, symptoms can be treated with non-steroidal anti-inflammatory drugs. The administration of high-titre IVIG has proven successful in the treatment of patients with chronic infection but this is expensive and remission may be temporary in the immunocompromised host (Kurtzman et al., 1989b; Fukushige et al., 1995; Lui et al., 2001). In addition, IVIG treatment does not work in all cases and no data is available on the actual protective level of B19 IgG although levels greater than 6 IU/ml are thought to be protective (Searle et al., 1997). For cases of foetal infection, intrauterine blood transfusions may be beneficial especially in the case of hydrops but this procedure does involve additional risks to the outcome of pregnancy (Berry et al., 1992; Cameron et al., 1997; Bousquet et al., 2000; Enders et al., 2004).

If B19 infection occurs during pregnancy, the pregnancy should be allowed to proceed but carefully monitored. In cases of mild hydrops or with evidence of resolution of hydrops, foetuses should be closely monitored by ultrasound to detect any signs of hydrops, oedema, ascites and effusions (Morgan-Capner and Crowcroft, 2002). If hydrops worsens, a diagnostic cordocentesis and foetal blood transfusion should be considered. Currently, primary management of hydropic foetuses is cordocentesis to assess foetal haemoglobin and reticulocyte count, and intrauterine transfusion, if necessary (Markenson et al., 1998). A reticulocyte count in a foetal blood sample could provide evidence of bone marrow recovery. At present there is no reliable way to predict prognosis for individual foetuses and termination of pregnancy should not be recommended (Barrett et al., 1994). At delivery, examination of the cord blood for B19 IgM will reveal whether the virus has crossed the placenta and infected the foetus. The child should be carefully followed up for several weeks to check for any delayed sequelae.

The administration of high-titre IVIG has proven successful in treating foetal hydrops in some cases (Selbing et al., 1995; Alger, 1997). Alternatively, clinical symptoms of infection have been treated effectively by intrauterine blood transfusions (Schwarz et al., 1988; Hansmann et al., 1989). A study by Wattré reported two cases where intrauterine blood transfusions led to the cessation of symptoms and to the birth of normal babies (Wattre et al., 1998). In a separate study, 38 cases of B19-associated foetal hydrops were reported, 12 of whom received intrauterine blood transfusion. Although three of these foetuses subsequently died, the probability of death among fetuses that did not receive a blood transfusion was significantly higher (Fairley et al., 1995). In addition, spontaneous resolution of hydrops without intervention has been reported thus suggesting that treatment is not always necessary (Pryde et al., 1992).

Infection with B19 and rubella can be detrimental to the foetus if the mother is infected during pregnancy. However, primary infection with rubella in the first trimester of pregnancy is associated with a high risk of congenital abnormalities (Gibbs and Sweet, 1994; Pastuszak, 1994) unlike B19 infection, which is most likely to affect the foetus adversely during the second or third trimester (Tolfvenstam et al., 2001a). As both infections present with similar symptoms, it is essential to distinguish between the two infections to decide upon the appropriate course of action.

The major finding that intrauterine foetal transfusion to treat severe foetal hydrops was associated with 85% foetal survival and that no foetal survival was apparent in the absence of intrauterine transfusion (Enders et al., 2004) is perhaps the most compelling evidence that this therapeutic strategy should be given serious consideration should B19 infection occur during pregnancy.

As of 2005, there is no effective vaccine against B19 infection available for either seronegative pregnant women or for immunosuppressed individuals. A possible candidate vaccine comprising baculovirus-expressed B19 empty virus-like particles (VLP) is presently under evaluation which is the first B19 vaccine to reach human trials and is sponsored by MedImmune, Inc (Gaithersburg, MD) (Bansal et al., 1993). Ballou et al. (2003) have recently shown that the recombinant vaccine (MEDI-491; Medimmune), comprises B19 VP1 and VP2 capsid proteins, could elicit neutralising antibody titres in volunteer adults ($n = 24$). Sera from immunised individuals was also shown to be capable of inhibiting *in vitro* B19 replication. The efficacy of this formulation to prevent infection with parvovirus B19 remains to be established, nonetheless it is an encouraging and welcome advance in the fight against this insidious pathogen.

Acknowledgements

The authors wish to acknowledge both the European Union (Grant number: QLK2-CT-2001-00877) and the Irish Health Research Board for financial support (1998–2004). Biotrin Limited is also acknowledged for granting permission to include previously unpublished data.

References

Aberham C, Pendl C, Gross P, Zerlauth G, Gessner MA. Quantitative, internally controlled real-time PCR assay for the detection of parvovirus B19 DNA. J Virol Methods 2001; 92: 183–191.

Alger LS. Toxoplasmosis and parvovirus B19. Infect Dis Clin North Am 1997; 11: 55–75.

Anderson LJ, Gillespie SM, Torok TJ, Hurwitz ES, Tsou CJ, Gary GW. Risk of infection following exposures to human parvovirus B19. Behring Inst Mitt 1990; 85: 60–63.

Anderson MJ, Higgins PG, Daies LR, Willman JS, Jones SE, Kidd IM, Pattison JR, Tyrell DAJ. Experimental parvovirus infection in humans. J Infect Dis 1985; 153: 257–265.

Anderson MJ, Jones SE, Fisher-Hoch SP, Lewis E, Hall SM, Bartlett CLR, Cohen BJ, Mortimer PP, Pereira MS. Human parvovirus, the cause of erythema infectiosum (fifth disease). Lancet 1983; 1: 1378.

Ballou WR, Reed JL, Noble W, Young NS, Koenig S. Safety and immunogenicity of a recombinant parvovirus B19 vaccine formulated with MF59C.1. J Infect Dis 2003; 187: 675–678.

Bansal GP, Hatfield JA, Dunn FE, Kramer AA, Brady F, Riggin CH, Collett MS, Yoshimoto K, Kajigaya S, Young NS. Candidate recombinant vaccine for human B19 parvovirus. J Infect Dis 1993; 167: 1034–1044.

Barrett J, Ryan G, Morrow R, Farine D, Kelly E, Mahony J. Human parvovirus B19 during pregnancy. J Soc Obstet Gynaecol Can 1994; 16: 1253–1258.

Bataille R, Barlogie B, Lu ZY, Rossi JF, Lavabre-Bertrand T, Beck T, Wijdeness J, Brochier J, Klein B. Biologic effects of anti-interleukin-6 murine monoclonal antibody in advanced multiple myloma. Blood 1995; 86: 685–691.

Beersma MF, Claas EC, Sopaheluakan T, Kroes AC. Parvovirus B19 viral loads in relation to VP1 and VP2 antibody responses in diagnostic blood samples. J Clin Virol 2005; 34: 71–75.

Bernstein IM, Capeless EL. Elevated maternal serum alpha-fetoprotein and hydrops fetalis in association with fetal parvovirus B-19 infection. Obstet Gynecol 1989; 74: 456–457.

Berry PJ, Gray ES, Porter HJ, Burton PA. Parvovirus infection of the human fetus and newborn. Semin Diagn Pathol 1992; 9: 4–12.

Blumel J, Schmidt I, Effenberger W, Seitz H, Willkommen H, Brackmann HH, Lower J, Eis-Hubinger AM. Parvovirus B19 transmission by heat-treated clotting factor concentrates. Transfusion 2002; 42: 1473–1481.

Blundell MC, Beard C, Astell CR. *In vitro* identification of a B19 parvovirus promoter. Virology 1987; 157: 534–538.

Bousquet F, Segondy M, Faure JM, Deschamps F, Boulot P. B19 parvovirus-induced fetal hydrops: good outcome after intrauterine blood transfusion at 18 weeks of gestation. Fetal Diagn Ther 2000; 15: 132–133.

Brown CS, Salimans MMM, Noteborn MHM, Weiland HT. Antigenic parvovirus B19 coat proteins VP1 and VP2 produced in large quantities in a baculovirus expression system. Virus Res 1990; 15: 197–212.

Brown KE, Anderson SM, Young NS. Erythrocyte P antigen: cellular receptor for B19 parvovirus. Science 1993; 262: 114–117.

Brown KE, Hibbs JR, Gallinella G, Anderson SM, Lehman ED, McCarthy P, Young NS. Resistance to parvovirus B19 infection due to lack of virus receptor (erythrocyte P antigen). N Engl J Med 1994; 330: 1192–1196.

Brown KE, Young NS. Human parvovirus B19 infections in infants and children. Adv Pediatr Infect Dis 1998; 13: 101–126.

Brown T, Anand A, Richie LD, Clewley JP, Reid TM. Intrauterine parvovirus infection associated with hydrops fetalis. Lancet 1984; 2: 1033–1034.

Bültmann BD, Klingel K, Nabauer M, Wallwiener D, Kandolf R. High prevalence of viral genomes and inflammation in peripartum cardiomyopathy. Am J Obstet Gynecol 2005; 193: 363–365.

Caillet-Fauquet P, Draps ML, Di Giambattista M, de Launoit Y, Laub R. Hypoxia enables B19 erythrovirus to yield abundant infectious progeny in a pluripotent erythroid cell line. J Virol Methods 2004; 121: 145–153.

Cameron AD, Swain S, Patrick WJ. Human parvovirus B19 infection associated with hydrops fetalis. Aust NZ J Obstet Gynaecol 1997; 37: 316–319.

Candotti D, Etiz N, Parsyan A, Allain JP. Identification and characterization of persistent human erythrovirus infection in blood donor samples. J Virol 2004; 78: 12169–12178.

Carrington D, Whittle MJ, Gibson AAM, Brown T, Field AM, Gilmore DH, Aitken D, Patrick WJA, Caul EO, Clewley JP, Cohen BJ. Maternal serum alpha-fetoprotein-a marker of fetal aplastic crisis during intrauterine human parvovirus infection. Lancet 1987; 1: 433–435.

Cassinotti P, Bas S, Siegl G, Vischer TL. Association between human parvovirus B19 infection and arthritis. Ann Rheum Dis 1995; 54: 498–500.

Cassinotti P, Siegl G. Quantitative evidence for persistence of human parvovirus B19 DNA in an immunocompetent individual. Eur J Clin Microbiol Infect Dis 2000; 19: 886–887.

Cassinotti P, Weitz M, Siegl G. Human parvovirus B19 infections: routine diagnosis by a new nested polymerase chain reaction assay. J Med Virol 1993; 40: 228–234.

A. Corcoran, S. Doyle

Chen MY, Hung CC, Fang CT, Hsieh SM. Reconstituted immunity against persistent parvovirus B19 infection in a patient with acquired immunodeficiency syndrome after highly active antiretroviral therapy. Clin Infect Dis 2001; 32: 1361–1365.

Chipman PR, Agbandje-McKenna M, Kajigaya S, Brown KE, Young NS, Baker TS, Rossmann MG. Cryo-electron microscopy studies of empty capsids of human parvovirus B19 complexed with its cellular receptor. Proc Natl Acad Sci USA 1996; 93: 7502–7506.

Clewley JP. Biochemical characterisation of a human parvovirus. J Gen Virol 1984; 65: 241–245.

Clewley JP, Cohen BJ, Field AM. Detection of parvovirus B19 DNA, antigen, and particles in the human fetus. J Med Virol 1987; 23: 367–376.

Cohen BJ, Bates CM. Evaluation of 4 commercial test kits for parvovirus B19-specific IgM. J Virol Methods 1995; 55: 11–25.

Cohen BJ, Buckley MM. The prevalence of antibodies to human parvovirus B19 in England and Wales. J Med Microbiol 1988; 25: 151–153.

Corcoran A, Crowley B, Dewhurst C, Pizer BL, Doyle S. Establishment of functional B cell memory against parvovirus B19 capsid proteins may be associated with resolution of persistent infection. J Med Virol 2005a; 78: 125–128.

Corcoran A, Doyle S, Allain JP, Candotti D, Parsyan A. Evidence of serological cross-reactivity between genotype 1 and genotype 3 erythrovirus infections. J Virol 2005b; 79: 5238–5239.

Corcoran A, Doyle S, Waldron D, Nicholson A, Mahon BP. Impaired gamma interferon responses against parvovirus B19 by recently infected children. J Virol 2000; 74: 9903–9910.

Corcoran A, Mahon BP, McParland P, Davoren A, Doyle S. *Ex vivo* cytokine responses against parvovirus B19 antigens in previously infected pregnant women. J Med Virol 2003; 70: 475–480.

Cooling LL, Koerner TA, Naides SJ. Multiple glycosphingolipids determine the tissue tropism of parvovirus B19. J Infect Dis 1995; 172: 1198–1205.

Cossart YE, Field A, Cant B, Widdows D, Parvovirus-like particles in human sera. Lancet 1975; 1: 72–73.

Cotmore SF, Tattersall P. Characterization and molecular cloning of a human parvovirus genome. Science 1984; 226: 1161–1165.

Coulombel L, Morinet F, Mielot F. Parvovirus infection, leukemia and immunodeficiency. Lancet 1989; 1: 101–102.

Crowley B, Kokai G, Cohen B. Human parvovirus B19 and fetal death. Lancet 2001; 358: 1180–1181.

Daly P, Corcoran A, Mahon BP, Doyle S. High-sensitivity PCR detection of parvovirus B19 in plasma. J Clin Microbiol 2002; 40: 1958–1962.

Davenport R, Geohas G, Cohen S, Beach K, Lazo A, Lucchesi K, Pehta J. Phase IV study of Plas + ᴿSD:Hepatitis A (HAV) and parvovirus B19 (B19) safety results. Blood 2000; 96: 1942.

Dieck D, Schild RL, Hansmann M, Eis-Hubinger AM. Prenatal diagnosis of congenital parvovirus B19 infection: value of serological and PCR techniques in maternal and fetal serum. Prenat Diagn 1999; 19: 1119–1123.

Doyle S, Kerr S, O'Keeffe G, O'Carroll D, Daly P, Kilty C. Detection of parvovirus B19 IgM by antibody capture enzyme immunoassay: receiver operating characteristic analysis. J Virol Methods 2000; 90: 143–152.

Enders G, Biber M. Parvovirus B19 infections in pregnancy. Behring Inst Mitt 1990; 85: 74–78.

Enders M, Weidner A, Zoellner I, Searle K, Enders G. Fetal morbidity and mortality after acute human parvovirus B19 infection in pregnancy: prospective evaluation of 1018 cases. Prenat Diagn 2004; 24: 513–518.

Ennis O, Corcoran A, Kavanagh K, Mahon BP, Doyle S. Baculovirus expression of parvovirus B19 (B19V) NS1: utility in confirming recent infection. J Clin Virol 2001; 22: 55–60.

Erdman DD, Anderson BC, Torok TJ, Finkel TH, Anderson LJ. Possible transmission of parvovirus B19 from intravenous immune globulin. J Med Virol 1997; 53: 233–236.

Erdman DD, Usher MJ, Tsou C, Caul EO, Gary GW, Kajigaya S, Young NS, Anderson LJ. Human parvovirus B19 specific IgG, IgA, and IgM antibodies and DNA in serum specimens from persons with erythema infectiosum. J Med Virol 1991; 35: 110–115.

European Pharmacopoeia. European Pharmacopoeia monograph of human anti-D immunoglobulin. Document 01:0557. European Pharmacopoeia, Strasbourg, France; 2004.

Eurostat. Statistics in focus: population and social conditions. ISSN 1024-4352. Cat. No.: CA-NK-98-001-EN-C; 1998.

Fairley CK, Smoleniec JS, Caul OE, Miller E. Observational study of effect of intrauterine transfusions on outcome of fetal hydrops after parvovirus B19 infection. Lancet 1995; 346: 1335–1337.

Ferguson M, Walker D, Cohen B. Report of a collaborative study to establish the international standard for parvovirus B19 serum IgG. Biologicals 1997; 25: 283–288.

Foto F, Saag KG, Scharosch LL, Howard EJ, Naides SJ. Parvovirus B19-specific DNA in bone marrow from B19 arthropathy patients: evidence for B19 virus persistence. J Infect Dis 1993; 167: 744–748.

Franssila R, Auramo J, Modrow S, Mobs M, Oker-Blom C, Kapyla P, Soderlund-Venermo M, Hedman K. T helper cell-mediated interferon-gamma expression after human parvovirus B19 infection: persisting VP2-specific and transient VP1u-specific activity. Clin Exp Immunol 2005; 142: 53–61.

Franssila R, Hokynar K, Hedman K. T helper cell-mediated *in vitro* responses of recently and remotely infected subjects to a candidate recombinant vaccine for human parvovirus B19. J Infect Dis 2001; 183: 805–809.

Frickhofen N, Abkowitz JL, Safford M, Berry JM, Antunez-de-Mayolo J, Astrow A, Cohen R, Halperin I, King L, Mintzer D, et al. Persistent B19 parvovirus infection in patients infected with human immunodeficiency virus type 1 (HIV-1): A treatable cause of anemia in AIDS. Ann Intern Med 1990; 113: 926–933.

Fukushige J, Takahashi N, Ueda K, Okada K, Miyazaki C, Maeda Y. Kawasaki disease and human parvovirus B19 antibody: role of immunoglobulin therapy. Acta Paediatr Jpn 1995; 37: 758–760.

Gallinella G, Manaresi E, Zuffi E, Venturoli S, Bonsi L, Bagnara GP, Musiani M, Zerbini M. Different patterns of restriction to B19 parvovirus replication in human blast cell lines. Virology 2000; 278: 361–367.

Gibbs RS, Sweet RL. Clinical disorders. In: Maternal Fetal Medicine (Creasy RK, Resnik R, editors). 3rd ed. Philadelphia: W.B. Saunders; 1994; pp. 671–752.

Graesslin O, Andreoletti L, Dedecker F, Grolier F, Quereux C, Gabriel R. Successful *in utero* treatment of parvovirus B19-induced fetal hydrops in a case of twin pregnancy. Prenat Diagn 2005; 25: 336–337.

Grilli EA, Anderson AJ, Hoskins TW. Concurrent outbreaks of influenza and Parvovirus B19 in a boys boarding school. Epidemiol Infect 1989; 103: 359–369.

Hall SM, Cohen BJ, Mortimer PP, Caul EO, Cradock-Watson J. Prospective study of human parvovirus (B19) infection in pregnancy. Br Med J 1990; 300: 1166–1170.

Hansmann M, Gembruch U, Bald R. New therapeutic aspects in non-immune hydropsfetalis based on four hundred and two prenatally diagnosed cases. Fetal Diagn Ther 1989; 4: 29–36.

Hedrick J. The effects of human parvovirus B19 and cytomegalovirus during pregnancy. J Perinat Neonatal Nurs 1996; 10: 30–39.

Heegaard ED, Hornsleth A. Parvovirus: the expanding spectrum of disease. Acta Paediatr 1995; 84: 109–117.

Heegaard ED, Jensen IP, Christensen J. Novel PCR assay for differential detection and screening of erythrovirus B19 and erythrovirus V9. J Med Virol 2001; 65: 362–367.

Heegaard ED, Petersen BL, Heilmann CJ, Hornsleth A. Prevalence of parvovirus B19 and parvovirus V9 DNA and antibodies in paired bone marrow and serum samples from healthy individuals. J Clin Microbiol 2002a; 40: 933–936.

Heegaard ED, Petersen BL, Heilmann CJ, Hornsleth A, Heegaard ED, Rasksen CJ, Christensen J. Detection of parvovirus B19 NS1-specific antibodies by ELISA and western blotting employing recombinant NS1 protein as antigen. J Med Virol 2002b; 67: 375–383.

Hemauer A, Gigler A, Searle K, Beckenlehner K, Raab U, Broliden K, Wolf H, Enders G, Modrow S. Seroprevalence of parvovirus B19 NS1-specific IgG in B19-infected and un-infected individuals and in infected pregnant women. J Med Virol 2000; 60: 48–55.

Henriques I, Monteiro F, Meireles E, Cruz A, Tavares G, Ferreira M, Araujo F. Prevalence of parvovirus B19 and hepatitis A virus in Portuguese blood donors. Transfus Apher Sci 2005; 33: 305–309.

Hokynar K, Norja P, Laitinen H, Palomaki P, Garbarg-Chenon A, Ranki A, Hedman K, Soderlund-Venermo M. Detection and differentiation of human parvovirus variants by commercial quantitative real-time PCR tests. J Clin Microbiol 2004; 42: 2013–2019.

Hokynar K, Soderlund-Venermo M, Pesonen M, Ranki A, Kiviluoto O, Partio EK, Hedman K. A new parvovirus genotype persistent in human skin. Virology 2002; 302: 224–248.

Jawad ASM. Persistent arthritis after human parvovirus infection. Lancet 1993; 341: 494.

Jindal HK, Yong CB, Wilson GM, Tam P, Astell CR. Mutations in the NTP-binding motif of minute virus of mice (MVM) NS-1 protein uncouple ATPase and DNA helicase functions. J Biol Chem 1994; 269: 3283–3289.

Johnson DR, Fisher RA, Helwick JJ, Murray DL, Patterson MJ, Downes FP. Screening maternal serum alpha-fetoprotein levels and human parvovirus antibodies. Prenat Diag 1994; 14: 455–458.

Jones LP, Erdman DD, Anderson LJ. Prevalence of antibodies to human parvovirus B19 nonstructural protein in persons with various clinical outcomes following B19 infection. J Infect Dis 1999; 180: 500–504.

Jordan JA. Identification of human parvovirus B19 infection in idiopathic nonimmune hydrops fetalis. Am J Obstet Gynecol 1996; 174: 37–42.

Jordan JA. Comparison of a baculovirus-based VP2 enzyme immunoassay (EIA) to an *Escherichia coli*-based VP1 EIA for detection of human parvovirus B19 immunoglobulin M and immunoglobulin G in sera of pregnant women. J Clin Microbiol 2000; 38: 1472–1475.

Jordan JA, DeLoia JA. Globoside expression within the human placenta. Placenta 1999; 20: 103–108.

Jordan JA, Huff D, DeLoia JA. Placental cellular immune response in women infected with human parvovirus B19 during pregnancy. Clin Diagn Lab Immunol 2001; 8: 288–292.

Kaikkonen L, Lankinen H, Harjunpaa I, Hokynar K, Soderlund-Venermo M, Oker-Blom C, Hedman L, Hedman K. Acute-phase-specific heptapeptide epitope for diagnosis of parvovirus B19 infection. J Clin Microbiol 1999; 37: 3952–3956.

Kajigaya S, Fujii H, Field A, Anderson S, Rosenfeld S, Anderson LJ, Shimada T, Young NS. Self assembled B19 parvovirus capsids, produced in a baculovirus system, are antigenically and immunogenically similar to native virions. Proc Natl Acad Sci USA 1991; 88: 4646–4650.

Kajigaya S, Shimada T, Fujita S, Young NS. A genitically modified cell line that produces empty capsids of B19 (human) parvovirus. Proc Natl Acad Sci USA 1989; 86: 7601–7605.

Kerr JR, Curran MD, Moore JE, Coyle PV, Ferguson WP. Persistent parvovirus B19 infection. Lancet 1995a; 345: 1118.

Kerr JR, O'Neill HJ, Deleys R, Wright C, Coyle PV. Design and production of a target-specific monoclonal antibody to parvovirus B19 capsid proteins. J Immunol Methods 1995b; 180: 101–106.

Kerr S, O'Keeffe G, Kilty C, Doyle S. Undenatured parvovirus B19 antigens are essential for the accurate detection of parvovirus B19 IgG. J Med Virol 1999; 57: 179–185.

Kinney JS, Anderson LJ, Farrar J, Strikas RA, Kumar ML, Kliegman RM, Sever JL, Hurwitz ES, Sikes RK. Risk of adverse outcomes of pregnancy after human parvovirus B19 infection. J Infect Dis 1988; 157: 663–667.

Klouda PT, Corbin SA, Bradley BA, Cohen BJ, Woolfe AD. HLA and acute arthritis following human parvovirus infection. Tissue Antigens 1986; 28: 318–319.

Knoll A, Louwen F, Kochanowski B, Plentz A, Stussel J, Beckenlehner K, Jilg W, Modrow S. Parvovirus B19 infection in pregnancy: quantitative viral DNA analysis using a kinetic fluorescence detection system (TaqMan PCR). J Med Virol 2002; 67: 259–266.

Koch WC, Adler SP. Human parvovirus B19 infections in women of childbearing age and within families. Pediatr Infect Dis J 1989; 8: 83–87.

Komischke K, Searle K, Enders G. Maternal serum alpha-fetoprotein and human chorionic gonadotropin in pregnant women with acute parvovirus B19 infection with and without fetal complications. Prenat Diagn 1997; 17: 1039–1046.

Kurpad C, Mukherjee P, Wang XS, Ponnazhagan S, Li L, Yoder MC, Srivastava A. Adeno-associated virus 2-mediated transduction and erythroid lineage-restricted expression from parvovirus B19p6 promoter in primary human hematopoietic progenitor cells. J Hematother Stem Cell Res 1999; 8: 585–592.

Kurtzman GJ, Cohen BJ, Field AM, Oseas R, Blaese RM, Young NS. The immune response to B19 parvovirus and an antibody defect in persistent viral infection. J Clin Invest 1989a; 84: 1114–1123.

Kurtzman GJ, Cohen BJ, Meyers P, Amunullah A, Young NS. Persistent B19 parvovirus infection as a cause of severe chronic anemia in children with acute lymphocytic leukaemia. Lancet 1988; 2: 1159–1162.

Kurtzman GJ, Frickhofen N, Kimball J, Jenkins DW, Nienhuis AW, Young NS. Pure red-cell aplasia of 10 years' duration due to persistent parvovirus B19 infection and its cure with immunoglobulin therapy. N Engl J Med 1989b; 321: 519–523.

Kurtzman GJ, Ozawa K, Cohen BJ. Chronic bone marrow failure due to persistent B19 parvovirus infection. N Engl J Med 1987; 317: 287–294.

Lehmann HW, Knoll A, Kuster RM, Modrow S. Frequent infection with a viral pathogen, parvovirus B19, in rheumatic diseases of childhood. Arthritis Rheum 2003; 48: 1631–1638.

Lee PR. Arthritis and rubella. Br Med J 1962; 2: 925.

Levy R, Weissman A, Blomberg G, Hagay ZJ. Infection by parvovirus B 19 during pregnancy: a review. Obstet Gynecol Surv 1997; 52: 254–259.

Li X, Rhode III SL. Mutation of lysine 405 to serine in the parvovirus H-1 NS1 abolishes its function for viral DNA replication, late promoter trans activation and cytotoxicity. J Virol 1990; 64: 4654–4660.

Liefeldt L, Plentz A, Klempa B, Kershaw O, Endres AS, Raab U, Neumayer HH, Meisel H, Modrow S. Recurrent high level parvovirus B19/genotype 2 viremia in a renal transplant recipient analyzed by real-time PCR for simultaneous detection of genotypes 1 to 3. J Med Virol 2005; 75: 161–169.

Lui SL, Luk WK, Cheung CY, Chan TM, Lai KN, Peiris JS. Nosocomial outbreak of parvovirus B19 infection in a renal transplant unit. Transplantation 2001; 71: 59–64.

Luo W. A novel protein encoded by small RNAs of parvovirus B19. Virology 1993; 195: 448–455.

Lyon DJ, Chapman CS, Martin C, Brown KE, Clewley JP, Flower AJ. Symptomatic parvovirus B19 infection and heat-treated factor IX concentrate [Letter]. Lancet 1989; 1: 1085.

Manaresi E, Gallinella G, Zerbini M, Venturoli S, Gentilomi G, Musiani M. IgG immune response to B19 parvovirus VP1 and VP2 linear epitopes by immunoblot assay. J Med Virol 1999; 57: 174–178.

Manaresi E, Gallinella G, Zuffi E, Bonvicini F, Zerbini M, Musiani M. Diagnosis and quantitative evaluation of parvovirus B19 infections by real-time PCR in the clinical laboratory. J Med Virol 2002; 67: 275–281.

Manaresi E, Zuffi E, Gallinella G, Gentilomi G, Zerbini M, Musiani M. Differential IgM response to conformational and linear epitopes of parvovirus B19 VP1 and VP2 structural proteins. J Med Virol 2001; 64: 67–73.

Markenson GR, Yancey MK. Parvovirus B19 infections in pregnancy. Semin Perinatol 1998; 22: 309–317.

Marton T, Martin WL, Whittle MJ. Hydrops fetalis and neonatal death from human parvovirus B19: an unusual complication. Prenat Diagn 2005; 25: 543–545.

McCarthy DM, Ni TH, Muzyczka N. Analysis of mutations in adeno-associated virus Rep protein *in vivo* and *in vitro*. J Virol 1992; 66: 4050–4057.

Miki NPH, Chantler JK. Non-permissiveness of synovial membrane cells to human parvovirus *in vitro*. J Gen Virol 1992; 73: 1559–1562.

Miller E, Fairley CK, Cohen BJ, Seng C. Immediate and long term outcome of human parvovirus B19 infection in pregnancy. Br J Obstet Gynaecol 1998; 105: 174–178.

Mitchell LA. Parvovirus B19 nonstructural (NS1) protein as a transactivator of interleukin-6 synthesis: common pathway in inflammatory sequelae of human parvovirus infections? J Med Virol 2002; 67: 267–274.

Mitchell LA, Leong R, Rosenke KA. Lymphocyte recognition of human parvovirus B19 non-structural (NS1) protein: associations with occurrence of acute and chronic arthropathy? J Med Microbiol 2001; 50: 627–635.

Moffatt S, Tanaka N, Tada K, Nose M, Nakamura M, Muraoka O, Hirano T, Sugamura K. A cytotoxic nonstructural protein, NS1, of human parvovirus B19 induces activation of interleukin-6 gene expression. J Virol 1996; 70: 8485–8491.

Momoeda M, Kawase M, Jane SM, Miyamura K, Young NS, Kajigaya S. The transcriptional regulator YY1 binds to the 5′-terminal region of B19 parvovirus and regulates P6 promoter activity. J Virol 1994a; 68: 7159–7168.

Momoeda M, Wong S, Kawase M, Young NS, Kajigaya S. A putative nucleoside triphosphate-binding domain in the nonstructural protein of B19 parvovirus is required for cytotoxicity. J Virol 1994b; 68: 8443–8446.

Morey AL, Ferguson DJ, Fleming KA. Ultrastructural features of fetal erythroid precursors infected with parvovirus B19 *in vitro*: evidence of cell death by apoptosis. J Pathol 1993; 169: 213–220.

Morey AL, Keeling JW, Porter HJ, Fleming KA. Clinical and histopathological features of parvovirus B19 infection in the human fetus. Br J Obstet Gynaecol 1992; 99: 566–574.

Morgan-Capner P, Crowcroft NS. PHLS Joint Working Party of the Advisory Committees of Virology and Vaccines and Immunisation. Guidelines on the management of, and exposure to, rash illness in pregnancy (including consideration of relevant antibody screening programmes in pregnancy). Commun Dis Public Health 2002; 5: 59–71.

Morita E, Nakashima A, Asao H, Sato H, Sugamura K. Human parvovirus B19 nonstructural protein (NS1) induces cell cycle arrest at G(1) phase. J Virol 2003; 77: 2915–2921.

Mortimer PP, Humphries RK, Moore JG, Purcell RH, Young NS. A human parvovirus-like virus inhibits haematopoietic colony formation *in vitro*. Nature 1983; 302: 426–429.

Müller J, Eis-Hubinger AM, Madlener K, Kuppers C, Herzig M, Potzsch B. Development and validation of a real-time PCR assay for routine testing of blood donations for parvovirus B19 DNA. Infus Ther Transfus Med 2002; 29: 254–258.

Musiani M, Zerbini M, Gentilomi G, Plazzi M, Gallinella G, Venturoli S. Parvovirus B19 clearance from peripheral blood after acute infection. J Infect Dis 1995; 172: 1360–1363.

Nguyen QT, Sifer C, Schneider V, Bernaudin F, Auguste V, Garbarg-Chenon A. Detection of an erythrovirus sequence distinct from B19 in a child with acute anemia. Lancet 1998; 352: 1524.

Nguyen QT, Wong S, Heegaard ED, Brown KE. Identification and characterization of a second novel human erythrovirus variant, A6. Virology 2002; 301: 374–380.

Nigro G, Bastianon V, Colloridi V, Ventriglia F, Gallo P, D'Amati G, Koch WC, Adler SP. Human parvovirus B19 infection in infancy associated with acute and chronic lymphocytic myocarditis and high cytokine levels: report of 3 cases and review. Clin Infect Dis 2000; 31: 65–69.

Norbeck O, Isa A, Pohlmann C, Broliden K, Kasprowicz V, Bowness P, Klenerman P, Tolfvenstam T. Sustained CD8 + T-cell responses induced after acute parvovirus B19 infection in humans. J Virol 2005; 79: 12117–12121.

Nunoue T, Kusuhara K, Hara T. Human fetal infection with parvovirus B19: maternal infection time in gestation, viral persistence and fetal prognosis. Pediatr Infect Dis J 2002; 21: 1133–1136.

Nyman M, Skjoldebrand-Sparre L, Broliden K. Non-hydropic intrauterine fetal death more than 5 months after primary parvovirus B19 infection. J Perinat Med 2005; 33: 176–178.

Ozawa K, Ayub J, Kajigaya T, Shimada T, Young NS. The gene encoding the non-structural protein of B19 (human) parvovirus may be lethal in transfected cells. J Virol 1988; 62: 2884–2889.

Ozawa K, Ayub J, Yu-Shu H, Kurtzman G, Shimada T, Young N. Novel transcription map for the B19 (human) pathogenic parvovirus. J Virol 1987; 61: 2395–2406.

Palmer P, Pallier C, Leruez-Ville M, Deplanche M, Morinet F. Antibody response to human parvovirus B19 in patients with primary infection by immunoblot assay with recombinant proteins. Clin Diagn Lab Immunol 1996; 3: 236–238.

Pastuszak AL. Outcome after maternal varicella infection in the first 20 weeks of pregnancy. N Engl J Med 1994; 330: 901–905.

Pereira L, Maidji E, McDonagh S, Tabata T. Insights into viral transmission at the uterine–placental interface. Trends Microbiol 2005; 13: 164–174.

PHLS. Prospective study of human parvovirus (B19) infection in pregnancy. Public Health Laboratory Service Working Party of Fifth Disease. BMJ 1990; 300: 1166–1170.

Pillet S, Le Guyader N, Hofer T, NguyenKhac F, Koken M, Aubin JT, Fichelson S, Gassmann M, Morinet F. Hypoxia enhances human B19 erythrovirus gene expression in primary erythroid cells. Virology 2004; 327: 1–7.

Prowse C, Ludlam CA, Yap PL. Human parvovirus B19 and blood products. Vox Sang 1997; 72: 1–10.

Pryde PG, Nugent CE, Pridjian G, Barr Jr. M, Faix RG. Spontaneous resolution of non-immune hydrops fetalis secondary to human parvovirus B19 infection. Obstet Gynecol 1992; 79: 859–861.

Raab U, Beckenlehner K, Lowin T, Niller HH, Doyle S, Modrow S. NS1 protein of parvovirus B19 interacts directly with DNA sequences of the p6 promoter and with the cellular transcription factors Sp1/Sp3. Virology 2002; 293: 86–93.

Rayment FB, Crosdale E, Morris DJ, Pattison JR, Talbot P, Clare JJ. The production of human parvovirus capsid proteins in *Escherichia coli* and their potential as diagnostic antigens. J Gen Virol 1990; 71: 2665–2672.

Reid DM, Reid TMS, Brown T, Rennie RAN. Human parvovirus associated arthritis: a clinical and laboratory description. Lancet 1985; 1: 422–425.

Rodis JF, Borgida AF, Wilson M, Egan JF, Leo MV, Odibo AO, Campbell WA. Management of parvovirus infection in pregnancy and outcomes of hydrops: a survey of members of the Society of Perinatal Obstetricians. Am J Obstet Gynecol 1998; 179: 985–988.

Rodis JF, Hovick Jr. TJ, Quinn DL, Rosengren SS, Tattersall P. Human parvovirus infection in pregnancy. Obstet Gynecol 1988; 72: 733–738.

Rodriguez MM, Bruce JH, Jimenez XF, Romaguera RL, Bancalari E, Garcia OL, Ferrer PL. Nonimmune hydrops fetalis in the liveborn: series of 32 autopsies. Pediatr Dev Pathol 2005; 8: 369–378.

Rodriguez MM, Chaves F, Romaguera RL, Ferrer PL, de la Guardia C, Bruce JH. Value of autopsy in nonimmune hydrops fetalis: series of 51 stillborn fetuses. Pediatr Dev Pathol 2002; 5: 365–374.

Saldanha J, Lelie N, Yu MW, Heath A, B19 Collaborative Study Group. Establishment of the first World Health Organization International Standard for human parvovirus B19 DNA nucleic acid amplification techniques. Vox Sang 2002; 82: 24–31.

Saller Jr. DN, Rogers BB, Canick JA. Maternal serum biochemical markers in pregnancies with fetal parvovirus B19 infection. Prenat Dign 1993; 13: 467–471.

Sanghi A, Morgan-Capner P, Hesketh L, Elstein M. Zoonotic and viral infection in fetal loss after 12 weeks. Br J Obstet Gynaecol 1997; 104: 942–945.

Santagostino E, Mannuci PM, Gringeri A, Azzi A, Morfini M. Eliminating parvovirus B19 from blood products. Lancet 1994; 343: 798–799.

Santagostino E, Mannucci PM, Gringeri A, Azzi A, Morfini M, Musso R, Santoro R, Schiavoni M. Transmission of parvovirus B19 by coagulation factor concentrates exposed to 100 degrees C heat after lyophilization. Transfusion 1997; 37: 517–522.

Sato H, Takakura F, Kojima E, Fukada K, Okochi K, Maeda Y. Screening of blood donors for human parvovirus B19. Lancet 1995; 346: 1237–1238.

Schneider B, Becker M, Brackmann HH, Eis-Hubinger AM. Contamination of coagulation factor concentrates with human parvovirus B19 genotype 1 and 2. Thromb Haemost 2004; 92: 838–845.

Schwarz TF, Roggendorf M, Hottentrager B, Deinhardt F, Enders G, Gloning KP, Schramm T, Hansmann M. Human parvovirus B19 infection in pregnancy. Lancet 1988; 2: 566–567.

Schwarz TF, Roggendorf M, Hottentrager B, Modrow S, Deinhardt F, Middeldorp J. Immunoglobulins in the prophylaxis of parvovirus B19 infection. J Infect Dis 1990; 162: 1214.

Searle K, Guilliard C, Enders G. Parvovirus B19 diagnosis in pregnant women—quantification of IgG antibody levels (IU/ml) with reference to the international parvovirus B19 standard serum. Infection 1997; 25: 32–34.

Searle K, Schalasta G, Enders G. Development of antibodies to the nonstructural protein NS1 of parvovirus B19 during acute symptomatic and subclinical infection in pregnancy: implications for pathogenesis doubtful. J Med Virol 1998; 56: 192–198.

Sebire NJ. Human parvovirus B19 and fetal death. Lancet 2001; 358: 1180.

Selbing A, Josefsson A, Dahle LO, Lindgren R. Parvovirus B19 infection during pregnancy treated with high-dose intravenous gammaglobulin. Lancet 1995; 345: 660–661.

Serjeant BE, Hambleton IR, Kerr S, Kilty CG, Serjeant GR. Haematological response to parvovirus B19 infection in homozygous sickle-cell disease. Lancet 2001; 358: 1779–1780.

Servant A, Laperche S, Lallemand F, Marinho V, De Saint Maur G, Meritet JF, Garbarg-Chenon A. Genetic diversity within human erythroviruses: identification of three genotypes. J Virol 2002; 76: 9124–9134.

Skjoldebrand-Sparre L, Tolfvenstam T, Papadogiannakis N, Wahren B, Broliden K, Nyman M. Parvovirus B19 infection: association with third-trimester intrauterine fetal death. BJOG 2000; 107: 476–480.

Sloots T, Devine PL. Evaluation of four commercial enzyme immunoassays for detection of immunoglobulin M antibodies to human parvovirus B19. Eur J Clin Microbiol Infect Dis 1996; 15: 758–761.

Soderlund M, Brown CS, Spaan WJ, Hedman L, Hedman K. Epitope type-specific IgG responses to capsid proteins VP1 and VP2 of human parvovirus B19. J Infect Dis 1995; 172: 1431–1436.

Soderlund M, von Essen R, Haapasaari J, Kiistala U, Kiviluoto O, Hedman K. Persistence of parvovirus B19 DNA in synovial membranes of young patients with and without chronic arthropathy. Lancet 1997; 349: 1063–1065.

St Amand J, Beard C, Humphries K, Astell CR. Analysis of splice junctions and *in vitro* and *in vivo* translation potential of the small, abundant B19 parvovirus RNAs. Virology 1991; 183: 133–142.

Thomas I, Di Giambattista M, Gerard C, Mathys E, Hougardy V, Latour B, Branckaert T, Laub R. Prevalence of human erythrovirus B19 DNA in healthy Belgian blood donors and correlation with specific antibodies against structural and non-structural viral proteins. Vox Sang 2003; 84: 300–307.

Toivanen P. Persistence of parvovirus B19 in synovial fluid and bone marrow. Ann Rheum Dis 1995; 54: 597–600.

Tolfvenstam T, Lundqvist A, Levi M, Wahren B, Broliden K. Mapping of B-cell epitopes on human parvovirus B19 non-structural and structural proteins. Vaccine 2000; 19: 758–763.

Tolfvenstam T, Oxenius A, Price DA, Shacklett BL, Spiegel HM, Hedman K, Norbeck O, Levi M, Olsen K, Kantzanou M, Nixon DF, Broliden K, Klenerman P. Direct *ex vivo* measurement of CD8(+) T-lymphocyte responses to human parvovirus B19. J Virol 2001a; 75: 540–543.

Tolfvenstam T, Papadogiannakis N, Norbeck O, Petersson K, Broliden K. Frequency of human parvovirus B19 infection in intrauterine fetal death. Lancet 2001b; 357: 1494–1497.

Tolfvenstam T, Ruden U, Broliden K. Evaluation of serological assays for identification of parvovirus B19 immunoglobulin M. Clin Diagn Lab Immunol 1996; 3: 147–150.

Torok TJ. Human parvovirus B19 infections in pregnancy. Pediatr Infect Dis J 1990; 9: 772–776.

Tuckerman JG, Brown T, Cohen BJ. Erythema infectiosum in a village primary school: clinical and virological studies. J R Coll Gen Pract 1986; 36: 267.

Valeur-Jensen AK, Pedersen CB, Westergaard T, Jensen IP, Lebech M, Andersen PK, Aaby P, Pedersen BN, Melbye M. Risk factors for parvovirus B19 infection in pregnancy. JAMA 1999; 281: 1099–1105.

van Elsacker-Niele AM. Human parvovirus B19-clinical consequence of infection. PhD Thesis; Leiden, The Netherlands; 1998.

van Elsacker-Niele AM, Kroes AC. Human parvovirus B19: relevance in internal medicine. Neth J Med 1999; 54: 221–230.

Venturoli S, Gallinella G, Manaresi E, Gentilomi G, Musiani M, Zerbini M. IgG response to the immunoreactive region of parvovirus B19 nonstructural protein by immunoblot assay with a recombinant antigen. J Infect Dis 1998; 178: 1826–1829.

Von Landenberg P, Lehmann HW, Knoll A, Dorsch S, Modrow S. Antiphospholipid antibodies in pediatric and adult patients with rheumatic disease are associated with parvovirus B19 infection. Arthritis Rheum 2003; 48: 1939–1947.

von Poblotzki A, Gerdes C, Reischl H, Wolf H, Modrow S. Lymphoproliferative response after infection with human parvovirus B19. J Virol 1996; 70: 7327–7330.

von Poblotzki A, Gigler A, Lang B, Wolf H, Modrow S. Antibodies to parvovirus B19 NS-1 protein in infected individuals. J Gen Virol 1995a; 76: 519–527.

von Poblotzki A, Hemauer A, Gigler A, Puchhammer-Stockl E, Heinz FX, Pont J, Laczika K, Wolf H, Modrow S. Antibodies to the nonstructural protein of parvovirus B19 in persistently infected patients: implications for pathogenesis. J Infect Dis 1995b; 172: 1356–1359.

Vuorinen T, Lammintausta K, Kotilainen P, Nikkari S. Presence of parvovirus B19 DNA in chronic urticaric and healthy human skin. J. Clin Virol 2002; 25: 217–221.

Wagner AD, Goronzy J, Matteson E, Weyland C. Systemic monocyte and T cell activation in a patient with human parvovirus B19 infection. Mayo Clin Proc 1995; 70: 261–265.

Wakamatsu C, Takakura F, Kojima E, Kiriyama Y, Goto N, Matsumoto K, Oyama M, Sato H, Okochi K, Maeda Y. Screening of blood donors for human parvovirus B19 and characterization of the results. Vox Sang 1999; 76: 14–21.

Wattre P, Dewilde A, Subtil D, Andreoletti L, Thirion V. A clinical and epidemiological study of human parvovirus B19 infection in fetal hydrops using PCR Southern blot hybridization and chemiluminescence detection. J Med Virol 1998; 54: 140–144.

Weigel-Kelley KA, Yoder MC, Srivastava A. Recombinant human parvovirus B19 vectors: erythrocyte P antigen is necessary but not sufficient for successful transduction of human hematopoietic cells. J Virol 2001; 75: 4110–4116.

Weigel-Kelley KA, Yoder MC, Srivastava A. $\alpha 5\beta 1$ integrin as a cellular co-receptor for human parvovirus B19: requirement of functional activation of $\beta 1$ integrin for viral entry. Blood 2003; 102: 3927–3933.

Wegner CS, Jordan J. Human parvovirus B19 VP2 empty capsids bind to human villous trophoblast cells *in vitro* via the globoside receptor. Infect Dis Obstet Gynecol 2004; 12: 69–78.

White DG, Mortimer PP, Blake DR, Woolf AD, Cohen BJ, Bacon PA. Human parvovirus arthropathy. Lancet 1985; I: 419–421.

Williams MD, Cohen BJ, Beddall AC, Pasi KJ, Mortimer PP, Hill FGH. Transmission of human parvovirus B19 by coagulation factor concentrates. Vox Sang 1990; 58: 177–181.

Woolf AD, Campion GV, Chishick A, Wise S, Cohen BJ, Kloeida PT, Caul O, Dieppe PA. Clinical manifestations of human parvovirus B19 in adults. Arch Intern Med 1989; 149: 1153–1156.

Woolf AD, Cohen BJ. Parvovirus B19 and chronic arthritis—causal or casual association? Ann Rheum Dis 1995; 54: 535–536.

Woolf AD, Hall ND, Giulding NJ. Predictors of the long-term outcome of early synovitis: a 5-year follow-up study. Br J Rheumatol 1991; 30: 251–254.

Wolff K, Broliden K, Marsk A, Tolfvenstam T, Papadogiannakis N, Westgren M. One stillborn and one severely hydropic twin due to parvovirus B19 infection; successful outcome of the surviving twin. Acta Obstet Gynecol Scand 2005; 78: 828–830.

Wright C, Hinchliffe SA, Taylor C. Fetal pathology in intrauterine death due to parvovirus B19 infection. Br J Obstet Gynaecol 1996; 103: 133–136.

Yaegashi N. Pathogenesis of nonimmune hydrops fetalis caused by intrauterine B19 infection. Tohoku J Exp Med 2000; 190: 65–82.

Yaegashi N, Niinuma T, Chisaka H, Uehara S, Okamura K, Shinkawa O, Tsunoda A, Moffatt S, Sugamura K, Yajima A. Serologic study of human parvovirus B19 infection in pregnancy in Japan. J Infect 1999; 38: 30–35.

Yaegashi N, Okamura K, Yajima A, Murai C, Sugamura K. The frequency of human parvovirus B19 infection in nonimmune hydrops fetalis. J Perinat Med 1994; 22: 159–163.

Yaegashi N, Shiraishi H, Tada K, Yajima A, Sugamura K. Enzyme-linked immunosorbent assay for IgG and IgM against human parvovirus B19, use of monoclonal antibodies and viral antigen propagated *in vitro*. J Virol Methods 1989; 26: 171–181.

Yoto Y, Kudoh T, Haseyama K, Suzuki N, Oda T, Katoh T, Takahashi T, Sekiguchi S, Chiba S. Incidence of human parvovirus B19 DNA detection in blood donors. Br J Haematol 1995; 91: 1017–1018.

Congenital and Other Related Infectious
Diseases of the Newborn
Isa K. Mushahwar (Editor)
© 2007 Elsevier B.V. All rights reserved
DOI 10.1016/S0168-7069(06)13011-6

Rubella Virus: Molecular Composition, Pathogenesis, Diagnosis, and Control

Isa K. Mushahwar

Abbott Laboratories, Congenital Infectious Diseases, Abbott Park, IL 60064, USA

Molecular composition

Rubella virus (RV) is a member of the genus Rubivirus in the family of Togaviridae (Porterfield et al., 1978). It is a spherical particle of about 60–70 nm in diameter. The particle is enveloped with a single-stranded polyadenylated genomic RNA of positive polarity composed of 9757 nucleotides in length, excluding the poly (A) tail and has a very high G/C content of 69.5% (Dominguez et al., 1990). The virus is encapsulated by a capsid protein (C) and is contained within a lipid bilayer envelope (E) in which the two virus-specific envelope proteins, E1 and E2 are embedded (Ho-Terry etal., 1984; Oker-Blom, 1984; Waxham and Wolinsky, 1983). The virus contains two forms of E2 (E2a and E2b) which differ in the structure of their oligosaccharide side chain (Kalkkinen et al., 1984). The RV genomic RNA encodes two long open-reading frames (ORFs), a 5′-proximal ORF of 6656 nucleotides that codes for the non-structural proteins that are involved in replication and transcription, and a 3′-proximal ORF of 3189 nucleotides which encodes the structural protein (Dominguez et al.,1990). The virus non-structural protein ORF contains two global amino acid motifs conserved in a large number of positive polarity RNA viruses, a motif indicative of helicase activity, and a motif indicative of replicase (RNA-dependent RNA polymerase) activity (Dominguez et al., 1990). Also, a papain-like protease domain is found in the non-structural protein ORF (Garbalenga et al., 1991).

Several investigators (Wolinsky et al., 1991) have localized domains in the mid portion of the E1 glycoprotein that are critical for infectivity and hemagglutinating functions of the virus (Garbalenga et al., 1991). A second neutralization domain resides on the E2 glycoprotein.

Rubella genotypes

Phylogenetic analysis of a collection of over 100 gene sequences from viruses isolated from several countries between 1961 and 2000 verified the existence of at least two main genotypes (Zheng et al., 2003): rubella genotype I (RGI) isolates from Japan, and the Western Hemisphere, and rubella genotype II (RG II) which showed greater genetic diversity than did RG I. RG II viruses are limited to Asia. Of interest, is that RG I viruses also present in most of the countries where RG II viruses are isolated (Zheng et al., 2003). Antigenically, RG I and II are cross reactive and immunization with either virus results in immunity to all rubella viruses.

Clinical manifestations

The virus is transmitted from one individual to another through aerosols from the naso-pharynx of infected individuals. The virus is shed in the naso-pharynx for approximately 7 days before and after a rash is visible. Rubella is contagious from 7 days before to 5–7 days after the rash is visible. In most cases of rubella, symptoms appear within 12–23 days, and 20–50% of cases are asymptomatic. Besides naso-pharynx droplets, the virus is also present in blood, feces, and urine during the clinical illness (Edlich et al., 2005).

The incubation period is usually from 10 to 21 days, generally about 18 days (Best and Bantavala, 1990; Haukenes et al., 1990). Communicability period starts generally from the onset of catarrhal symptoms for at least 4 days, but not more than 7 days.

Congenital rubella

Infection with RV during the first 12 weeks of pregnancy results in congenital infection and/or miscarriage in 80–90% of cases (Edlich et al., 2005). This infection is often associated with severe physical and mental defects of the developing fetus. Rubella during pregnancy still occur at an estimated frequency of 1 case per 6000–10,000 life births in industrialized countries (Enders, 1994; Pustowoit and Liebert, 1998). Transmission of RV during early pregnancy can lead to severe birth defects known as congenital rubella syndrome or CRS (Cutts and Vynnycky, 1999). The major manifestations seen in children with CRS are: central nervous system involvement (Frey, 1997; Neto et al., 2004) that include three distinct neurological syndromes (Frey, 1997), namely, post-infectious encephalitis after acute infection, or a range of neurological manifestations after congenital infection, and an extremely rare neurodegenerative disorder that progresses to rubella panencephalitis (Kuroda and Matsui, 1997), that can follow either congenital or post-natal infection (Frey, 1997).

Among other defects seen in children as a result of CRS are growth retardation (Gleghorn, 1989), ventriculitis (Cary et al., 1987), ophthalmic manifestations (Given et al., 1993), congenital hearing impairment (Rahman et al., 2002), hyperthyroidism and diabetes mellitus (Floret et al., 1980).These defects seen in children may be manifested singly or in multiple form.They also may be transient, progressive, or permanent (Kalvenes et al., 1995).

Diagnosis

Hemagglutination inhibition (HAI) was the first serological assay to be used in clinical laboratories and remained for some time the standard against which many of the newer assays were compared (Dille et al., 2005). The HAI assay is no longer required when screening for protective maternal immunity. During the last 15 years, the HAI assay has been replaced entirely by more sensitive, specific, and technically less demanding enzyme-linked immunosorbent assay (ELISA) and microparticle enzyme immunoassay (MEIA) (Abbott et al., 1990).

Serodiagnosis of primary rubella infection

The appearance of antibodies of different classes as a response to rubella infection was reported by several investigators (Kalimo et al., 1976; Meurman et al., 1977; Meurman and Ziola, 1978). The first antibodies appearing after infection are IgM class, and these are eventually replaced by IgG class antibodies which persist as markers of immunity. The determination of antibody class can serve to distinguish current infection (primary IgM immune response) from long-term acquired immunity (IgG).

Solid-phase radioimmunoassay (Kalimo et al., 1976; Meurman et al., 1977) were the first assays to replace complement fixation, immunofluorescence and counter-immune electrophoresis (CIE) for the detection of antibodies to RV because they were more sensitive and less cumbersome. Radioimmunoassays in turn were replaced by ELISA. Many direct and indirect ELISA for the detection of antibodies to RV have been reported in the literature (Voller and Bidwell, 1975, 1976; Gravell et al., 1977; Matter et al., 1994; Hudson and Morgan-Capner, 1996; Tipples et al., 2004).

Several commercial kits for the detection of rubella IgM antibodies have been compared (Matter et al., 1994; Hudson and Morgan-Capner, 1996; Tipples et al., 2004). One of the most reliable and reproducible ELISA for the detection of anti-Rubella IgM is an anti-u capture assay as illustrated by the following three steps (Mushahwar and Overby, 1983):

I   SP-Abu + IgM → SP-Abu.IgM
II SP-Abu.IgM + RV → SP-Abu.IgM.RV
III SP-Abu.IgM.RV + *AbRV → SP.Abu.IgM.RV.*AbRV

Where, SP-Abu is a solid-phase surface coated with u chain-specific goat anti-human antibody. In step I, if anti-RV IgM is present in a patient's serum it will be bound by the u chain-specific solid-phase antibody. In step II, RV will be attached to it to form the complex SP-Abu.IgMRV. This complex is then detected in step III by incubation with probe antibody, *AbRV, an enzyme-linked human anti-RV IgG. The resulting absorbancy of the multiple-layer product SP-Abu.IgMR-V.*AbRV is in proportion to anti-RV IgM concentration in the patient's serum. This test was shown to be highly reproducible and sensitive.

These assays for IgM and IgG employing anti-human u and anti-human gamma globulins have some problems with specificity. Unless the anti-u and -gamma immunoglobulins are of exceptional purity and specificity, cross reactions prevent a clear distinction of IgM and IgG in pathologic serum. An exceptionally high titer of IgG, for example could give significant cross reactions with other anti-u reagent. Second, false-positive reactions have been observed (Meurman and Ziola, 1978; Mushahwar and Overby, 1983) when analyzing for IgM in elevated rheumatoid factor (RF) positive sera. RF is an antibody primarily of the IgM class that reacts with the Fc portion of bound IgG. It is found in a high percentage of persons with rheumatoid arthritis and related connective tissues and is also found in varying degrees in people with sub-acute bacterial endocarditis, chronic liver disease, parasitic infections, and tuberculosis as well as during pregnancy and among apparently normal healthy persons, particularly neonates and the elderly (Meurman, 1983; Fuccillo et al., 1992). Transient appearance of RF has been associated with acute parvovirus B19, measles virus, rubella virus, and cytomegalovirus infections and also, following prophylactic vaccination (Erdman, 2000).

The false-positive results that have been described already can be eliminated by absorption of the serum to be analyzed with aggregated gamma globulin or with anti-human IgG or by using labeled F(ab') fragments as detector antibody, thereby eliminating the Fc portion of the IgG molecule that binds RF (Mushahwar and Overby, 1983; Erdman, 2000).

Besides the problems with high-titered IgG and RF false positivity, IgM assays for a variety of viruses in general and for RV in particular have other disadvantages, such as persistence for over 4 months, and it may remain detectable for much longer intervals in a majority of patients (Pattison et al., 1975; Thomas et al., 1992; Matter et al., 1994), and also after apparent rubella reinfection and vaccination (Morgan-Capher et al., 1983). These types of problems can occur in both direct and indirect IgM assays (Erdman, 2000).

Because of the persistence of RV IgM antibodies over a long period of time, it is sometimes very difficult to differentiate between a recent (acute) and remote infection utilizing commercially available IgM immunoassays. It has been reported several years ago (Inouye et al., 1984; Lehtonen et al., 1989) that the avidity of specific IgG antibody is low in primary acute viral infections and it increases with time. Thus, the IgG avidity index may be useful in distinguishing acute from pre-existing immunity, including RV reinfection (Hedman and Rousseau, 1989).

The avidity index is calculated by measuring absorbencies in the presence or absence of protein denaturing agents, such as diethylamine, guanidine, thiocyanate, SDS, or urea. The avidity index is calculated by dividing the absorbancy value with denaturing agent by the absorbancy value without denaturing agent. Avidity indices of 0.50 or less are considered low.

By use of RV-specific IgG avidity index assay together with a specific IgM positive samples from patients with clinical symptoms of a RV infection (rash), the diagnosis of infection with RV in early pregnancy has been improved significantly. The avidity assay for such patients is a reliable assay for the exclusion of a recently acquired infection with RV (less than 4 months) in pregnant women (Hedman and Sappala, 1988; Enders and Knotek, 1989; Hedman and Rousseau, 1989).

Two main problems of RV avidity test however, are (1) low-avidity indices may persist for a long time just as RV IgM antibodies (Meurman, 1978; Thomas et al., 1992; Thomas et al., 1993), and in some cases it has been reported of persistence over 6.5 months (Thomas et al., 1992), and (2) at present there is no gold standard avidity assay that is available commercially. Standardizations of these assays are of critical importance.

Based on these observations, it is obvious that at present, there is not a single immunoassay that is sufficiently reliable by itself to diagnose a recently acquired (acute) RV infection although it is generally agreed that the appearance of virus-specific IgG in serum of pregnant women who were previously seronegative is one of the best tests to diagnose a primary RV infection. This, however, is hard to achieve and implement since rubella IgG testing is not performed routinely, which is the case in most industrialized countries.

In order to diagnose a primary RV infection in pregnant women without clinical symptoms, a battery of tests are required. These tests are an anti-rubella IgM test, a quantitative RV anti-rubella IgG test, an IgG avidity test, an immunoplot anti-rubella E2-specific test (under non-reducing conditions), and in cases of fetal exposure to RV, a reverse transcriptase-polymerase chain reaction (RT-PCR) test. Pustowoit and Liebert (1998) proposed a practical algorithm for the use of these tests through a rational stepwise serological diagnosis of RV infection during pregnancy. Based on their evaluation of 798 serum samples from 499 patients either without clinical signs of RV infection or after vaccination, their findings were as follows:

(1) Acute RV infection:
   - Rubella IgG less than 10–25 IU/ml
   - Positive Rubella IgM test
   - Low index RV IgG avidity test
   - Negative RV E2-specific antibody test
(2) Immunity to RV following vaccination or infection:
   - Rubella IgG more than 25 IU/ml
   - High index RV IgG avidity test
   - Positive RV E2-specific antibody test
(3) Reinfection with RV:
   - Positive rubella IgM test
   - High index RV IgG avidity test
   - Positive RV E2-specific antibody test

It is obvious from these findings that a positive RV E2-specific antibody test and a high index RV IgG avidity test are of a tremendous help in confirming a remote (past) infection with RV. In general, antibody to RV-E2 specific test is detectable only after 12 weeks post-RV infection (Pustowoit and Liebert, 1998), hence its usefulness for the exclusion of a recent acute RV infection. Unfortunately, RV E2 protein is not available commercially. Methods to prepare this protein have been described (Kalkkinen et al., 1984; Yang et al., 1998).

Serodiagnosis of congenital rubella syndrome

In comparison to maternal IgG, maternal IgM antibody induced by a primary rubella infection does not cross the intact plasma. The infected fetus develops IgM antibody to the virus and detection of that antibody in the neonate aids in the diagnosis of CRS. A sample should be drawn from the neonate as soon as possible following parturition. Comparison of IgG antibody in the neonate at the time of birth with the IgG antibody 6 months later also aids in the diagnosis of CRS. A significant drop in over that time interval suggests decreasing maternal antibody in the absence of perinatal or pre-natal infection. Pre- or perinatal infection should be suspected if stable or increasing IgG antibody levels are detected (Dille et al., 2005). Also a positive RT-PCR result in amniocentesis during the 12th until 22nd week of pregnancy indicates a fetal exposure with RV (Bosma et al., 1995) as does the detection of RV-specific IgM antibody after the 22nd week of gestation in fetal blood obtained by cordocentesis (Pustowoit and Liebert, 1998).

Immune status

Objective results are generally obtained using IgG-specific ELISA or MEIA assays. In order to avoid dependence on cumbersome HAI, all specific IgG anti-rubella assays are standardized using World Health Organization (WHO) reference preparations of rubella antiserum The comparison of the rubella IgG ELISA tests with the HAI assay (Pustowoit and Liebert, 1998) showed that HAI titers < 1:32 correlated with IgG values below 25 IU/ml. Values greater than 25 IU/ml are sufficient to protect an individual from clinical reinfection. Values less than 10 IU/ml are considered non-protective and may not prevent clinical rubella after exposure. Sera with titers between 10 and 25 IU/ml are considered intermediate and of questionable protective ability (Pustowoit and Liebert, 1998).

RT-PCR

Several RT-PCR assays for the detection of RV RNA have been described in the literature (Bosma et al., 1995; Revello et al., 1997; Katow, 1998; Steininger et al., 2001; Vyse and Jin, 2002; Mace et al., 2004; Cooray et al., 2006) and so far no RT-PCR assays for RV RNA are available commercially. The best-biological samples for RV RT-PCR analysis are blood, naso-pharyngeal aspirates, throat swabs, urine and three types of fetal tissue, namely chorionic villi, amniotic fluid, and umbilical cord blood. Primer pairs for RV RT-PCR are derived either from a variable region of the E1 gene (Vyse and Jin, 2002; Cooray et al., 2006) or from the highly 5′-non-coding region (Steininger et al., 2001). Caution however, should be taken when selecting primer pairs from this region of the genome because of the close homology between RV and enterovirus genomes. The sequence of the primers chosen by Steininger et al. (2001) for RT and the first step of the PCR, amplifying a fragment of 106 base pairs, was as follows: cDNA, 5′-CCC CTG AAT G(CT)G GCT AAC CT-3′; reverse, 5′-CGG ACA CCC AAA GTA GT(CT) GGT CC-3′. For nested PCR, primers amplifying a fragment of 93 base pairs were used: cDNA, 5′-GAA TG(CT) GGC TAA CCT TAA (AC)CC-3′; reverse, 5′-CAA AGT AGT (CT)GG TCC C(AG)T CC-3′.

By utilizing these sequences, Steininger et al. (2001) developed a sensitive, rapid and an RV-specific nested RT-PCR assay and used it to test naso-pharyngeal aspirates from 556 patients presenting with acute respiratory tract infections. RV RNA was detected by nested PCR in all 52 samples that were RV positive by virus isolation methods, but also in 124 of 367 samples that were negative by virus isolation methods and ELISA. The utilization of primers from the E1 gene for the detection of RV RNA from pharyngeal swabs by Bosma et al. (1995) showed 100% agreement with virus isolation.

A reverse transcription nested PCR assay was also developed (Cooray et al., 2006) and evaluated for the detection of RV RNA directly from clinical specimens. This RT-PCR utilized primers that amplified 592 nucleotides of a variable region within the E1 gene. RV RNA was detected in pre- and post-natal congenital rubella samples and samples from patients with acute rubella.

Successful detection of RV RNA from amniotic fluid has been reported by three groups of investigators (Revello et al., 1997; Katow, 1998; Steininger et al., 2001). All assays showed 100% sensitivity and specificity for pre-natal diagnosis of RV infection.

Rubella vaccine

It is well known that in order to reduce the number of patients with German measles or with CRS, immunization is the most effective strategy that any department or ministry of health, of any country should adopt. Several strains of live-attenuated rubella vaccines have been developed and introduced into immunization programs in many industrialized countries (Katow, 2004). The WHO has recognized that a reliable immunization program can be combined with the measles immunization program. Inclusion of rubella in the expanded program of immunization of measles would be ideal in many Asian, African, and Middle Eastern countries, as it would be efficient and cost effective to administer one injection containing a three-combined vaccine. This has been discussed in detail by Katow (2004).

Rubella vaccine was licensed first in the United States in 1969. About 95% of those who receive the rubella vaccine develop protective immunity. To date, vaccine protection lasts life long for most persons. Most of the currently licensed vaccines use live-attenuated RA 27/9 strain of RV propogated in human diploid cells. One dose is given by either the intramuscular or subcutaneous route. Generally, no booster is required. The vaccine RA 27/9 is highly efficacious. In clinical trials, 95–100% of susceptible persons aged 12 months and older developed protective rubella antibodies by 21–28 days after vaccination (see Rubella Vaccines: World Health Organization position paper, 2000). According to the United States Center for Disease Control and Prevention (CDC), the following individuals should get the rubella vaccine:

- Adults born in 1957 or later, who do not have a medical contraindication should receive the vaccine.
- College and university students, healthcare personnel, non-pregnant women of childbearing age, childcare workers such as teachers and day care personnel, and international travelers.

A report summarizing the history and accomplishments of the rubella vaccination program in the United States and the Western Hemisphere and the challenges posed by rubella for the future has been published (CDC, 2005):

> In October 2004, CDC convened an independent panel of internationally recognized authorities on public health, infectious disease, and immunization to assess progress toward elimination of rubella and CRS in the United States, a national health objective for 2010. Since rubella vaccine licensure in 1969, substantial declines in rubella and CRS have occurred, and the absence of endemic-transmission in the United States is supported by recent data: (1) fewer than 26 reported rubella cases each year since 2001, (2) at least 95% vaccination coverage among school-aged children, (3) estimated 91% population immunity, (4) adequate surveillance to detect rubella outbreaks, and (5) a pattern of virus genotypes consistent with virus originating in other parts of the world. Given the available data, panel members concluded unanimously that rubella is no longer endemic in the United States

In summary, a safe, effective rubella vaccine is available, and there are proven vaccination strategies for preventing rubella and CRS. At present, a total of 124 of 214 countries (58%) are implementing rubella vaccination (Robertson et al., 2004). Rubella vaccine use varies by the stage of economic development: 100% for industrialized countries, 71% for countries with economics in transition, and 48% for developing countries (Robertson et al., 2004). Ministries of Health of developing countries with some help from the WHO should encourage the introduction of rubella vaccine and its universal use by their governments and emphasize that the introduction of rubella vaccine in the long run is cost-effective and cost-beneficial.

References

Abbott GG, Safford JW, McDonald RG, Craine M, Applegren RR. Development of automated immunoassays for immune status screening and serodiagnosis of rubella infection. J Virol Methods 1990; 27: 227–240.

Best JM, Bantavala JE. Congenital virus infections. Br Med J 1990; 300: 1151–1152.

Bosma TJ, Corbett KM, O'Shea S, Banatvala JE, Best JM. Polymerase chain reaction of rubella virus RNA in clinical samples. J Clin Microbiol 1995; 33: 1075–1079.

Cary BM, Arthur RJ, Houlsby WT. Ventriculitis in congenital rubella syndrome: ultrasound demonstration. Pediat Radiol 1987; 17: 358–368.

Centers for Disease Control and Prevention (CDC). Elimination of rubella and congenital rubella syndrome—United States, 1969–2004. MMW 2005; 54: 279–282.

Cooray S, Warner L, Jin L. Improved RT-PCR for diagnosis and epidemiological surveillance of rubella. J Clin Virol 2006; 35: 73–80.

Cutts FT, Vynnycky E. Modelling the incidence of congenital rubella syndrome in developing countries. Int J Epidemiol 1999; 28: 1176–1184.

Dille BJ, Safford JW, Mushahwar IK. Congenital diseases of microbiological origin. In: The Immunoassay Handbook (Wild D, editor). 3rded. London: Elsevier; 2005; pp. 746–755.

Dominguez G, Wang CY, Frey TK. Sequence of the genome RNA of rubella virus: evidence for genetic rearrangement during togavirus evolution. Virology 1990; 177: 225–238.

Edlich RF, Winters KL, Long WB, Gubler KD. Rubella and congenital rubella (German measles). J Long Term Eff Med Implants 2005; 15: 319–328.

Enders, G. Infektionen und impfungen in der Schwangerschaft. Munich: Urban & Schwarzenberg; 1994; pp. 9–35.

Enders G, Knotek F. Rubella IgG total antibody avidity and IgG subclass-specific antibody avidity assay and their role in the differentiation between primary rubella and rubella reinfection. Infection 1989; 17: 218–226.

Erdman E. Immunoglobulin M determinations. In: Clinical Virology Manual (Specter S, Hodinka RL, Young SA, editors). 3rd ed. Washington, DC: ASM Press; 2000; pp. 146–153.

Floret D, Rosenberg D, Hage GN, Monnet P. Hyperthyroidism, diabetes mellitus and congenital rubella syndrome. Acta Pediatt Scan 1980; 69: 259–261.

Frey TK. Neurological aspects of rubella virus infection. Intervirology 1997; 40: 167–175.

Fuccillo DA, Vacante DA, Sever JL. Rapid viral diagnosis. In: Manual of Clinical Laboratory Immunology (Rose NR, deMacario EC, Fahey L, Friedman H, Penn GM, editors). 4th ed. Washington, DC: ASM Press; 1992; pp. 445–445.

Garbalenga AE, Konin EV, Lai MN. Putative papain-related thiol proteases of positive-strand RNA viruses. Identification of rubi- and apathovirus proteases and delineation of a novel conserved domain associated with proteases of rubi-1x alpha- and coronaviruses. FEBS Lett 1991; 288(1–2): 201–205.

Given KT, Lee DA, Jones T, Ilstrop DM. Congenital rubella syndrome: ophthalmic manifestations and associated systemic disorders. Br J Opthalmol 1993; 77: 358–363.

Gleghorn EE. Growth of children with congenital rubella syndrome. J Pediat 1989; 115: 922–925.

Gravell M, Dorsett PH, Gutenson O, Ley AC. Detection of antibody to rubella virus by enzyme-linked immunosorbent assay. J Infect Dis 1977; 136(Suppl 1): S300.

Haukenes G, Matre R, Tondor O, Myrmel H, Schrumpf E. Measles and rubella antibodies in patients with chronic liver disease. J Hepatol 1990; 11: 389.

Hedman K, Rousseau SA. Measurement of avidity of specific IgG for verification of recent primary rubella. J Med Virol 1989; 27: 288–292.

Hedman K, Sappala I. Recent rubella virus infection indicated by low avidity of specific IgG. J Clin Immunol 1988; 8: 214–221.

Ho-Terry L, Cohen A, Landesborough P. Rubella virus wild type and RA 27/3 strains: a comparison by polyacrylamide-gel electrophoresis and radioimmune precipitation. J Med Microbiol 1984; 15: 393–398.

Hudson P, Morgan-Capner P. Evaluation of 15 commercial immunoassays for the detection of rubella-specific IgM. Clin Diag Virol 1996; 5: 21–26.

Inouye S, Hasegawa A, Matsuno S, Katow S. Changes in antibody avidity after virus infection: detection by an immunosorbent assay in which a mild protein-denaturing agent is employed. J Clin Microbiol 1984; 20: 525–529.

Kalimo KOK, Meurman OH, Halonen PE, Ziola BR. Solid-phase radioimmunoassay of rubella virus immunoglobulin G and immunoglobulin M antibodies. J Clin Microbiol 1976; 4: 117–123.

Kalkkinen N, Oker-Blom C, Pattersson RF. Three genes code for rubella virus structural proteins E1, E2a, E2b and C. J Gen Virol 1984; 65: 1549–1557.

Kalvenes MB, Haukenes G, Nysaeter G, Kalland KH, Myrmel H. Raised levels of antibodies to human viruses at the clinical onset of autoimmune chronic active hepatitis. J Viral Hepat 1995; 2: 159–164.

Katow H. Rubella virus genome diagnosis during pregnancy and mechanism of congenital rubella. Intervirology 1998; 41: 163–169.

Katow S. Molecular epidemiology of rubella virus in Asia: utility for reduction in the burden of diseases due to congenital rubella syndrome. Pediat Int 2004; 46: 207–213.

Kuroda Y, Matsui M. Progressive rubella panencephalitis. Nippon Rinsho 1997; 55: 922–925.

Lehtonen OP, Meurman OH. An ELISA for the establishment of high-avidity and total specific IgG and IgM antibodies of recent primary rubella. J Med Virol 1989; 27: 288–292.

Mace M, Cointe D, Six C, Levy-Bruhl D, Parent du Chatalet I, Ingrand D, Grangeot-Keros L. Diagnosis value of reverse transcription-PCR of amniotic fluid for prenatal diagnosis of congenital rubella infection in pregnant women with confirmed primary rubella infection. J Clin Microbiol 2004; 42: 4818–4820.

Matter L, Gorgierski-Hrisoha M, Germann D. Comparison of four ELISAs for detection of IgM antibodies against rubella virus. J Clin Microbiol 1994; 32: 2134–2139.

Meurman OH. Persistence of immunoglobulin G and immunoglobulin M after postnatal rubella infection determined by radioimmunoassay. J. Clin. Microbiol. 1978; 7: 34–38.

Meurman OH. Detection of antiviral IgM antibodies and its problems—a review. Curr Top Microbiol Immunol 1983; 104: 101–131.

Meurman OH, Viljanen MK, Granfors K. Solid-phase radioimmunoassay of rubella virus immunoglobulin M antibodies: comparison with sucrose density gradient centrifugation test. J Clin Microbiol 1977; 5: 257–262.

Meurman OH, Ziola BR. IgM class rheumatoid factor interference in the solid-phase radioimmunoassay of rubella-specific IgM antibodies. J Clin Pathol 1978; 31: 483–487.

Morgan-Capher P, Burgess C, Ireland RM, Sharp JC. Clinically apparent rubella reinfection with a detectable rubella specific IgM response. Br Med J 1983; 2816: 1616.

Mushahwar IK, Overby LO. Radioimmne assays for diagnosis of infectious diseases. In: Radioimmunoassays (Ashkar FS, editor). Boca Raton, FL: CRC Press; 1983; pp. 167–194.

Neto EC, Rubin R, Schulte J, Giugliani R. Screening for congenital infectious diseases. Emer Infect Dis 2004; 10: 1068–1073.

Oker-Blom C. The gene order of rubella virus structural proteins is NH2-C-E2-E1-COOH. J Virol 1984; 31: 354–358.

Pattison JR, Dane DS, Mace JE. Persistence of specific IgM after natural infection with rubella virus. Lancet 1975; 1: 185–187.

Porterfield JS, Casals J, Chumakuv MP, Gaidamovich SY, Hannoun IH, Horzinek MC, Mussgay M, Oker-Blom N, Russell PK, Trent DW. Togaviridae. Intervirology 1978; 9: 129–148.

Pustowoit B, Liebert UG. Predictive value of serological tests in rubella virus infection during pregnancy. Intervirology 1998; 41: 176–177.

Rahman MM, Khan AM, Hafiz MM, Ronny FM, Ara S, Chowdhury SK, Nazir SS, Khan WI. Congenital hearing impairment associated with rubella: lessons from Bangladesh. Southeast Asian J Trop Med Pub Health 2002; 33: 811–817.

Revello MG, Baldanti F, Sarasini A, Zavattoni M, Torsellini M, Gerna G. Prenatal diagnosis of rubella virus infection by direct detection and semiquantitation of viral RNA in clinical samples by reverse transcription-PCR. J Clin Microbiol 1997; 55: 708–713.

Robertson SE, Featherstone DA, Gacic-Dobo M, Hersh BS. Rubella and congenital rubella syndrome: global update. Rev Panam Salus Publica 2004; 15: 145–146.

Rubella vaccines: World Health Organization position paper. Wkly Epidem Record 2000; 75: 161–169.

Steininger C, Aberle SW, Popow-Kraup T. Early detection of acute Rhiovirus infection by rapid reverse transcription-PCR assay. J Clin Microbiol 2001; 39: 129–133.

Thomas HI, Morgan-Capner P, Cradock-Watson JG, Enders G, Best JM, O'Shea S. Slow maturation of IgG1 avidity and persistence of specific IgM in congenital rubella: implication for diagnosis and immunopathology. J Med Virol 1993; 41: 196–200.

Thomas HI, Morgan-Capner P, Enders G, O'Shea S, Caldicott D, Best JM. Persistence of specific IgM and low avidity specific IgG1 following primary rubella infection. J Virol Methods 1992; 39: 149–155.

Tipples GA, Hamkar R, Mokhtari AT, Gary M, Ball J, Head C, Ratnam S. Evaluation of rubella IgM immunoassays. J Clin Virol 2004; 30: 233–238.

Voller A, Bidwell DE. A simple method for detecting antibodies to rubella. Br J Exp Pathol 1975; 56: 338–339.

Voller A, Bidwell DE. Enzyme-immunoassay for antibodies to measles, cytomegalovirus infections and after rubella vaccination. Br J Exp Pathol 1976; 57: 243–247.

Vyse AJ, Jin L. An RT-PCR assay using oral fluid samples to detect rubella virus genome for epidemiological surveillance. Mol Cell Probes 2002; 16: 93–97.

Waxham MN, Wolinsky JS. Immunochemical identification of rubella virus hemagglutination. Virology 1983; 126: 194–203.

Wolinsky JS, McCarthy M, Allen-Cannady O, Moore WT, Jin R, Cao SN, Lovett A, Simmons D. Monoclonal antibody-defined epitope map of expressed rubella virus protein domain. J Virol 1991; 67: 3986–3994.

Yang D, Hwang D, Qiu Z, Gillam S. Effects of mutations in the rubella virus E1 glycoprotein E1–E2 interaction and membrane fusion activity. J Virol 1998; 72: 8747–8755.

Zheng DP, Frey TK, Icenogle J, Katow S, Abernathy ES, Song KJ, Xu WB, Yarulin V, Desjatskova RG, Aboudy Y, Enders G, Croxon M. Global distribution of rubella virus genotypes. Emerg Infect Dis 2003; 9: 1523–1530.

Congenital and Other Related Infectious
Diseases of the Newborn
Isa K. Mushahwar (Editor)
DOI 10.1016/S0168-7069(06)13012-8

Congenital Chagas Disease

Alejandro Gabriel Schijman

*Laboratorio de Biología Molecular de la Enfermedad de Chagas (LABMECH),
Instituto de Investigaciones en Ingeniería Genética y Biología Molecular (INGEBI),
Consejo Nacional de Ciencia y Tecnología (CONICET), Vuelta de Obligado 2490,
Buenos Aires, 1428, Argentina*

Abstract

Chagas disease, a antropozoonosis caused by the protozoan *Trypanosoma cruzi*, is
one of the main parasitic diseases to threaten public health in the world. More than
any other parasitic disease, Chagas disease is closely related to social and economic
development. *T. cruzi* infection may be acquired through the triatomid insect vector, blood transfusion, and the transplacental route causing congenital Chagas
disease. The success in the control of vector-transmitted Chagas'disease and
screening programs in blood banks has uncovered the public health relevance of
congenital transmission, which has been gradually emerging in vector-free suburban areas and non-endemic cities, contributing to the urbanization of the infection.
It has been estimated that congenital transmission is responsible for 8000–16,000
annual cases in the endemic countries of America. It is a consensus that congenital
Chagas disease will be a pressing public health concern until the pool of infected
women of childbearing age decreases to insignificant levels, which may happen only
30 years onwards, at least in the Southern Cone countries.
Congenital transmission may occur at any time of pregnancy, in successive gestations and may affect twins. The infection may produce pathology in the growing
foetus. The consequences on the newborn are variable, ranging from asymptomatic
to severe clinical manifestations. The prevalence of *T. cruzi* infection in women of
childbearing age, congenital transmission rates, clinical forms of disease, and mortality vary largely according to the geographical areas under study. Host conditions, such as the immunological, genetic, and nutritional status of the mothers,
age, obstetrical history, and maternal stage of the disease, as well as parasite strains,
histotropism and maternal parasitaemia may account as risk factors for pregnancy
outcome and incidence of congenital Chagas disease. Congenital transmission

cannot be prevented, but early diagnosis of the newborn enables prompt treatment, achieving cure rates close to 100% and thus avoiding progression to chronic Chagas disease.

In this chapter, epidemiological, clinical, and inmunological aspects as well as mechanisms of transmission, host and parasitic risk factors are described and discussed. Finally, consensus recommendations of strategies for diagnosis and treatment of congenital Chagas disease are presented in detail.

Background on *Trypanosoma cruzi* infection and Chagas disease

Introduction

Chagas disease, an antropozoonosis caused by the protozoan *Trypanosoma cruzi*, is one of the main parasitic diseases to threaten worldwide public health (WHO, 2002). It affects approximately 20 million persons; other 90 millions are at risk of acquiring the infection, and 1 million new cases and more than 45,000 deaths are recorded annually primarily in Central and South America (Schmuñis, 1999; WHO, 2002). Chagas' disease contributes an annual losss of approximately 2,740,000 disability-adjusted life years, four times the overall burden of malaria, schistosomiasis, leprosy, and leishmaniasis in the Continent (Schmuñis, 1999). The economic loss due to early deaths and disabilities caused by Chagas disease in the productive human population has been estimated to be 8,156,000 US dollars, which corresponds to the 2.5% of the external debt of America in 1995 (WHO, 2002).

The disease was named after the Brazilian physician and infectologist Carlos Justiniano Ribeiro das Chagas, who first described it in 1909 (Chagas, 1909). Chagas discovered that the intestines of Triatomidae harboured a flagellate protozoan, a new species of the *Trypanosoma* genus, named *Schizotrypanum cruzi* (later renamed to *T. cruzi*), after Oswaldo Cruz, the distinguished Brazilian physician and epidemiologist. Chagas was able to prove experimentally that the infection could be transmitted into marmoset monkeys, which were bitten by the infected bug. Chagas' work is unique in the history of medicine, because he was the only researcher so far to discover the pathogen in the vector, before describing the epidemiological and clinical features of the human disease. Later on, in 1926, the Argentinean physician Salvador Mazza, corroborated Dr Chagas' findings revealing that the disease was endemic in the Americas.

It was speculated that Charles Darwin might have suffered from Chagas disease as a result of a bite of a triatomine bug. The episode was reported by him in his diaries of the *Voyage of the Beagle* as occurring in March 1835 near Mendoza in Argentina. In 1837, almost a year after he returned to England, he began to suffer intermittently from strange symptoms that incapacitated him for much of the rest of his life. Attempts to test Darwin's remains at the Westminster Abbey by using Polymerase Chain Reaction (PCR) techniques were rejected by the Abbey's curator.

The parasite is transmitted to humans mostly by domiciliated hematophagous insects of the subfamily Triatominae (Family Reduviidae). Once *T. cruzi* enters the body, the infection passes through two successive stages: an acute and a chronic phase. The acute phase may last between six and eight weeks. Once this subsides, most infected patients appear without clinical signs and symptoms of disease. This form is known as the indeterminate phase, which is life-long in most patients. However, several years after the chronic phase is ensued, 10–40% of infected individuals, depending on the geographical area, will develop irreversible lesions in the heart, oesophagus, colon, and the nervous system. This symptomatic chronic phase lasts for the rest of the life of the infected individual (WHO, 2002).

More than any other parasitic disease, Chagas disease is closely linked to social and economic under-development: poor living conditions, limited access to health care and poor housing of rural endemic areas or on the outskirts of urban centres. A determining factor is the abundance of domestic animals, livestock enclosures, clay-walled vegetable plots, chicken runs and wood-burning stoves. However, the epidemiological picture of Chagas disease has changed over the last decades; it is no longer restricted to rural areas of endemicity, as migration to urban centres has opened up new modes of transmission, mainly via blood transfusion and congenitally.

Trypanosoma cruzi

Taxonomy, developmental stages and life cycle

T. cruzi belongs to the Kinetoplastida order and the Trypanosomatidae family. It is classified into a special section, designated Stercoraria, because it is the only human trypanosome to be transmitted by the faeces of its invertebrate vector. This protozoan is widespread in the Americas, from the Great Lakes of the United States of America to the southern Patagonia of Argentina (approximately 42°N–46°S).

Four main evolutive forms can be identified during the parasite life cycle: (1) The trypomastigote is the infective flagellate form of the parasite, which is found in (a) the bloodstream of the mammalian host, known as blood trypomastigote and (b) in the terminal portion of the digestive and urinary tracts of the vectors, named as metacyclic trypomastigote; (2) The epimastigote is the replicative form of the parasite in the reduviid bug as well as in the acellular culture medium; (3) The amastigote is the intracellular replicative form of the parasite in the vertebrate host; (4) The spheromastigote is the non-replicative form found in the stomach of the vector.

T. cruzi amastigotes are transmitted from the redivuiid bug to the mammalian host via the vector faeces after a bug bite and can invade several types of host cells, where they differentiate into aflagellate amastigotes. The amastigotes develop into non-dividing extracellular trypomastigotes, which can initiate another round of host cell infection or infect a reduviid vector during feeding and differentiate into epismastigotes. A schematic view of the *T. cruzi* life cycle can be obtained at http://www.dpd.cdc.gov/dpdx/HTML/ TrypanosomiasisAmerican.htm or at http://www.who.int/tdr/diseases/chagas/lifecycle.htm.

Populational genetic structure of T. cruzi

T. cruzi is a paradigmatic case of predominantly clonal evolution (Tibayrenc et al., 1986) with "unequivocal evidence of genetic recombination", recently demonstrated in the laboratory (Gaunt et al., 2003). Long-term clonal evolution together with episodes of genetic exchange led to the individualization of six lineages, designated as *T. cruzi* I, *T. cruzi* IIa, *T. cruzi* IIb, *T. cruzi* IIc, *T. cruzi* IId and *T. cruzi* IIe, which include all typed strains and cloned stocks thus far isolated (Brisse et al., 2003; Tibayrenc, 2003). On the basis of sequence analysis from nuclear and mitochondrial genes, it has been estimated that the major extant lineages of *T. cruzi* have diverged during the Miocene or early Pliocene (3–16 million years ago) (Machado and Ayala, 2001; Brisse et al., 2003). It has been proposed that ancestral *T. cruzi* I and *T. cruzi* IIb strains gave rise to a heterozygous hybrid that homogenized its genome to become the homozygous progenitor of lineages *T. cruzi* IIa and *T. cruzi* IIc; a second hybridization event between *T. cruzi* IIb and *T. cruzi* IIc strains generated *T. cruzi* lineages IId and IIe (Westenberger et al., 2005). This ability for genetic exchange is relevant concerning the potential spreading of pathogenic strains and drug-resistant genotypes.

   T. cruzi lineages appear to be distributed differentially among triatomine and host species and habitats in different geographical areas (Higo et al., 2004; Yeo et al., 2005). Although all *T. cruzi* populations cause the human disease, epidemiological studies suggest that *T. cruzi* IIb, IId and IIe are more related to anthroponotic environments and chronic Chagas disease patients, *T. cruzi* lineages IIa and IIc to sylvatic environments, and *T. cruzi* lineage I to both (Yeo et al., 2005). These host and geographic specificities are associated with different biological properties, such as growth rate, histotropism, antigenicity, pathogenicity, infectivity of potential insect vectors, drug susceptibility, chromosome number and DNA content, which are likely to represent key determinants in transmission and pathogenesis of Chagas disease (Macedo and Pena, 1998; Macedo et al., 2004). The identification of lineages, natural isolates and strains of *T. cruzi* has been established by a plethora of biochemical and molecular markers from parasite isolates (Brisse et al., 2000; Tibayrenc, 2003; Macedo et al., 2004), and more recently, directly from clinical and vector specimens (Freitas et al., 2005; Burgos et al., 2005; Burgos, 2006; Marcet et al., 2006).

   In 1994, the Strategic Research Branch of the Special Programme for Research and Training in Tropical Diseases (TDR) of the World Health Organization (WHO) founded the *T. cruzi* Genome Network. The characterization of the gene content and genome architecture of *T. cruzi*, as well as a whole-organism proteomic analysis of its four life cycle stages has been recently achieved (El-Sayed et al., 2005). Based on the assembly of a whole genome shotgun, the parasite diploid genome size has been estimated to range between 106.4 and 110.7 M bp and it has been predicted to contain 23,022 protein coding genes of which 12,574 represent allelic pairs and 704 RNA genes. More than 50% is conformed by repetitive sequences. A proteome of about 6200 genes organized in large polycistronic gene clusters has been identified (El-Sayed et al., 2005). Peptides mapping to 2784 proteins in 1168 protein groups from the annotated genome have been identified across the four life cycle stages. Protein products have been identified from more than 1000 genes annotated as "hypothetical" in the sequenced genome (Atwood et al., 2005). Future comparative genomics of different strains may identify genes associated with pathogenecity and lead to prognostic markers. This source of genomic and proteomic data constitutes a powerful tool to design novel strategies for diagnosis, epidemiological control and management of the infection, as well as for development of vaccines and identification of new drug targets for innovative aetiological therapies.

Modes of transmission of human T. cruzi infection

Transmission by vectors

The main epidemiological way of infection occurs through infected triatomine bugs, when they puncture the skin to feed on blood and simultaneously eject their faeces or urine containing metacyclic trypomastigotes. The parasites make contact with the mucous membrane of eyes, nose, mouth or injured skin of the mammalian host (Dias, 1979). Direct skin penetration seems more difficult and generally the itching caused by the bite leads to scratching, allowing the parasites to enter the circulation through the microlesions thus created. Alternatively, during scratching, parasites can also be transferred to the conjunctiva, leading to the Romaña sign (Romaña, 1935), which is typical of 20–50% of acute vectorial cases. Most cases of Chagas disease can be attributed to the principal domiciliated insect species, namely *Panstrongylus megistus, Rhodnius prolixus, Triatoma brasiliensis, T. dimidiata* and *T. infestans* (WHO, 2002).

Transfusional transmission

Transfusion of infected blood, containing trypomastigotes, is responsible for 5–20% of the human cases of Chagas disease (Schmuñis, 1999). The migratory movements in Latin America during the past decades, from rural endemic areas to non-endemic centres and countries have changed the traditional epidemiological picture of Chagas disease transmission (WHO, 2002). A Southern Cone Initiative (Schofield and Dias, 1999) has promoted the interruption of vectorial and transfusional Chagas disease in Uruguay since 1997, in Chile since 1999, in central and southern Brazil since 2001, in four endemic provinces of Argentina since 2002, and in one department of Paraguay since 2003. This succesful initiative has spawned an Andean Pact control programme, a Central America Control programme and a surveillance programme to protect the Amazon basin from incursion by domestic vectors (WHO, 2002).

Oral transmission

Oral transmission of Chagas disease has been recorded in many microepidemics of acute Chagas disease in Brazil, Colombia and Mexico, after ingestion of food contaminated with infected triatomines or their dejections (Shikanai-Yasuda et al., 1991; WHO, 2002).

Transmission from donor organ transplantation to uninfected recipients

Kidney, heart, bone marrow, pancreas and liver transplantation, from both dead and live donors are the causes of *T. cruzi* transmissions (WHO, 2002).

Sexual transmission

The presence of *T. cruzi* in menstrual blood of chronic Chagas disease women as well as in the genitalia of patients with AIDS implies the possibility of transmission through sexual intercourse (Concetti et al., 2000; Rocha et al., 1994).

Accidental transmission

Accidental transmission of human Chagas disease has been reported in many situations, in laboratories, hospitals and research laboratories handling different sources of contaminated materials, namely triatomine dejections, parasite cultures and infected blood of human and animals. All personnel manipulating *T. cruzi*-infected biological samples or triatomines must follow safety precautions for laboratory work (WHO, 2002).

Congenital transmission

Congenital transmission of *T. cruzi* infection, leading to congenital Chagas disease (CCD) can be suspected in any child born to a *T. cruzi*-infected pregnant woman, regardless of her stage of *T. cruzi* infection. The parasite may be transmitted into some or all siblings of successive gestations (Bittencourt et al., 1992; Freilij and Altcheh, 1995; Russomando et al., 1998; Torrico et al., 2004) and may also affect twins (Hoff et al., 1978). Moreover, CCD of second generation has been recorded in non-endemic areas (Schenone et al., 1987; Freilij et al., 1994; Sanchez Negrette et al., 2005).

Epidemiological, clinical and inmunological aspects, mechanisms of transmission and risk factors, strategies of diagnosis and treatment of CCD are presented in the following section.

Congenital *T. cruzi* infection

Epidemiological aspects

The first documentation of CCD in humans was raised by Carlos Chagas in 1911, with the follow-up of two newborns with convulsive episodes who died after six and eight days of life, respectively, revealing parasites in their necropsies (Chagas, 1911). Four decades later, Dao (1949) described a *T. cruzi* infection in a newborn from Venezuela. Jörg (1953) published the first record of CCD in Argentina, Howard (1957) in Chile and Rezende (1959) and Bittencourt (1960) in Brazil (Freilij et al., 1994). All these records were based on severe clinical manifestations. In the 1970s, histopathological studies by Bittencourt and coworkers (1972), demonstrated the presence of *T. cruzi* in necropsies from foetuses and stillbirths. However, prospective studies of siblings born to seropositive women have revealed that most CCD cases were asymptomatic.

CCD has also been reported in Bolivia, Colombia, Guatemala, Honduras, Paraguay, Uruguay and recently in Mexico (Guzman-Bracho et al., 1998). In addition, it has also been diagnosed in descendants from infected immigrant women born in non-endemic American and European countries (Woody and Woody, 1955; Pehrson et al., 1981; congenital infection with *T. cruzi*: from mechanisms of transmission to strategies for diagnosis and control. Rev Soc Bras Med Trop Nov–Dec, 2003; 36(6): 767–771).

The prevalence of Chagas disease in pregnant women of urban and rural areas of Latin America oscilates between 4 and 52% (WHO, 2002). In recent years, the success in the control of vector-transmitted Chagas' disease and screening programs in blood banks has reduced the prevalence of infected pregnant women, most of which were infected by the vectorial route. Most pregnant women infected with *T. cruzi* do not show signs and symptoms of Chagas disease. The lack of electrocardiographic and clinical signs in women of reproductive age is likely due to the fact that the onset of cardiac manifestations of chronic Chagas disease occurs more frequently at older ages.

It is a consensus that CCD will be a pressing public health concern until the pool of infected women of childbearing age decreases to insignificant levels, which may happen only 30 years onwards, at least in the Southern Cone countries (WHO, 2002).

The transmission rates of CCD vary in different geographical regions, ranging from 0.1% in regions of Brazil and Argentina to 7% or more in some areas of Bolivia, Chile and Paraguay (Schenone, 1985; Lorca et al., 1987; Zaidenberg and Segovia, 1993; Freilij and Altcheh, 1995; Russomando et al., 1998; Blanco et al., 1999; Gûrtler et al., 2003; Torrico et al., 2004; Mora et al., 2005; Mendoza Ticona et al., 2005).

The control of vectorial and transfusional transmission has uncovered the Public Health importance of CCD.

Pinto Diaz has estimated that congenital transmission is responsible for 8000–16,000 annual cases in America (INCOSUR Report, 2001); recent estimations from Argentina have indicated that the rate of CCD is 10 times higher than that of acute vectorial cases (Gürtler et al., 2003).

Owing to the migration from endemic areas to vector-free suburban and urban centres, CCD is becoming increasingly responsible for the urbanization of Chagas disease.

Mechanisms of transmission

Transplacental transmission

The maternal trypomastigotes at the intervillous space penetrate actively through the trophoblast. They differentiate to amastigotes and multiply mainly within the Hofbauer cells. Rupture of these nests or pseudocysts spreads the parasites and cellular contents in the interstitium, where they provoke an inflammatory reaction and necrosis of the placental villi. Intact trypomastigotes, which may also be released, invade other cells and/or may reach the foetal circulation, leading to congenital infection (Bittencourt, 1963, 1992).

The mechanisms by which the trophoblastic layer prevents foetal infection are not well understood. It has been shown that lysosomal enzymes expressed by the trophoblasts might restrict parasite propagation (Fretes and De Fabro, 1995; Frank et al., 2000). Otherwise, a pathogenetic role for human placental alkaline phosphatase (PLAP) in CCD has been proposed. PLAP is a trophoblast plasma membrane protein anchored to the outer leaflet of the cell membrane lipid bilayer by a glycosylphosphatidylinositol (GPI) molecule and it has been suggested that it is important for maternal acceptance of the foetal autograft. Sartori et al. (1997) have postulated that a decrease in PLAP activity from 36 to 40 weeks of gestation in women with Chagas disease is related to congenital transmission. PLAP is modified in the sera of seropositive pregnant women (Sartori et al., 1997) and in placental villi cultured with *T. cruzi* (Sartori et al., 2002). PLAP participates in the process of *T. cruzi* invasion into placental syncytiotrophoblast cells by a mechanism that involves hydrolysis of the GPI molecule, the activation of tyrosine kinase proteins, increase of cytosolic calcium and finally the rearrangement of active filaments of the host cells.

Placental inflammation always represents a primary immune response of the foetus to *T. cruzi* because the placenta is the first foetal organ to encounter the parasite in the maternal circulation. Immunohistochemical characterization of placental villitis caused by *T. cruzi* infection has revealed CD68+ macrophages and CD8+ T lymphocytes as the predominant cell populations. Interestingly, differences in the pattern of the inflammatory reaction have been observed between live and stillbirths (Altemani et al., 2000). In live births, the villitis is focal with few parasite nests, whereas in stillbirths it is diffused and severe with high quantities of parasite cells. Other placental features of stillbirths are frequent trophoblastic necrosis, MAC 387+ macrophages and CD15+ granulocytes at sites of trophoblastic necrosis, the lowest CD4+ : CD8+ ratios in 75% of cases and increased numbers of S-100 protein + macrophages in the villous stroma (Altemani et al., 2000).

In other histopathological studies, placental parasitism has been mainly detected in chorionic fibroblasts, and in the subamniotic mesenchyma of the marginal sinus, where the placental membranes attach to the chorionic plate, in the absence of villitis or intervillitis lesions, suggesting transference of parasites via the chorionic route without direct invasion of the trophoblast.

Placental parasitism and severity of histologic changes in placenta are not necessarily associated with foetal infection (Rassi et al., 1958; Moya et al., 1979; Moretti et al., 2005).

Extra-placentary transmission

The literature describes CCD with parasitism of the chorion and amnium of extraplacental membranes without invasion of chorionic villi, suggesting trans-membrane transmission of parasites without transplacental passage (Moya et al., 1979; Azogue et al., 1985). However, the mentioned works have not detailed the number of placental tissue sections analysed. On the basis of the higher blood supply reaching the placenta (half litre/minute) compared to the extra-placental membranes, it is unlikely that congenital infection may occur via extra-placental membranes without transplacental transmission. The simultaneous detection of parasites in foetal alveolar walls causing pneumonitis, in amniotic fluid of extraplacentary membranes and in amniotic epithelium of the umbilical cord (Bittencourt, 1988), has also been reported. However, these cases have only been detected in cases of pneumonitis; thus, transmission can be originated from the passage of parasites invading the foetal lungs to the amniotic fluid with subsequent parasitic invasion of the umbilical cord surface and extra-placentary membranes.

Congenital transmission can also take place at time of delivery in the birth canal. This mechanism of transmission could occur in parasitologically negative newborns that become parasitologically positive several weeks after birth (Moya et al., 1989; Blanco et al., 2000).

Breast-feeding transmission

There have been two published cases of Chagas disease in which breast milk was the suspected route of infection. The first case occurred in Salta, Argentina, in 1936 (Mazza et al., 1936) and the second one in Bahia, Brazil, in 1983 (Bittencourt et al., 1988). Following the second case, studies were carried out to determine if milk could transmit the infection. In one of them, when 100 milk or colostrum samples from 78 nursing mothers with acute Chagas disease were examined, the results showed that all were negative. A serological study of 97 breast-fed babies born free of infection did not detect seropositivity. The few cases of neonates free of infection who became infected during breast-feeding were associated with bleeding lesions of their mothers' nipples, thus oral transmission could not be discarded (Jörg, 1992).

In the murine model, a low number of non-infected neonatal mice nursed by female mice with acute Chagas disease acquired the infection during breast-feeding (Miles, 1972). Based on these findings, the WHO does not recommend that chagasic women restrict breast-feeding, except in cases of nipple bleeding (WHO, 2002).

Clinical aspects

Without treatment, *T. cruzi* infection is life-long. The outcome of infection in a particular individual is the result of complex interactions among the host genetic background, the genetic constitution of the parasite and environmental and social factors (Campbell et al., 2004).

There is no specific clinical marker of CCD. Congenital cases are frequently asymptomatic, passing unnoticed unless specific tests are made (Bittencourt, 1988; Freilij and Altcheh, 1994, 1995).

The symptoms of CCD are frequently prematurity, displaying low birth weight, hepatomegaly, splenomegaly, symptoms of acute respiratory distress, probably related to prematurity and/or anasarca. Bronchopneumonitis, digestive manifestations, transient ocular involvement central nervous system compromise intracranial calcification with signs of early foetal injury and microcephaly have been recorded (Pehrson et al., 1982; Atias et al., 1985; Muñoz et al., 1992). The clinical signs currently associated with CCD are not due to the so-called TORCH coinfections, conformed by (T)oxoplasmosis, (O)ther agents, (R)ubella, (C)ytomegalovirus and (H)erpes simplex (Klein and Remington, 2001). Differences among clinical manifestations of CCD newborns are observed in studies performed in diverse endemic and non-endemic regions. Indeed, in Salta, Northern Argentina, of a total of 102 CCD patients, 33.3% were asymptomatic, 28.4% premature, 58.8% had hepatomegaly, 42.1% splenomegaly, 40.2% jaundice, 39.2% anaemia, 4.9% hydrops foetalis and 3.9% meningoencephalitis (Zaidenberg, 1999). In Buenos Aires, among 168 patients, 75.6% were aymptomatic and only 8.6% showed hepatosplenomegaly, 1.32% sepsis, 2.3% myocarditis and 2.3% hepatitis (Freilij and Altcheh, 1995). These differences may depend on the nutritional and immunological status of the mother, the parasite strain and other factors yet to be identified. In cases of perinatal coinfection with HIV, signs of acute myocarditis or meningoencephalitis have been more frequently described (Freilij and Altcheh, 1995; Freilij et al., 1995). The coinfected neonates present higher levels of parasitaemia than HIV-negative ones. Double-infected children may have a poor clinical outcome, despite a good parasitologic response to trypanomicidal treatment (Freilij et al., 1995).

Around the seventh month of life congenitally infected patients depict their own IgG humoral response and subpatent parasitaemia, evolving to the so-called indeterminate phase of disease (Freilij et al., 1994). In this phase, neurologic sequelae and chronic cardiopathy have been detected (Arteaga-Fernandez et al., 1987; Bittencourt, 1988). In those patients who evolve to the chronic phase of disease, cardiac involvement is the most frequent and serious clinical form; it typically leads to complex arrhythmias, cardiac failure, thromboembolism and sudden death (Rosenbaum, 1964; Rassi et al., 2000; WHO, 2002). However, a multivariate analysis of aged-matched chronic Chagas disease patients from Argentina has shown that congenitally infected patients present a lower prevalence of cardiopathy, and when they do present cardiopathy, there is a lower prevalence of dilation when compared to patients infected by the vectorial route and residing in endemic areas (Storino et al., 2002).

The digestive forms can lead to megaesopaghus and/or megacolon, with an associated cardiopathy in a proportion of cases (Atias, 1994; WHO, 2002).

The acquired immunodeficiency syndrome (AIDS) pandemic, with 1.4 million infected people in endemic regions for Chagas disease, may lead to reactivation of quiescent chronic *T. cruzi* infections. We have recently reported the diagnosis and follow-up of a congenital Chagas disease patient born in Buenos Aires city, non-endemic for *T. cruzi* infection, who acquired HIV infection at 29 years of life; his infection with *T. cruzi* was diagnosed when the patient was hospitalized with presumptive diagnosis of cerebral toxoplasmosis, which was later defined as cerebral Chagas disease reactivation. This stresses out the public health importance of surveying all newborns to seropositive mothers in both endemic and non-endemic areas for *T. cruzi* infection (Burgos et al., 2005).

Immunological aspects

Pregnancy is known to induce a transient depression of maternal cell-mediated immunity to prevent rejection of the foetus, which can increase the susceptibility to infections with pathogens.

Mothers who transmit CCD to their offspring have shown depressed production of parasite-specific interferon-γ by blood cells that persist after delivery (Hermann et al., 2004). Moreover, a significant correlation between *T. cruzi*-specific production of IFN-γ and either the age or the parity of infected mothers was observed. This indicates that younger infected mothers with fewer previous pregnancies produced less IFN-γ than did the older infected mothers with a higher number of previous pregnancies.

Flow cytometry has demonstrated that T cells and monocytes of transmitting mothers stimulated with *T. cruzi* lysate are less activated than those of non-transmitting mothers (Hermann et al., 2004).

Maternal–foetal transfer of antigens might influence the capacity of the progeny to respond to infection through modulation of the foetal immune system. *T. cruzi* infection in mothers induces deep alterations in the cytokine response of their uninfected neonates. The possibility of maternal in uterus modulation of the innate and/or of adaptive immune responses of uninfected newborns from *T. cruzi*-infected mothers has been investigated by studying the capacity of their white blood cells to produce cytokines in response to parasite lysate or lipopolysaccharide-plus-phytohaemagglutinin (LPS–PHA) stimulation (Vekemans et al., 2000). Cells of uninfected newborns occasionally release gamma interferon

(IFN-γ) and no interleukin-2 (IL-2) and IL-4 upon specific stimulation, while their mothers' cells produce IFN-γ, IL-2, and IL-4. In maternal cells and, remarkably, in cells from their uninfected neonates, the delivery of proinflammatory (IL-1β, IL-6, and tumour necrosis factor alpha (TNF-α]) and anti-inflammatory (IL-10 and soluble TNF receptor) cytokines or factors is upregulated in the presence of LPS-PHA and/or parasite lysate (Vekemans et al., 2000). Such maternal influence on neonatal innate immunity might have protective effects, contributing to limit the rate and severity of CCD.

Cord blood cells from CCD newborns display a predominant activation and oligoclonal expansion of CD8+ T lymphocytes producing interferon-γ, indicating a foetal immunologic response against *T.cruzi*. By contrast, non-infected newborns show an overactivation of their innate immunity, since their cord blood cells produce higher levels of inflammatory cytokines when stimulated with *T. cruzi*.

The analysis of IgM and IgG specificities against recombinant antigens in sera from chagasic mothers and their newborns has allowed the detection of new specificities in CCD, mostly targeted to shed acute-phase antigen (SAPA) and, less frequently, to other parasite antigens, undetectable in the mothers and in non-infected controls (Reyes et al., 1990). These findings led to propose these antigens as indicators of congenital transmission, but further work has revealed their presence in a proportion of chronic Chagas disease patients (Vergara et al., 1991).

Risk factors for congenital transmission

The prevalence of *T. cruzi* infection in women of childbearing age, the transmission rate and the morbidity and mortality of congenitally infected cases vary largely according to the geographical areas under study. Host conditions, such as the immunological, genetic and nutritional status of the women, age, obstetrical history and maternal stage of the disease, as well as parasitic characteristics, such as the strain of *T. cruzi* or the parasitic load, may account as risk factors for pregnancy outcome and congenital transmission (Bittencourt, 1992). Information on the effects of chronic *T. cruzi* infection on foetal growth, and health of uninfected babies born to infected mothers remains contradictory. Indeed, some studies have mentioned that maternal infection induces an increased risk of pregnancy loss or prematurity (de Castilho and de Silva, 1976; Hernandez-Matheson et al., 1983; Schenone et al., 1985), whereas other investigations have not detected any significant difference (Oliveira et al., 1966; Bittencourt, 1992; Blanco et al., 2000).

Pregnancy outcome

Studies carried out in endemic areas of Brazil and Bolivia (Oliveira et al., 1966; Azogue et al., 1985) have shown that in the absence of CCD transmission, maternal *T. cruzi* infection has no effect on gestational outcome, does not induce premature delivery or foetal growth retardation and does not affect the general health of newborns. In contrast, in Argentina and Chile, a positive correlation between abortion histories and maternal *T. cruzi* seropositivity has been reported (Schenone et al., 1985; Freilij et al., 1994). Studies of the experimental *T. cruzi* infection might reinforce our knowledge of materno–foetal interactions. *T. cruzi* acute infection deeply impairs the reproductive capacity of mice, compromising implantation and favouring placental parasitism and injury leading to foetal growth retardation and death, in the absence of CCD. Mjihdi et al. (2002) have found that acutely infected mice exhibit a reduction in fecundity associated to higher maternal parasitaemia. In fact, infected mated females do not become gravid and do not show implantation scars, suggesting that the reproductive failure occurs before implantation. Such "in-uterus" harmful effects may be triggered by a strong inflammatory response, the release of cytokines such as interferon-γ and TNF-α, which may in turn shed potent proinflammatory parasitic molecules (Laucella et al., 1996). Such maternal systemic inflammatory response might also contribute to induce resorptions, because a similar association is observed between the proportion of resorptions and maternal parasitaemia, whereas no parasites are detected in the uteroplacental units at an early step of gestation. Foetal mortality has been detected in late gestation, which is associated with high parasitism of uteroplacental units, particularly in decidua, without foetal transmission (Andrade, 1982; Mjihdi et al., 2002). Late placental parasitism has been related to placenta vascularization, increase of maternal parasitaemia and local release of type 2 cytokines and transforming growth factor-β, which antagonized the type 1 response that controls local intracellular parasite proliferation. Besides, transforming growth factor-β might favour the invasion of trypomastigotes to host cells by activating a specific signalling pathway for parasitic invasion (Hall and Pereira, 2000). The absence of congenital infection in foetuses, despite the massive parasite invasion in placenta and maternal blood, underlines the efficacy of the placental trophoblastic layer to block mother-to-foetus parasitic passage (Delgado and Santos-Buch, 1978; Andrade, 1982; Mjihdi et al., 2002). Placental injury, aggravated by the local inflammation caused by parasite persistence, might drastically limit the materno–foetal exchanges, leading to foetal death, as strongly suggested by the positive correlation between foetal death and placental parasitic load.

The higher frequency of premature rupture of membranes observed in mothers with Chagas disease who delivered CCD siblings might be related to the frequent chorioamnionitis detected in their placentas (Torrico et al., 2004). A higher frequency of premature births has been found among congenitally infected cases (Bittencourt et al., 1972). A comparison made between premature (30–37 weeks of gestation) and mature (38–40 weeks of gestation) newborns to seropositive mothers has shown a higher infection rate in premature (50.0%) than in mature children (8.7%; $p = 4.1 \times 10^{-6}$) (Sanchez Negrette et al., 2005). The correlation between birth weight and infection is strongly determined by the correlation between birth weight and gestational age. Even when excluding premature children, the association of weight at birth and congenital transmission is still highly significant. Thus, low birth weight and prematurity are independent risk factors for foetal infection with *T. cruzi*. Studies in Bahia, Brazil, from stillbirths, livebirths and mortinates have shown a higher frequency of congenital transmission during weeks 22 and 26 of gestation (Bittencourt, 1992). In a Bolivian study that included only livebirths, a higher frequency of transmission has been found between weeks 26 and 37 of gestation (Azogue and Darras, 1991).

Maternal age and family clustering

A higher incidence of CCD has been observed in infants born to younger *T. cruzi*-infected women with a lower number of previous pregnancies (Torrico et al., 2004). This might be related to the fact that parasitaemia decreases during the natural evolution of the infection to the chronic phase (Hoff et al., 1979). The decline of parasitaemia with age also argues for an improvement in immunity against *T. cruzi* infection over time. This is in line with data obtained in placental malaria studies highlighting the presence of higher levels of immunosuppressive corticosteroids in primigravidae (Rasheed et al., 1993) as well as the immunoenhancing effect of multiparity (Fievet et al., 2002).

Family clustering of CCD has been reported (Freilij and Altcheh, 1995; Sanchez Negrette et al., 2005; Burgos, 2006). The transmission rate in siblings of CCD patients selected as index cases is remarkably higher than that of siblings born to seropositive mothers who delivered all uninfected children. These findings have demonstrated that siblings of a CCD infant are at high risk for infection and, even in the absence of symptoms, should also be screened for infection (Sanchez Negrette et al., 2005). No influence on the proportion of CCD children has been detected regarding gender of the child (Sanchez Negrette et al., 2005).

CCD transmission from pregnant women with acute Chagas disease

Owing to the higher parasitaemia observed during acute Chagas disease, the risk of CCD transmission from mothers with acute infection appears to be higher than that from women with indeterminate or chronic Chagas disease. However, there are few reports on acute infections in pregnant women.

The first case in Brazil was described by Rassi and coworkers in 1958. At least 11 acute cases have been already reported in Brazil and Argentina, six of which have led to congenital transmission (Bittencourt, 1988; Moretti et al., 2005). Out of the three reported Argentinean pregnant women with acute Chagas disease (Moretti et al., 2005), the one who transmitted CCD had acquired *T. cruzi* infection at an early stage of her pregnancy, whereas the two non-transmitting women became infected during the third trimester, suggesting that the gestational period in which the mother acquires acute Chagas disease could be a risk factor for vertical transmission.

CCD transmission from pregnant women with chronic Chagas disease

Most studies targeted to elucidate the mechanisms of vertical transmission have been conducted in mothers at the indeterminate phase of the infection. Physiological immunomodulation occurring during pregnancy could lead to changes in the parasite populations. Xenodiagnosis-based follow-up has demonstrated an increase of the parasitaemia during pregnancy in women with indeterminate Chagas disease, particularly towards the last trimester (Storni and Bolsi, 1979). Moreover, an evaluation of the parasitemic profiles of 119 chronic Chagas disease women by means of xenodiagnosis during and after pregnancy, has shown a high frequency of positive xenodiagnosis during pregnancy (Menezes et al., 1992). Otherwise, the frequency of infected triatomines used for xenodiagnosis is more elevated during pregnancy, indicating higher parasitaemic levels in this period (Menezes et al., 1992). The association between higher maternal parasitaemia and higher CCD transmission has also been detected by means of haemoculture (Hermann et al., 2004) and PCR analysis (Burgos, 2006).

CCD transmission from pregnant women with T. cruzi and HIV co-infection

Exacerbation of *T. cruzi* parasitaemia may occur in immunosuppressed patients (Sartori et al., 2002a). *T. cruzi* parasitaemia is more frequently detected in HIV-positive than in HIV-negative subjects; HIV-positive subjects also exhibit higher parasitaemic levels (Sartori et al., 2002b). The follow-up of pregnant women with indeterminate Chagas disease has shown a higher frequency of HIV coinfected women among those who transmit CCD than among those who do not (Burgos, 2006). Moreover, parasite populations from HIV-coinfected CCD patients exhibit higher diversity in their minicircle signatures (Fig. 1B, F3) suggesting that immunosuppression might favour the proliferation of emergent *T. cruzi* variants, as recently detected in a CCD adult patient who suffered an episode of cerebral Chagas reactivation indicator of AIDS (Burgos et al., 2005).

Parasite histotropism and CCD

Studies performed in Chile have revealed that the distribution of parasite strains among CCD patients depends on the endemicity of the region; in highly endemic regions, CCD patients were exclusively infected with clonet 39 (*T. cruzi* IId), whereas in low endemic regions CCD patients were infected with clonet 39 and clonet 19/20 (*T. cruzi* I) in a low proportion (Garcia et al., 2001). Recent molecular fingerprinting of bloodstream *T. cruzi* populations in chagasic mothers from Argentina and Bolivia have identified, in all cases, *T. cruzi* IId, which corresponded to the lineage detected in their CCD newborns (Burgos et al., 2004; Burgos, 2006). Interestingly, one CCD newborn with perinatal HIV co-infection was dually infected with *T. cruzi* I and *T. cruzi* II lineages (Burgos et al., 2005). These novel findings are in agreement with the predominance of *T. cruzi* IId lineage in these endemic areas (Montamat et al., 1991; Breniere et al., 1998; Schijman, 2005). Previous research has demonstrated that the high variability of *T. cruzi* minicircle sequences may be useful for the characterization of genetic diversity at the infra-lineage level and directly in clinical or biological specimens (Vago et al., 1996).

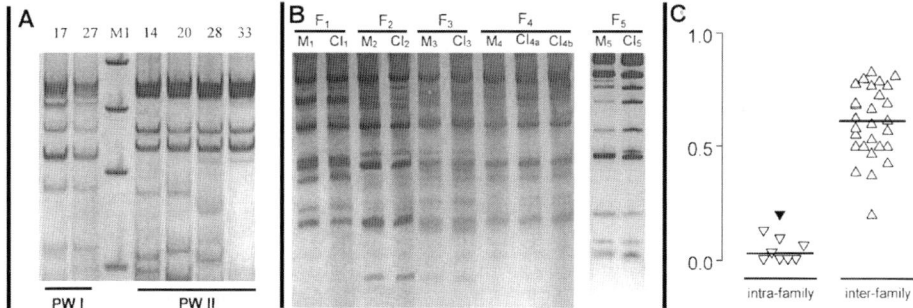

Fig. 1 Minicircle signatures of maternal and neonatal bloodstream *Trypanosoma cruzi* populations implicated in CCD. 10% Polyacrylamide gels showing MspI—RsaI minicircle RFLP-based profiles from 330 bp kinetoplastid DNA amplicons obtained from peripheral blood samples of: (A) Two infected pregnant women (PWI and PWII) analysed at different gestational weeks of second and third trimesters of pregnancy, indicated by the numbers at the top. M1: 100 bp molecular weight marker. (B) Five families composed by infected mothers (M) and their CCD infants (CI). Family 4 is conformed by two CCD twins, CI4a and CI4b. Blood samples were collected at time of CCD diagnosis: F1 and F2: 2 months; F3: 48 h; F4: 16 days and F5: 12 months after delivery, respectively. C: Jaccard Genetic distances among the minicircle signatures between each paired mother–infant (intra-family) and among the mothers of nine families (inter-family) are shown. It was calculated as: $D = -(a/(a+b+c))$, where a is the number of bands that are common to the two compared profiles, b the number of specific bands of the first profile and c the number of specific bands of the second profile. The intra-family JD median value was 0.056 (min 0–max 0.2) with the highest value for F5 pair (▼), the inter-family JD median value was (0.605, min 0.2–max 0.83) ($p < 0.05$) (Burgos, 2006).

Accordingly, we carried out RFLP–PCR of the 330 bp variable regions of the minicircles from the kinetoplastid genome obtained from consecutive peripheral blood samples collected at different gestational weeks during pregnancy, and found that the *T. cruzi* genetic profiles were different among each *T. cruzi* IId-infected pregnant woman (Fig. 1A, PWI and PWII). However, for each tested woman, a similar profile was detected along gestation, suggesting the persistence of the bloodstream parasite populations, with the exception of slight fluctuations of minor minicircle fragments (Fig. 1A, PWII, weeks 14, 20, 28 and 33) (Burgos et al., 2004; Burgos, 2006). Moreover, in the same work, comparative fingerprinting of minicircle signatures between maternal and neonatal parasite populations indicates almost identical profiles within each paired mother–neonate case (Fig. 1B and 1C, intra-family Jaccard Genetic Distances), including populations infecting CCD twins (Fig. 1B, CI 4a, and CI 4b of F4). A lower degree of similarity was observed in a pair of mother—infant whose blood samples were characterized one year after delivery (Fig. 1B, F5 and Fig. 1C, ▼). This PCR-based strategy demonstrates that the predominant populational structure of maternal bloodstream parasites persisted in their CCD babies at least during the first year of life. Noteworthy, similar minicircle profiles have been observed in blood collected from a pair of CCD sisters, born in consecutive gestations, confirming that pregnancy does not induce changes in the predominant parasite populations (Burgos, 2006; Schijman, 2005).

The parasite strain has also been implicated in the congenital infection in the experimental model. In a study performed by Andrade (1982), where pregnant female mice were infected with *T. cruzi* strains that differed according to several parameters, clear-cut differences were noted in the incidence of placental parasitism and in the localization of amastigotes in the vascular sinus of the placenta among the animals in the acute phase with different strains. No parasitism of the foetal tissues was seen. The incidence of placental parasitism reached 98% for the Colombian strain, 18.4% for the Peruvian strain, 17% for the Y strain and 13.2% for the Honorina strain (isolated from a woman who transmitted the infection to twins). The presence of parasites in the vascular part of the placenta was outstanding with the Colombian strain and infrequent with the others (Andrade, 1982).

In another study performed by Solana et al. (2002) where C3H/HeN female mice were infected with parasite strains of different lineages and histotropism (RA strain, *T. cruzi* II, pantropic/reticulotropic and K98 clone of CA-I strain, *T. cruzi* I, myotropic) differences in inflammatory compromise of the genital tract, in pregnancy outcome and incidence of congenital transmission were observed (Solana et al., 2002). The group of mice infected with the myotropic clone depicted lymphomononuclear infiltrates in pelvian fat and uterus interstitium, *T. cruzi* DNA and moderate oophoritis, perioophoritis and vasculitis. Fertility was significantly diminished and foetal resorptions increased but no cases of CCD were produced. In contrast, female mice infected with the pantropic–reticulotropic strain, showed, at mating time, mild oophoritis in the absence of inflammatory foci and parasite DNA in utero. It is worth to note that pregnant mice infected with this pantropic/reticulotropic strain transmitted CCD to 4% of their offspring (Solana et al., 2002).

On the basis of the above mentioned findings, it can be hypothesized that CCD patients become infected with the parasite populations predominating in maternal blood, which may not have a tropism for placental tissues and are more likely to actively penetrate from the intervillous space through the trophoblast layer reaching the foetal circulation originating CCD. Further studies comparing the molecular signatures of *T. cruzi* amastigotes detected in placental tissues with trypomastigotes circulating in maternal and CCD neonatal blood will shed more light regarding the role of the parasitic tropism in the incidence of congenital transmission.

Diagnosis of congenital T. cruzi infection

There is a consensus to define a case of CCD, namely: (i) the child has to be born to a mother with positive serology for *T. cruzi*, (ii) parasites must be identified at birth, or (iii) parasites and/or non-maternal-specific antibodies must be detected later after birth, providing that previous blood transfusion and vectorial contamination is discarded.

Parasitological diagnosis

Direct methods.   The microscopical observation of fresh blood between slide and coverslip can easily disclose the presence of the parasites because of their motility. Thin- and thick-stained blood smears allow detection of the morphological characteristis of the parasite, even to differentiate *T. cruzi* from *T. rangeli.* When the parasite load is low, a concentration method is required, namely the Strout and the microhaematocrit methods. The latter has been proved to be very sensitive in infants under 6 months of age (Freilij and Altcheh, 1995) and it is the most recommended parasitological method for assessment of CCD (Fig. 2).

Indirect methods.   Xenodiagnosis and haemoculture are traditional indirect parasitological methods, whose sensitivity much depends on the parasitic load of the sample. These techniques can only be performed in specialized laboratories. Owing to the fact that some patients present bug bite skin reaction, artificial xenodiagnosis is recommended, which has a higher positivity than the routine method (Dos Santos et al., 1995; Schenone, 1999).

Molecular methods.   PCR detection of *T. cruzi* DNA has been evaluated in different types of samples such as cord blood, peripheral blood and serum samples, from neonates and infants suspected of having CCD (Russomando et al., 1992; Schijman et al., 2003; Virreira et al., 2003; Mora et al., 2005; Burgos, 2006). Moreover, congenital *T. cruzi* infection was detected by PCR in amniotic fluid from an infected mother with a premature delivery (Nilo et al., 2000).

Most PCR procedures are targeted to the 330 bp four-high variable region of the minicircle parasite genome (Sturm et al., 1989; Avila et al., 1991; Britto et al., 1995) or the 195-bp satellite repeat (Moser et al. 1989), which depict the highest analytical sensitivities, and are capable of detecting *T. cruzi* DNA of any lineage from blood samples containing around 2×10^{-2} parasite genomic equivalents (Schijman et al., 2003; Virreira et al., 2003). The sensitivity of PCR for diagnosis of CCD has been evaluated in comparison with conventional parasitological methods in single and serial samples (Schijman et al., 2003; Solari et al., 2003; Virreira et al., 2003; Mora et al., 2006). PCR carried out from 1998 to 2000 in 152 children born to infected mothers in Buenos Aires showed a sensitivity of 100% in infants younger than 6 months of age where that of microhaematocrit was 82.4%. PCR specificity was 97% and that of the microhaematocrit was 100%. The PCR positivity decreased to 73.8% in CCD patients at the indeterminate CCD phase in which serodiagnosis was the gold standard (Schijman et al., 2003). In an active transmission area of Bolivia, the PCR depicted a sensitivity of 93.6% among infected children (Wincker et al., 1997). Russomando et al. (1998) evaluated the PCR for early diagnosis of CCD in newborns from Paraguay; the rate of CCD was 3% using direct microscopic observation but it increased to 10% by means of PCR, which corresponded to the incidence rate detected later by serologic monitoring at the indeterminate phase. The diversity of the operational characteristics of the PCR in different epidemiologic settings makes it compelling to establish multicentre studies for

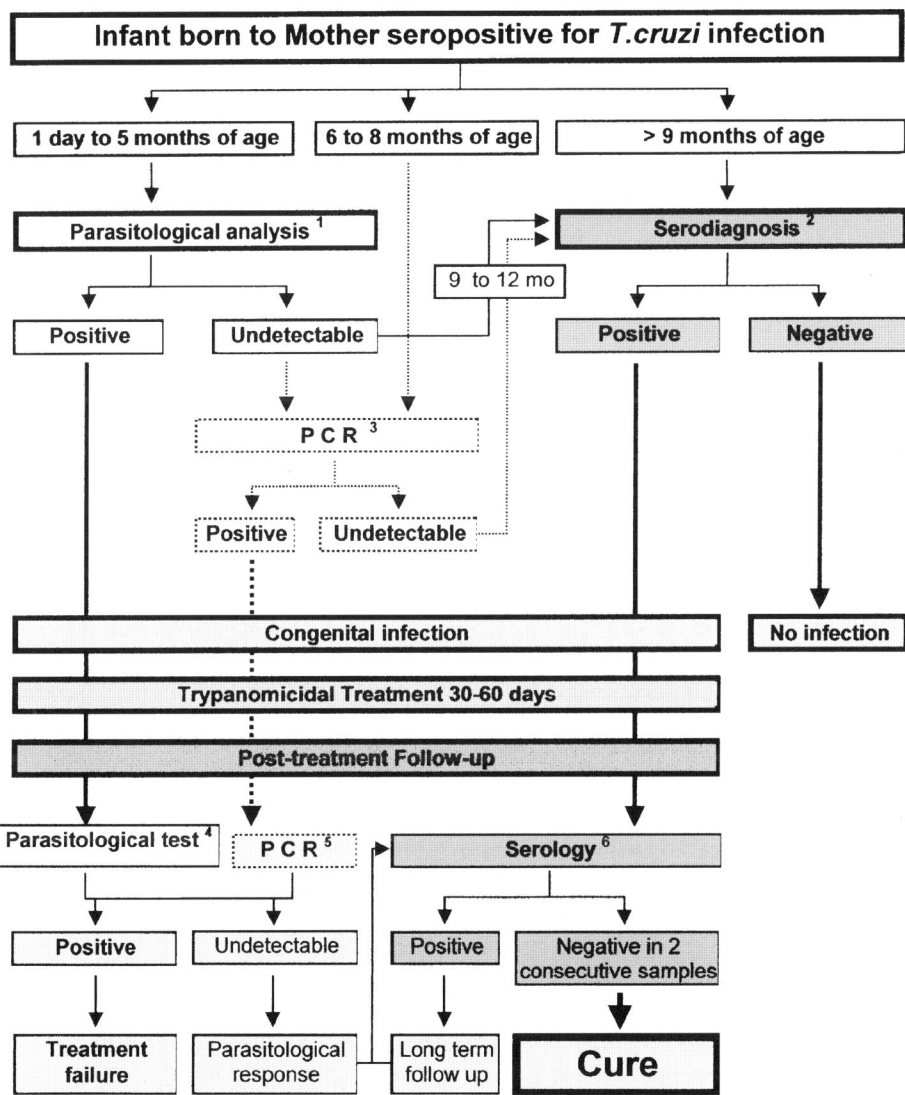

Fig. 2 Algorithm of laboratory diagnosis, treatment and follow-up of congenital Chagas disease. This algorithm is based on the consensus recommendations published by a WHO expert committee (WHO, 2002).

(1) Microhaematocrit is recommended as parasitological method.

(2) Two serological techniques must be positive for reliable diagnosis.

(3) Standardized PCR is required for reliable diagnosis.

(4) It is recommended to perform serial microhaematocrit analysis every 7–15 days after therapy.

(5) PCR follow-up analysis may be performed at the end of treatment and every 3 months during the first year after treatment.

(6) Serological follow-up should be performed every three months during the first year after treatment.

standardization of this technique that should be carried out only by skilled personnel in specialized laboratories. As in other infections acquired by vertical transmission, PCR positive findings in two consecutive clinical samples or concordant PCR-positive results obtained by amplifying different regions of the parasite genome could be considered as a reliable diagnosis of *T. cruzi* infection. Once standardized, PCR might be a valuable diagnosis tool for rapid diagnosis of CCD at birth or during the first months of life, avoiding the delay of treatment when the child is at the indeterminate chronic phase of CCD (Fig. 2).

Immunodiagnosis

Conventional serological assays.   Three conventional IgG-based serological tests are widely used, namely indirect haemagglutination (IHA), indirect immunofluorescence (IIF) and enzyme-linked immunoassay (ELISA). In most conventional tests, either a complex mixture of antigens (IHA and ELISA) or the entire parasite (IIF) is employed. This increases the likelihood of detecting infection even when the antibody levels are low. On the other hand, the probability of cross reactivity with *Leishmania* spp. or *T. rangeli* infections increases, thus leading to false-positive diagnosis in overlapping endemic areas.

IHA is rapid, takes about 2 h, easy to perform and its sensitivity ranges from 96 to 98%. IIF has a sensitivity of 99%, but its reading is subjective and must be carried out by skilled personnel; in addition, a special ultraviolet light microscope is required and the procedure implies several steps. Titration of conjugates is essential as control of reagents. ELISA sensitivity and specificity may oscillate between 97% and 100%, and 93% and 100%, respectively, depending on the area under study. Accuracies among different comercial assays range from 93% to 100% (Oelemann et al., 1998). ELISA takes several hours to perform, requires skilled technicians and a spectrophotometer, which avoids subjectivity and can be automated. It is useful for large-scale screening of samples. Borderline results can be obtained, which make it difficult to establish the criteria of diagnosis. In 95% of sera from *T. cruzi*-infected individuals, concordance is obtained with all three serological tests. When two of them disagree, it may indicate a technical mistake or a characteristic of the serum sample. In these cases, it is necessary to repeat the tests and in case of repetitive discordant findings, non-conventional tests should be used or the serum should be submitted to a reference laboratory.

Non-conventional serological tests.   These tests have been developed mostly at Universities and Research Institutes with the aim of increasing specificity and avoiding cross reactivity with *Leishmania* spp. or *T. rangeli*, which share endemic areas with *T. cruzi*. They are mostly based on ELISA using recombinant proteins, purified antigens or synthetic peptides. For example, the Shed Acute Phase Antigen (SAPA) protein (Reyes et al., 1990) has been proposed as an unequivocal antigen for the diagnosis of CCD; however, it has also been detected in 32% of cases with chronic infection (Vergara et al., 1991). New matrixes have been deviced for the use in antigen immobilization, such as strips for immunochromatographic assays, coloured beads, immuno- and Western blots. These tests are easy and rapid to perform and therefore most suitable for field studies, small laboratories and emergencies in the countryside of endemic areas, although they give only qualitative information. Recombinant proteins used as mixtures of several components (Umezawa et al., 2004) as well as artificially engineered recombinant antigens containing tandem sequences of *T. cruzi*-specific peptides (Ferreira et al., 2001), have also been developed. Several of them have been validated in multicentre studies (Levin et al., 1991; Luquetti et al., 2003; Umezawa et al., 2004; Ponce et al., 2005).

Compliance with good laboratory practice, including the implementation of quality control procedures and periodical evaluation of laboratory performance, together with legislation requiring reagents to be evaluated before they are marketed, is the only means to guarantee that the results of diagnosis are truthful.

Consensus recommendations for laboratory diagnosis of CCD

The most recent multicentre consultation on management of CCD, held in Montevideo, Uruguay in 2004 underlined the following recommendations for diagnosis of CCD.

Diagnostic procedures recommended to ascertain congenital infection at birth

This strategy has the advantage that, in case of a positive diagnosis, it gives the physicians the possibility of informing the mother while she is still at the maternity service and of explaining to her about the need to start antiparasitic treatment of the newborn. Moreover, it reduces the risk to lose contact with the mother and her baby, if they do not go back to the further appointments, which is something frequently observed in regions and countries in which health care is not well organized. In this situation, cord blood can be recommended, since it is easy to collect without physical or psychological traumatism for the baby and its mother. If cord blood sampling is not possible, blood can be collected from heel or peripheral venous puncture of the neonate. The direct examination of blood parasites using the microhaematocrit concentration method is recommended. Other options are Microstrout, haemoculture and/or artificial xenodiagnosis, or molecular examination of cord blood by reliable PCR techniques. In the case of negative direct parasitological tests in babies with strong clinical suspicion of CCD, it is suggested that these tests should be repeated.

Diagnostic procedures not recommended to ascertain congenital infection at birth

(a) *T. cruzi*-specific IgG serology has a low positive predictive value because the presence of anti-*T. cruzi* IgG antibodies in the newborn may be due to passive transfer of IgG maternal antibodies, which in the non-infected infant would normally disappear around the sixth month of age (Freilij and Altcheh, 1995).

Moreover, a small proportion of infected neonates may present false negative or conflicting *T. cruzi*-specific IgG results because of specific immune complexes (Corral et al., 1987) or because the infection was acquired just before or during delivery (Freilij and Altcheh, 1995). Therefore, this procedure can be applied when IgG specific antibodies of non-maternal origin are found, which usually occurs eight months after delivery.

(b) *T. cruzi*-specific IgM serology is not sensitive in every case and may also give false-positive results in uninfected babies born to infected mothers, possibly due to rheumatoid factor and/or materno–foetal transfer of parasitic antigens or IgM antibodies from placenta (Freilij and Altcheh, 1995; Russomando et al., 1998; Blanco et al., 2000).

(c) *T. cruzi*-specific IgA serology does not reach adequate sensitivity (Di Pentima and Edwards 1999).

Diagnostic procedures to be applied after birth

If the laboratory diagnosis cannot be performed at birth, and whatever the time after birth, it is important to discard possible contamination by other routes such as blood transfusion and vectorial contamination, before ascertaining CCD in infants.

Diagnosis during the first 6 months of life.   Since the early diagnosis of CCD is highly desirable, parasitological methods such as microhaematocrit or microstrout concentration methods, xenodiagnosis, haemoculture, inoculation into suckling mice should be performed. Out of them, microhaematocrit has been recommended by the WHO. In cases of negative findings, reliable PCR assays could be applied, since they present higher sensitivity (Fig. 2).

Diagnosis after 9 months of life.   There is a consensus that after nine months of age, antibodies passively transmitted from the mother disappear; so, positive serological findings indicate *T. cruzi* infection of the infant. Any combination of two serological techniques can be accepted. In terms of Public Health programmes, it is advisable to use conventional serology in children between 9 and 12 months (Fig. 2).

Trypanomicidal treatment

The crucial role of the parasite in the outcome of the disease has been demonstrated by successful treatment that has prevented its progress, particularly in the early stages of the infection. The only effective treatments are nifurtimox and benznidazole, the same drugs that have been used for the last 30 years

In cases of CCD patients with clinical signs of the disease, treatment has allowed marked clinical improvement (Freilij and Altcheh, 1995; De Andrade et al., 1996). The fundamental standards for the treatment of CCD are basically those recently established by the World Health Organization (WHO, Control of Chagas Disease. WHO Technical Report Series No. 905, Geneva, 2002), which indicate the soonest possible administration of either 5–10 mg/kg/day of benznidazole or 10–15 mg/kg/day of nifurtimox for 30–60 days, in all congenital cases. Benznidazole treatment may start with a dose of 5 mg/kg/daily and, if after three days of treatment there is neither leukopenia nor thrombocytopenia, the dose should be increased to 10 mg/kg daily (WHO, 2002). These drugs have proved to be effective with good efficacy and tolerance in several studies in Argentina (Freilij and Altcheh, 1995; Sosa Estani et al., 1998; Schijman et al., 2003), Chile (Solari et al., 2003) and Paraguay (Russomando et al., 1998). The follow-up of Argentinean cohorts with both drugs has not shown differences in toxicity, clinical, serological or PCR outcomes (Schijman et al., 2003). It is expected that all CCD infants could be cured with a 100% success if the treatment is performed before the first year of life (Freilij and Altcheh, 1995; Blanco et al., 2000; Schijman et al., 2003).

Common adverse effects of benznidazole include photosensitive skin rashes, headaches, peripheral neuritis, anorexia, nausea, dizziness, weight loss, asthenia and haematological alterations. Most common adverse effects of nifurtimox include weakness, anorexia, nausea, vomiting and abdominal pain. Less-common adverse effects include skin rashes, toxic hepatitis, central and peripheral nervous system symptoms. Haemolysis can occur in patients with Glucose-6-Phosphate Dehydrogenase deficiency. Children tolerate the drugs better than adults and preliminary findings of chromosomal aberrations need confirmation. A severe skin manifestation, the Lyell syndrome, may occur in children older than 10 years.

Specific treatment of chagasic mothers during pregnancy is not performed since the teratogenic risk of the available drugs is not known and its efficiency in chronically infected individuals is low. In the words of neonatologist Juan M. Jijena, from the Hospital of Tarija, Bolivia: "if we treat the girls, we will in turn be preventing their children from being infected when they become mothers" (Médecins sains frontières, 2005).

For decades now, Chagas disease has not been considered in the new drugs research and development programmes undertaken by the main pharmaceutical companies.

Indicators of treatment outcome

After aetiological treatment, the criterion of cure relies on serological conversion into negative of the anti-*T. cruzi* antibody response (WHO, 2002), but in patients initiating therapy at the indeterminate phase, seroconversion usually occurs several years after treatment, requiring long-term follow-up. However, when treatment is initiated at an early stage, parasitological tests should be used to follow-up parasitological response (Fig. 2).

Parasitological follow-up

Xenodiagnosis and haemoculture are hampered by their low sensitivity, since more than half of untreated individuals have a negative result; microhaematocrit is highly sensitive in infants up to 6 months of age; if a child starts treatment with a positive microhaematocrit result it is advisable to perform serial microhematocrit analysis every 7–15 days after therapy. A negative finding indicates a favourable parasitological response and is generally observed around the second and third weeks of therapy (Freilij and Altcheh, 1995). Once treatment is completed, serological control must be carried out every 3–6 months; seroconversion to negative in at least two consecutive samples should be taken as criterion of cure (Fig. 2).

PCR-based follow-up

PCR performance as an early marker of parasitological response to treatment has been evaluated after 3–4 years of post-treatment follow-up (Wincker et al., 1994; Russomando et al., 1998; Solari et al., 1998; Galvao et al., 2003; Schijman et al., 2003). In the Chilean cohort, parasitological cure in 0–10-year-old children is variable, and several months are required to obtain a prolonged negative result by PCR, even though xenodiagnosis rapidly turns negative after three months in all geographical areas studied, probably due to its lower sensitivity (Solari et al., 1998). The early xenodiagnosis conversion indicates that a large fraction of live parasites are rapidly eliminated from blood, but PCR becomes negative several months after xenodiagnosis, thus suggesting that persistent shedding of parasitic kDNA into the blood from infected cells might occur in treated patients. This explanation is based on the assumption that PCR amplifies DNA from viable parasites and also from lysed parasites from infected cells (polymorphonuclear cells and/or muscle fibres), which is in agreement with the finding of *T. cruzi* DNA in sera of chagasic patients (Russomando et al., 1992). In the Argentinean cohorts, serological cure has been achieved early after treatment in those infants who started the therapy during their first months of life. This is consistent with the results obtained by PCR monitoring, in which a decrease of parasitaemia to undetectable levels at the end of treatment or at the first post-treatment controls has been observed (Schijman et al., 2003). Among those patients treated at the indeterminate phase of CCD, short-term evaluation of cure has been difficult since conventional serology usually remains positive for many years. In fact, in that three-year follow-up study, seroconversion occurred in 66.7% of infants aged 7–20 months, but in only 12.5% of those initiating the therapy at an older age ($p = 0.023$) (Schijman et al., 2003). Interestingly, out of the latter patients, the few cases that became seronegative before the three-year follow-up were PCR negative in their pre-therapy samples, persisting PCR negative. This observation has led to the hypothesis that indeterminate phase CCD patients with undetectable parasitic loads by PCR might have a better treatment outcome than those with patent parasitemias. Dissociation between post-treatment persistent negative PCR results with positive conventional serology after the three-year follow-up was observed in 20 out of 30 CCD patients; in agreement with previous studies that show persistence of conventional seroreactivity with clearance of lytic antibodies (Galvao et al., 1993, Gomez et al., 1999).

Attempts to measure parasite loads for monitoring CCD treatment response have been performed by using competitive PCR, which have shown a parasite load decrease after 30 days of treatment with benznidazole that became undetectable after 60 days of therapy (Schijman et al., 2003).

Modern real-time PCR strategies are promising tools to develop reliable quantitative PCR tests for treatment monitoring (Cummings and Tarleton, 2003).

Parasitological tests are also of vital importance in demonstrating therapeutic failure during the follow-up. In this respect, PCR can be used as an early marker of resistance to specific chemotherapy, years before a conclusion can be drawn by serological analysis, providing a rapid information that might allow switching to an alternative drug.

Serological follow-up

At least two serological tests are recommended for treatment follow-up. The persistence of antibody responses both in treated and parasitologically cured chagasic patients could be explained by the presence of parasite antigens from lysed parasites for long periods in the lymph nodes (Schijman et al., 2003; Solari et al., 2003). However, the therapeutic effectiveness as assessed by serological cure seems to depend on the delay between infection and the start of treatment (Ahmed and Gray, 1996).

The F2/3 antigenic fraction isolated from trypomastigotes contains epitopes recognized by antibodies, that are representative of active infection (Altcheh et al., 2003). In that work, the kinetics of conventional seronegativity and clearance of anti-F2/3 response were compared in 21 CCD patients after receiving benznidazole. Patients < 8 months at intiation of treatment were seronegative at 6.6 months (CI 95 3.4–9.8 months) and 4 months (CI 95 0.9–7.1 months) for conventional and anti-F2/3 serodiagnosis respectively (p = non-significant). However, CCD patients initiating treatment at age > 9 months exhibited conventional seroconversion at 63.1 months (CI 95 42.1–84.2 months) and clearance of anti-F2/3 response at 21.9 months. (CI 95 5.7–38.1 months) ($p = 0.0025$). Consequently, the absence of anti-F2/3 antibody response could be taken as an early indication of cure, particularly in CCD cases with prolonged time of infection (Altcheh et al., 2003).

Consensus strategies for epidemiological control and management of congenital *T. cruzi* infection

International colloquia aiming to update the situational diagnosis of *CCD* and its management were organized both in Cochabamba, Bolivia in 2002 (Congenital Infection from *T.cruzi*: From Mechanisms of Transmission to Strategies for Diagnosis and Control (Rev. Soc. Bras. Med. Trop. 2003, 36 (6): 767–771) and in Montevideo, Uruguay in 2004 (PAHO Consultation on Congenital Chagas Disease, Its Epidemiology and Management). Groups of researchers, clinicians, and experts in disease-management programmes, mostly from the Southern Cone of

America participated in these events and prepared guidelines with strategies for effective and sustainable actions against CCD. A summary of the recommendations addressed by the Advisory groups is outlined below:

(1) Congenital T. cruzi infection occurs in all the endemic areas with different intensities and characteristics in each subregion, as well as in nonendemic areas. Therefore, it requires particular and institutional attention from the government of each country affected, in terms of Public Health Policy and investigation.

(2) All plans and operations developed for screening, diagnosis, treatment and monitoring of CCD should be incorporated into the national health system at all levels of complexity and integrated into Primary Health Care (PHC). Programmes to educate and train human resources should be set up to guarantee that recommended actions persist.

(3) Vector control programmes and serological screening of blood donors must be implemented since these are the most effective ways for preventing congenital transmission. In regions where control of vectorial and transfusional transmission of Chagas disease has been achieved or improved, congenital transmission constitutes the principal and most persistent form of the parasitosis in the human population.

(4) Because specific treatment of the mother during pregnancy should not be performed with the currently available drugs, research on new drugs for the specific and safe treatment of T. cruzi infection during gestation is strongly recommended.

(5) Since no specific direct prevention of congenital T. cruzi infection is available, the best strategies concerning this problem are: (i) the systematic and effective control of the basic primary transmission routes of the infection in endemic areas (mainly the vectorial and transfusional routes), in order to reduce the prevalence rate of infected women; and (ii) the early and correct diagnosis of congenital cases, in order to treat infected newborns/neonates, and thus avoid CCD-related mortality and morbidity in the neonatal period or later in life.

(6) In communities with a high incidence of vectorial transmission and acute infection during pregnancy, regardless of relevance, the possibility should be explored to provide universal testing for T. cruzi infection among all newborns. In countries with a high frequency of home deliveries, newborns should be tested during their first contact with the health system.

(7) Special attention must be paid to the diagnosis of CCD and its correlated public health implications, considering the following possibilities/strategies: (i) The ideal schedule is to institutionalize conventional serology for pregnant women in endemic areas and to perform a follow up of the infected ones and their babies, with the main objectives of providing adequate mother care and being able to perform an early detection and treatment of CCD; and (ii) For babies delivered from mothers serologically positive or with a known history of T. cruzi infection, or for all babies born in endemic areas where prenatal

mother examination is impossible, the suggestion is to perform laboratory diagnosis at birth.

(8) The babies with positive results derived from either direct or indirect parasitological examinations, reliable PCR or serology performed at 9–12 months of age must be treated with specific drugs. Negative babies for parasitological tests must be clinically followed until the age of nine months, when a new conventional serology must be performed. Negative cases at this time are considered non-infected (Fig. 2). Positive serology will mean active infection and the child will be treated.

(9) Concerning treatment, the Advisory Group recommended that the countries allocate resources to procure specific drugs (nifurtimox and benznidazole) available at uniform costs in all the concerned countries of Latin America, ideally in a paediatric formulation. The specific treatment with the currently available drugs (nifurtimox and benznidazole) is considered obligatory for all cases of congenital *T. cruzi* infection, since it presents a high degree of effectiveness and is very safe for the majority of treated children.

(10) The fundamental standards for the treatment of congenital *T. cruzi* infection are basically those already established by the WHO in a recent document (WHO, Control of Chagas Disease. WHO Technical Report Series No. 905, Geneva, 2002), which indicates the soonest possible administration of 5–10 mg/kg/day of benznidazole or 10–15 mg/kg/day of nifurtimox for 30–60 days, in all congenital cases.

(11) The treatment can be accomplished at an ambulatory level. However, it is very important to inform the parents and relatives about the correct administration of the drug to assure its best effectiveness and to avoid overdosage and collateral effects. Treated babies must be clinically and biologically followed, ideally every three months until one year after treatment. Cure assessment is established when conventional serology becomes persistently negative. In the rare congenital cases of therapeutic failure, re-treatment must be considered in each particular circumstance.

(12) Reinfection of treated and cured babies is possible and has been registered in endemic regions where housing infestation by triatomines occurs. So, an institutional programme against congenital *T. cruzi* infection in endemic areas must always be associated with regular activities of vector and blood banks control.

(13) Each detected case of congenital *T. cruzi* infection presupposes an epidemiological investigation in the whole family in terms of Public Health Policy, in order to detect other infected children and to make possible an epidemiological evaluation of the situation, also providing medical attention to other eventually infected relatives.

(14) In a particular way, infected mothers deserve special attention concerning future possible pregnancies because of the risk of repeated foetal infections in children of subsequent pregnancies. Moreover, it is reminded that the possibility of Chagas heart disease must be investigated in order to prevent complications during pregnancy and birth.

While we continue to be a semifeudal country based on an agricultural economy set up in the monoculture, we cannot talk seriously about the fight of tropical diseases. Tropical diseases are born in a different main disease, our delay. Our obsolete economy is the main responsible factor for schistosomiasis, leprosy, Chagas disease, malaria, smallpox, and other endemic and epidemic diseases of our poor land. Amado, 1985

Acknowledgements

I am grateful to Dr. Héctor Freilij and Dr. Mariano J. Levin for critically reading this manuscript.

I thank my collaborators Juan M. Burgos, Tomás Duffy and Margarita Bisio for their contributions and assistance.

References

Ahmed R, Gray D. Immunological memory and protective immunity: understanding their relation. Science 1996; 272: 54–60.

Altcheh J, Corral R, Biancardi MA, Freilij H. Anti-F2/3 antibodies as cure marker in children with congenital *Trypanosoma cruzi* infection. Medicina (B Aires) 2003; 63(1): 37–40.

Altemani AM, Bittencourt AL, Lana AM. Immunohistochemical characterization of the inflammatory infiltrate in placental Chagas' disease: a qualitative and quantitative analysis. Am J Trop Med Hyg 2000; 62(2): 319–324.

Amado J. Tenda dos milagres. 33ª Edition. Río de Janeiro, Brazil: ERCA Editora y Gráfica Ltda; 1985.

Andrade S. The influence of the strain of *T. cruzi* in placental infections in mice. Trans R Soc Trop Med Hyg 1982; 76: 123–128.

Arteaga-Fernandez E, Pereira Barretto AC, Ianni BM, Vianna Cde B, Mady C, Bellotti G, Pileggi F. Incidence of congenital transmission of Chagas' disease. Arq Bras Cardiol 1987; 49(1): 47–49.

Atias A. A case of congenital chagasic megaesophagus: evolution until death caused by esophageal neoplasm, at 27 years of age. Rev Med Chil 1994; 122(3): 319–322.

Atias A, Morales M, Munoz P, Barria M. Ocular involvement in congenital Chagas' disease. Rev Chil Pediatr 1985; 56(3): 137–141.

Atwood JA 3rd, Weatherly DB, Minning TA, Bundy B, Cavola C, Opperdoes FR, Orlando R, Tarleton RL. The *Trypanosoma cruzi* proteome. Science 2005; 309(5733): 473–476.

Avila HA, Sigman DS, Cohen LM, Millikan RC, Simpson LNO. Polymerase chain reaction amplification of *Trypanosoma cruzi* kinetoplast minicircle DNA isolated from whole blood lysates: diagnosis of chronic Chagas' disease. Mol Biochem Parasitol 1991; 48(2): 211–221.

Azogue E, Darras C. Prospective study of Chagas disease in newborn children with placental infection caused by *Trypanosoma cruzi* (Santa Cruz-Bolivia). Rev Soc Bras Med Trop 1991; 24(2): 105–109.

Azogue E, La Fuente C, Darras C. Congenital Chagas' disease in Bolivia: epidemiological aspects and pathological findings. Trans R Soc Trop Med Hyg 1985; 79(2): 176–180.

Bittencourt AL. American trypanosomiasis (Chagas' disease). In: Parasitic Infection in Pregnancy and the Newborn (Macleod C, editor). Oxford: Oxford Medical Publication; 1988; pp. 62–86.

Bittencourt AL. Possible risk factors for vertical transmission of Chagas' disease. Rev Inst Med Trop Sao Paulo 1992; 34(5): 403–408.

Bittencourt AL, Barbosa HS, Rocha T, Sodre I, Sodre A. Incidence of congenital transmission of Chagas' disease in premature births in the Maternidade Tsylla Balbino (Salvador, Bahia). Rev Inst Med Trop Sao Paulo 1972; 14(2): 131–134.

Bittencourt AL. Chagasic placentitis and congenital transmission of Chagas' disease. Rev Inst Med Trop Sao Paulo 1963; 5: 62–67.

Bittencourt AL, Sadigursky M, Da Silva AA, Menezes CA, Marianetti MM, Guerra SC, Sherlock I. Evaluation of Chagas' disease transmission through breast-feeding. Mem Inst Oswaldo Cruz 1988; 83(1): 37–39.

Blanco SB, Segura EL, Cura EN, Chuit R, Tulian L, Flores I, Garbarino G, Villalonga JF, Gurtler RE. Congenital transmission of *Trypanosoma cruzi*: an operational outline for detecting and treating infected infants in north-western Argentina. Trop Med Int Health 2000; 5(4): 293–301.

Blanco SB, Segura EL, Gurtler RE. Control of congenital transmission of *Trypanosoma cruzi* in Argentina. Medicina (B. Aires) 1999; 59(Suppl 2): 138–142.

Breniere SF, Bosseno MF, Telleria J, Bastrenta B, Yacsik N, Noireau F, Alcazar JL, Barnabé C, Wincker P, Tibayrenc M. Different behavior of two *Trypanosoma cruzi* major clones: transmission and circulation in young Bolivian patients. Exp Parasitol 1998; 89: 285–295.

Brisse S, Barnabé C, Tibayrenc M. Identification of six *Trypanosoma cruzi* phylogenetic lineages by random amplified polymorphic DNA and multilocus enzyme electrophoresis. Int J Parasitol 2000; 30: 35–44.

Brisse S, Henriksson J, Barnabe C, Douzery EJ, Berkvens D, Serrano M, De Carvalho MR, Buck GA, Dujardin JC, Tibayrenc M. Evidence for genetic exchange and hybridization in *Trypanosoma cruzi* based on nucleotide sequences and molecular karyotype. Infect Genet Evol 2003; 2(3): 173–183.

Britto C, Cardoso MA, Vanni CM, Hasslocher-Moreno A, Xavier SS, Oelemann W, Santoro A, Pirmez C, Morel CM, Wincker P. Polymerase chain reaction detection of *Trypanosoma cruzi* in human blood samples as a tool for diagnosis and treatment evaluation. Parasitology 1995; 110(Pt 3): 241–247.

Burgos JM, Begher S, Freitas JM, Bisio M, Duffy T, Altcheh J, Teijeiro R, Lopez Alcoba H, Deccarlini F, Freilij H, Levin MJ, Levalle J, Macedo A, Schijman AG. Molecular diagnosis and typing of *Trypanosoma cruzi* populations and lineages in cerebral Chagas disease in a patient with AIDS. Am J Trop Med Hyg 2005; 73(6): 1016–1018.

Burgos JM. Doctoral Thesis; College of Biological Sciences. Argentina: University of Buenos Aires; 2006.

Burgos JM, Bisio M, Seidenstein ME, Altcheh J, Talarico N, Pontoriero R, Marcellac M, Matzkin R, Freilij H, Macchi L, Levin MJ, Schijman AG. Congenital Chagas disease: detection and molecular typing of natural populations of *T. cruzi* involved in vertical transmission. BIOCELL 2004; 28: 330.

Campbell DA, Westenberger SJ, Sturm NR. The determinants of Chagas disease: connecting parasite and host genetics. Curr Mol Med 2004; 4(6): 549–562.

Chagas C. Nova trypanozomíaze humana. Estudos sobre a morfologia e cíclo evolutivo do *Schizotripanum cruzi* n. gen. n. sp., agente etiològico de nova entidade mórbida do homem.. Mem Inst Oswaldo Cruz 1909; 1(2): 159–218.

Chagas C. Nova entidade morbida do homem. Resumo geral de estudos etiológicos e clínicos.. Mem Inst Oswaldo Cruz 1911; 3: 219–275.

Concetti H, Retegui M, Perez G, Perez H. Chagas' disease of the cervix uteri in a patient with acquired immunodeficiency syndrome. Hum Pathol 2000; 31(1): 120–122.

Corral R, Freilij H, Grinstein S. Specific circulating immune complexes in acute Chagas' disease. Rev Inst Med Trop Sao Paulo 1987; 29(1): 26–32.

Cummings KL, Tarleton RL. Rapid quantitation of *Trypanosoma cruzi* in host tissue by real-time PCR. Mol Biochem Parasitol 2003; 129(1): 53–59.

De Andrade AL, Zicker F, de Oliveira RM, Almeida Silva S, Luquetti A, Travassos LR, Almeida IC, de Andrade SS, de Andrade JG, Martelli CM. Randomised trial of efficacy of benznidazole in treatment of early *Trypanosoma cruzi* infection. Lancet 1996; 348(9039): 1407–1413.

De Castilho E, da Silva GR. Maternal Chagas infection and prematurity. Rev Inst Med Trop Sao Paulo 1976; 18: 258–260.

Delgado MA, Santos-Buch CA. Transplacental transmission and fetal parasitosis of *Trypanosoma cruzi* in outbred white Swiss mice. Am J Trop Med Hyg 1978; 27(6): 1108–1115.

Di Pentima MC, Edwards MS. Enzyme-linked immunosorbent assay for IgA antibodies to *Trypanosoma cruzi* in congenital infection. Am J Trop Med Hyg 1999; 60(2): 211–214.

Dos Santos AH, da Silva IG, Rassi A. A comparative study between natural and artificial xenodiagnosis in chronic Chagas' disease patients. Rev Soc Bras Med Trop 1995; 28(4): 367–373.

El-Sayed NM, Myler PJ, Blandin G, Berriman M, Crabtree J, Aggarwal G, Caler E, Renauld H, Worthey EA, Hertz-Fowler C, Ghedin E, Peacock C, Bartholomeu DC, Haas BJ, Tran AN, Wortman JR, Alsmark UC, Angiuoli S, Anupama A, Badger J, Bringaud F, Cadag E, Carlton JM, Cerqueira GC, Creasy T, Delcher AL, Djikeng A, Embley TM, Hauser C, Ivens AC, Kummerfeld SK, Pereira-Leal JB, Nilsson D, Peterson J, Salzberg SL, Shallom J, Silva JC, Sundaram J, Westenberger S, White O, Melville SE, Donelson JE, Andersson B, Stuart KD, Hall N. Comparative genomics of trypanosomatid parasitic protozoa. Science 2005; 309(5733): 404–409.

Ferreira AW, Belem ZR, Lemos EA, Reed SG, Campos-Neto A. Enzyme-linked immunosorbent assay for serological diagnosis of Chagas' disease employing a *Trypanosoma cruzi* recombinant antigen that consists of four different peptides. J Clin Microbiol 2001; 39(12): 4390–4395.

Fievet N, Tami G, Maubert B, Moussa M, Shaw IK, Cot M, Holder AA, Chaouat G, Deloron P. Cellular immune response to Plasmodium falciparum after pregnancy is related to previous placental infection and parity. Malar J 2002; 26: 1–16 Epub 2002 Nov 26.

Frank F, Sartori MJ, Asteggiano C, Lin S, de Fabro SP, Fretes RE. The effect of placental subfractions on *T. cruzi*. Exp Mol Pathol 2000; 69(2): 144–151.

Freilij H, Altcheh J. Congenital Chagas'disease: diagnostic and clinical aspects. Clin Infect Dis 1995; 21: 551–555.

Freilij H, Altcheh J, Muchinik G. Perinatal human immunodeficiency virus infection and congenital Chagas' disease. Pediatr Infect Dis J 1995; 14(2): 161–162.

Freilij H, Altcheh J, Storino R. Chagas congénito. In: Enfermedad de Chagas (Storino R, Milei J, editors). Buenos Aires: Doyma; 1994; pp. 267–278.

Freitas JM, Lages-Silva E, Crema E, Pena SD, Macedo AM. Real time PCR strategy for the identification of major lineages of *T. cruzi* directly in chronically infected human tissues. Int J Parasitol 2005; 35(4): 411–417.

Fretes RE, De Fabro SP. *In vivo* and *in vitro* analysis of lysosomes and acid phosphatase activity in human chagasic placentas. Exp Mol Pathol 1995; 63(3): 153–160.

Galvão LM, Chiari E, Macedo AM, Luquetti AO, Silva SA, Andrade AL. PCR assay for monitoring *Trypanosoma cruzi* parasitemia in childhood after specific chemotherapy. J Clin Microbiol 2003; 41(11): 5066–5070.

Galvao LM, Nunes RM, Cancado JR, Brener Z, Krettli AU. Lytic antibody titre as a means of assessing cure after treatment of Chagas disease. Trans R Soc Trop Med Hyg 1993; 87(2): 220–223.

García HA, Bahamonde MMI, Verdugo BS, Correa SC, Pastene O, Solari A, Tassara OR, Lorca HM. Infección transplacentaria por *Trypanosoma cruzi*: Situación en Chile. Rev méd Chile 2001; 129(3): 330–332.

Gaunt MW, Yeo M, Frame IA, Stothard JR, Carrasco HJ, Taylor MC, Mena SS, Veazey P, Miles GAJ, Acosta N, Rojas de Arias A, Miles MA. Mechanism of genetic exchange in American trypanosomes. Nature 2003; 421: 936–939.

Gomez ML, Galvao LM, Macedo AM, Pena SD, Chiari E. Chagas disease diagnosis: comparative analysis of parasitologic, molecular and serologic methods. Am J Trop Med Hyg 1999; 60(2): 205–210.

Gûrtler RE, Segura EL, Cohen JE. Congenital transmission of *T. cruzi* infection in Argentina. Emerg Infect Dis 2003; 9: 29–35.

Guzman-Bracho C, Lahuerta S, Velasco-Castrejon O. Chagas disease. First congenital case report. Arch Med Res 1998; 29(2): 195–196.

Hall BS, Pereira MA. Dual role for transforming growth factor beta-dependent signaling in *Trypanosoma cruzi* infection of mammalian cells. Infect Immun 2000; 68(4): 2077–2081.

Hermann E, Truyens C, Alonso-Vega C, Rodriguez P, Berthe A, Torrico F, Carlier Y. Congenital transmission of *Trypanosoma cruzi* is associated with maternal enhanced parasitemia and decreased production of interferon-gamma in response to parasite antigens. J Infect Dis 1 2004; 189(7): 1274–1281.

Hernandez-Matheson IM, Frankowski RF, Held B. Foetomaternal morbidity in the presence of antibodies to *Trypanosoma cruzi*. Trans R Soc Trop Med Hyg 1983; 77: 405–411.

Higo H, Miura S, Horio M, Mimori T, Hamano S, Agatsuma T, Yanagi T, Cruz-Reyes A, Uyema N, Rojas de Arias A, Matta V, Akahane H, Hirayama K, Takeuchi T, Tada I, Himeno K. Genotypic variation among lineages of *Trypanosoma cruzi* and its geographic aspects. Parasitol Int 2004; 53(4): 337–344.

Hoff R, Mott KE, Milanesi ML, Bittencourt AL, Barbosa HS. Congenital Chagas's disease in an urban population: investigation of infected twins. Trans R Soc Trop Med Hyg 1978; 72: 247–250.

Hoff R, Mott KE, Silva JF, Menezes V, Hoff JN, Barrett TV, Sherlock I. Prevalence of parasitemia and seroreactivity to *Trypanosoma cruzi* in a rural population of Northeast Brazil. Am J Trop Med Hyg 1979; 28(3): 461–466.

INCOSUR Report. Congenital transmission should be included in the Southern Cone Initiative? IX Reunión de la Comisión Intergubernamental del Cono Sur contra la enfermedad de Chagas. Rev Patol Trop 2001; 30: 57.

Jörg ME. The transmission of *T. cruzi* via human milk. Rev Soc Bras Med Trop 1992; 25(1): 83.

Klein JO, Remington JS. Current concepts of infections of the fetus and newborn infant. In: Infectious Diseases of the Fetus and Newborn Infant (Remington JS, Klein JO, editors). Philadelphia: W.B. Saunders; 2001.

Laucella S, Salcedo R, Castanos-Velez E, Riarte A, de Titto EH, Patarroyo M, Orn A, Rottenberg ME. Increased expression and secretion of ICAM-1 during experimental infection with *Trypanosoma cruzi*. Parasite Immunol 1996; 18: 227–239.

Levin MJ, Franco da Silveira J, Frasch A, Camargo M, Lafon S, Degrave WM, Rangel-Aldao R. Recombinant *Trypanosoma cruzi* antigens and Chagas' disease diagnosis: analysis of a workshop. FEMS Microbiol Immunol 1991; 4(1): 11–19.

Lorca M, Beroiza A, Muñoz P, Guajardo U, Silva J, Canales M, Atías A. Estudio materno infantil de enfermedad de Chagas en zonas endémicas III: Salamanca, Valle del Choapa Chile. Parasitol día 1987; 11: 97–100.

Luquetti AO, Ponce C, Ponce E, Esfandiari J, Schijman A, Revollo S, Anez N, Zingales B, Ramgel-Aldao R, Gonzalez A, Levin MJ, Umezawa ES, Franco da Silveira J. Chagas' disease diagnosis: a multicentric evaluation of Chagas Stat-Pak, a rapid immunochromatographic assay with recombinant proteins of *Trypanosoma cruzi*. Diagn Microbiol Infect Dis 2003; 46(4): 265–271.

Macedo AM, Machado CR, Oliveira R, Pena SDJ. *Trypanosoma cruzi*: genetic structure of populations and relevance of genetic variability to the pathogenesis of Chagas disease. Mem Inst Oswaldo Cruz 2004; 99: 1–12.

Macedo AM, Pena SDJ. Genetic variability of *Trypanosoma cruzi*: implications for the pathogenesis of Chagas disease. Parasitol Today 1998; 14: 119–123.

Machado CA, Ayala FJ. Nucleotide sequences provide evidence of genetic exchange among distantly related lineages of *Trypanosoma cruzi*. Proc Natl Acad Sci 2001; 98(13): 7396–7401.

Marcet PL, Duffy T, Burgos JM, Cardinal MV, Levin MJ, Gurtler RE, Schijman AG. Molecular typing of Trypanosoma cruzi lineages in faeces from triatomines. Parasitology 2006; 132(Pt1): 57–65.

Mazza S, Montano A, Benitez C. Transmisión del *Schizotrypanum cruzi* al niño por leche de madre con enfermedad de Chagas. Publicaciones MEPRA 1936; 28: 41–46.

Médecines sains frontières. Chagas, a Silent Tragedy. 1st ed. Buenos Aires: Losada; 2005.

Mendoza Ticona CA, Córdova Benzaquen E, Ancca Juárez J, Saldaña Díaz J, Torres Choque A, Velásquez Talavera R, de los Ríos Álvarez J, Saldaña Díaz J, Vega Chirinos S, Sánchez Pérez R. The prevalence of Chagas' disease in puerperal women and congenital transmission in an endemic area of Peru. Rev Panam Salud Pública 2005; 17(3): 147–153.

Menezes CA, Bitterncourt AL, Mota E, Sherlock I, Ferreira J. The assessment of parasitemia in women who are carriers of *T. cruzi* infection during and after pregnancy. Rev Soc Bras Med Trop 1992; 25(2): 109–113.

Miles MA. *T. cruzi* milk transmission of infection and immunity from mother to young. Parasitology 1972; 65(1): 1–9.

Mjihdi A, Lambot MA, Stewart IJ, Detournay O, Noel JC, Carlier Y, Truyens C. Acute *Trypanosoma cruzi* infection in mouse induces infertility or placental parasite invasion and ischemic necrosis associated with massive fetal loss. Am J Pathol 2002; 161: 673–680.

Montamat EE, De Luca d'Oro G, Perret B, Rivas C. Characterization of *Trypanosoma cruzi* from Argentina by electrophoretic zymograms. Acta Trop 1991; 50(2): 125–133 Erratum in: Acta Trop (Basel) 1992; 51(2):173.

Mora MC, Sanchez Negrette O, Marco D, Barrio A, Ciaccio M, Segura MA, Basombrio MA. Early diagnosis of congenital *Trypanosoma cruzi* infection using PCR, hemoculture, and capillary concentration, as compared with delayed serology. J Parasitol 2005; 91(6): 1468–1473.

Moretti E, Basso B, Castro I, Carrizo Paez M, Chaul M, Barbieri G, Canal Feijoo D, Sartori MJ, Carrizo Paez R. Chagas disease: study of congenital transmission in cases of acute maternal infection. Rev Soc Bras Med Trop 2005; 38(1): 53–55.

Moser DR, Kirchhoff LV, Donelson JE. Detection of *Trypanosoma cruzi* by DNA amplification using the polymerase chain reaction. J Clin Microbiol 1989; 27(7): 1477–1482.

Moya P, Moretti E, Paolasso R, Basso B, Blanco S, Sanmartino C. Enfermedad de Chagas neonatal. Diagnostico de Laboratorio durante el primer año de vida. Medicina (B Aires) 1989; 49: 595–599.

Moya P, Villagia L, Risco JJ. Enfermedad de Chagas congénita. Hallazgos anatomopatológicos en placenta y cordón umbilical. Rev Fac Cienc Med Univ (Córdoba) 1979; 37: 21.

Muñoz P, Thiermann E, Atías A, Acevedo C. Enfermedad de Chagas congénita sintomática en recién nacidos y lactantes. Rev Chil Pediatr 1992; 65(4): 196–202.

Nilo ME, Alvarado J, Ramirez M, Espejo E. Clinical finding of trypomastigote in cytochemical study of amniotic fluid. Parasitol dia 2000; 24(1–2): 49–51.

Oelemann WM, Teixeira MD, Verissimo Da Costa GC, Borges-Pereira J, De Castro JA, Coura JR, Peralta JM. Evaluation of three commercial enzyme-linked immunosorbent assays for diagnosis of Chagas' disease. J Clin Microbiol 1998; 36(9): 2423–2427.

Oliveira FC, Chapadeiro E, Alonso MT, Lopes ER, Pereira FE. Chagas disease and pregnancy. Incidence of trypanosomiasis and spontaneous abortion in pregnant women with chronic Chagas disease. Rev Inst Med Trop Sao Paulo 1966; 8: 184–185.

Pehrson PO, Wahlgren M, Bengtsson E. Intracranial calcifications probably due to congenital Chagas' disease. Am J Trop Med Hyg 1982; 31(3 Pt 1): 449–451.

Pehrson PO, Walhlgren M, Bengsson E. Asymptomatic congenital Chagas disease in a five year old child. Scand J Infect Dis 1981; 13: 307–308.

Ponce C, Ponce E, Vinelli E, Montoya A, de Aguilar V, Gonzalez A, Zingales B, Rangel-Aldao R, Levin MJ, Esfandiari J, Umezawa ES, Luquetti AO, da Silveira JF. Validation of a rapid and reliable test for diagnosis of Chagas' disease by detection of *Trypanosoma cruzi*-specific antibodies in blood of donors and patients in Central America. J Clin Microbiol 2005; 43(10): 5065–5068.

Rasheed FN, Bulmer JN, Dunn DT, Menendez C, Jawla MF, Jepson A, Jakobsen PH, Greenwood BM. Suppressed peripheral and placental blood lymphoproliferative responses in first pregnancies: relevance to malaria. Am J Trop Med Hyg 1993; 48(2): 154–160.

Rassi A, Borges C, Koeberle F, De Paula OH. Sobre a transmissão congênita da doença de Chagas. Rev Goiania Med 1958; 4: 319–332.

Rassi Jr. A, Rassi A, Little WC. Chagas' heart disease. Clin Cardiol 2000; 23(12): 883–889.

Reyes B, Lorca M, Muñoz P, Frasch AC. Fetal IgG specificities against *Trypanosoma cruzi* antigens in newborns. Proc Natl Acad Sci 1990; 87: 2846–2850.

Rocha A, de Meneses AC, da Silva AM, Ferreira MS, Nishioka SA, Burgarelli MK, Almeida E, Turcato Junior G, Metze K, Lopes ER. Pathology of patients with Chagas' disease and acquired immunodeficiency syndrome. Am J Trop Med Hyg 1994; 50(3): 261–268.

Romaña C. Acerca de un síntoma inicial de valor para el diagnóstico de forma aguda de la enfermedad de Chagas. La conjuntivitis esquizotripanózica unilateral (Hipótesis sobre la puerta de entrada conjuntival de la enfermedad). Publicaciones MEPRA 1935; 22: 16–28.

Rosenbaum MB. Chagasic miocardiopathy. Prog Cardiovasc Dis 1964; 7: 199–225.

Russomando G, de Tomassone MM, de Guillen I, Acosta N, Vera N, Almiron M, Candia N, Calcena MF, Figueredo A. Treatment of congenital Chagas' disease diagnosed and followed up by the polymerase chain reaction. Am J Trop Med Hyg 1998; 59: 487–491.

Russomando G, Figueredo A, Almiron M, Sakamoto M, Morita K. Polymerase chain reaction-based detection of *Trypanosoma cruzi* DNA in serum. J Clin Microbiol 1992; 30: 2864–2868.

Sanchez Negrette O, Mora MC, Basombrío MÁ. High prevalence of congenital *Trypanosoma cruzi* infection and family clustering in Salta, Argentina. Pediatrics 2005; 115(6): e668–e672.

Sartori AM, Caiaffa-Filho HH, Bezerra RC, do S Guilherme C, Lopes MH, Shikanai-Yasuda MA. Exacerbation of HIV viral load simultaneous with asymptomatic reactivation of chronic Chagas' disease. Am J Trop Med Hyg 2002a; 67(5): 521–523.

Sartori AM, Neto JE, Nunes EV, Braz LM, Caiaffa-Filho HH, Oliveira Oda Jr. C, Neto VA, Shikanai-Yasuda MA. *Trypanosoma cruzi* parasitemia in chronic Chagas disease: comparison between human immunodeficiency virus (HIV)-positive and HIV-negative patients. J Infect Dis 2002b; 186(6): 872–875.

Sartori MJ, Lin S, Frank FM, Malchiodi EL, de Fabro SP. Role of placental alkaline phosphatase in the interaction between human placental trophoblast and *Trypanosoma cruzi*. Exp Mol Pathol 2002; 72(1): 84–90.

Sartori MJ, Lin S, Fretes RE, Ruiz Moreno L, Goldemberg L, de Fabro SP. Alkaline phosphatase activity in plasma of pregnant chagasic patients. Rev Fac Cien Med Univ Nac Cordoba 1997; 55(1–2): 5–8.

Schenone H. Xenodiagnosis. Mem Inst Oswaldo Cruz 1999; 94(Suppl 1): 289–294.

Schenone H, Contreras MC, Borgono JM, Rojas A, Villarroel F. Congenital Chagas' disease in Chile. Longitudinal study of the reproductivity of women with or without Chagas' disease and of some parasitological and clinical parameters of them and their corresponding children. Bol Chil Parasitol 1985; 40: 24–29.

Schenone H, Iglesias J, Schenone S, Contreras MC. Infección chagásica congénita de segunda generación. Bol chil Parasitol 1987; 42: 71–73.

Schijman AG. Caracterización molecular de poblaciones naturales de *T.cruzi* en distintos escenarios clínicos de la infección chagásica. Acta Bioq Clin Lat 2005; 3: 35–36.

Schijman AG, Altcheh J, Burgos JM, Biancardi M, Bisio M, Levin M, Freilij H. Aetiological treatment of congenital Chagas disease diagnosed and monitored by the polymerase chain reaction. J Antimicrob Chemother 2003; 52: 441–449.

Schmuñis GA. A Tripanossomíase Americana e seu impacto na saúde pública das Américas. In: *T. cruzi* e Doença de Chagas (Brener Z, Andrade ZA, Barral-Netto M, editors). Rio de Janeiro: Guanabara Koogan; 1999; pp. 1–15.

Schofield CJ, Dias JC. The Southern Cone initiative against Chagas disease. Adv Parasitol 1999; 42: 1–27.

Shikanai-Yasuda MA, Marcondes CB, Guedes LA, Siquiera GS, Barone AA, Dias JC, Amato Neto V, Tolezano JE, Peres BA, Arruda Jr. ER. Possible oral transmission of acute Chagas' disease in Brazil. Rev Inst Med Trop Sao Paulo 1991; 33(5): 351–357.

Solana ME, Celentano AM, Tekiel V, Jones M, Gonzalez Cappa SM. *Trypanosoma cruzi*: effect of parasite subpopulation on murine pregnancy outcome. J Parasitol 2002; 88(1): 102–106.

Solari A, Contreras MC, Lorca M, Garcia A, Salinas P, Ortiz S, Soto A, Arancibia C, Schenone H. Yield of xenodiagnosis and PCR in the evaluation of specific chemotherapy of Chagas' disease in children. Bol Chil Parasitol 1998; 53(1–2): 27–30.

Solari A, Ortíz S, Soto A, Arancibia C, Campillay R, Contreras M, Salinas P, Rojas A, Schenone H. Treatment of *T.cruzi*-infected children with nifurtimox: a 3 year follow-up by PCR. J Antimicrob Chemother 2003; 48(4): 515–519.

Sosa Estani S, Segura EL, Ruiz AM, Velazquez E, Porcel BM, Yampotis C. Efficacy of chemotherapy with benznidazole in children in the indeterminate phase of Chagas' disease. Am J Trop Med Hyg 1998; 9(4): 526–529.

Storino R, Auger S, Caravello O, Urrutia MI, Sanmartino M, Jörg M. Chagasic cardiopathy in endemic area versus sporadically infected patients. Rev. Saúde Pública 2002; 36(6): 755–758.

Storni P, Bolsi F. Embarazo y parasitemia por *T. cruzi*. Medicina (B Aires) 1979; 39: 193.

Sturm NR, Degrave W, Morel C, Simpson L. Sensitive detection and schizodeme classification of *Trypanosoma cruzi* cells by amplification of kinetoplast minicircle DNA sequences: use in diagnosis of Chagas' disease. Mol Biochem Parasitol 1989; 33(3): 205–214.

Tibayrenc M. Genetic subdivisions within *Trypanosoma cruzi* (discrete typing units) and their relevance for molecular epidemiology and experimental evolution. Kinetoplastid Biol Dis 2003; 2(1): 12.

Tibayrenc M, Ward P, Moya A, Ayala FJ. Natural populations of *Trypanosoma cruzi*, the agent of Chagas disease, have a complex multiclonal structure. Proc Natl Acad Sci USA 1986; 83(1): 115–119.

Torrico F, Alonso-Vega C, Suarez E, Rodríguez P, Torrico MC, Dramaix M, Truyens C, Carlier Y. Maternal *Trypanosoma cruzi* infection, pregnancy outcome, morbidity, and mortality of congenitally infected and non-infected nexborns in Bolivia. Am J Trop Med Hyg 2004; 70(2): 201–209.

Umezawa ES, Luquetti AO, Levitus G, Ponce C, Ponce E, Henriquez D, Revollo S, Espinoza B, Sousa O, Khan B, da Silveira JF. Serodiagnosis of chronic and acute Chagas' disease with *Trypanosoma cruzi* recombinant proteins: results of a collaborative study in six Latin American countries. J Clin Microbiol 2004; 42(1): 449–452.

Vago AR, Macedo AM, Oliveira RP, Andrade LO, Chiari E, Galvao LM, Reis D, Pereira ME, Simpson AJ, Tostes S, Pena SD. Kinetoplast DNA signatures of *Trypanosoma cruzi* strains obtained directly from infected tissues. Am J Pathol 1996; 149: 2153–2159.

Vekemans J, Truyens C, Torrico F, Solano M, Torrico M-C, Rodriguez P, Alonso-Vega C, Carlier Y. Maternal *Trypanosoma cruzi* infection upregulates capacity of uninfected neonate cells to produce pro- and anti-inflammatory cytokines. Infect Immun 2000; 68: 5430–5434.

Vergara U, Lorca M, Veloso C, Gonzalez A, Engstrom A, Aslund L, Pettersson U, Frasch AC. Assay for detection of *T. cruzi* antibodies in human sera based on reaction with synthetic peptides. J Clin Microbiol 1991; 29(9): 2034–2037.

Virreira M, Torrico F, Truyens C, Alonso-Vega C, Solano M, Carlier Y, Svoboda M. Comparison of PCR methods for reliable and easy detection of congenital *T. cruzi* infection. Am J Trop Med Hyg 2003; 68: 574–582.

Westenberger SJ, Barnabé C, Campbell D, Strum NR. Two hybridization events define the population structure of *Trypanosoma cruzi*. Genetics 2005; 171: 527–543.

Wincker P, Bosseno MF, Britto C, Yaksic N, Cardoso MA, Morel CM, Brenere SF. High correlation between Chagas' disease serology and PCR-based detection of *Trypanosoma cruzi* kinetoplast DNA in Bolivian children living in an endemic area. FEMS Microbiol Lett 1994; 124: 419–423.

Wincker P, Telleiria J, Bosseno MF, Cardoso MA, Marques P, Yaksic N, Aznar C, Liegeard P, Hontebeyrie M, Noireau F, Morel CM, Brenier SF. PCR-based diagnosis for Chagas'disease in Bolivian children living in an active transmission area: comparison with conventional serological and parasitological diagnosis. Parasitology 1997; 114(4): 367–373.

Woody NC, Woody HB. American trypanosomiasis (Chagas' disease); first indigenous case in the United States. J Am Med Assoc 1955; 159(7): 676–677.

World Health Organization (WHO). Control of Chagas disease. Report of a WHO expert committee. WHO Tech. Rep. Ser. 2002; 905: 1–109.

Yeo M, Acosta N, Llewellyn M, Sanchez H, Adamson S, Miles GA, Lopez E, Gonzalez N, Patterson JS, Gaunt MW, de Arias AR, Miles MA. Origins of Chagas disease: Didelphis species are natural hosts of *T. cruzi* I and armadillos hosts of *Trypanosoma cruzi* II, including hybrids. Int J Parasitol 2005; 35: 225–233.

Zaidenberg M. Congenital Chagas' disease in the province of Salta, Argentina, from 1980 to 1997. Rev Soc Bras Med Trop 1999; 32(6): 689–695.

Zaidenberg M, Segovia A. Enfermedad de Chagas congénita en la ciudad da Salta, Argentina. Rev Inst Med Trop Sao Paulo 1993; 35: 35–43.

Color Section

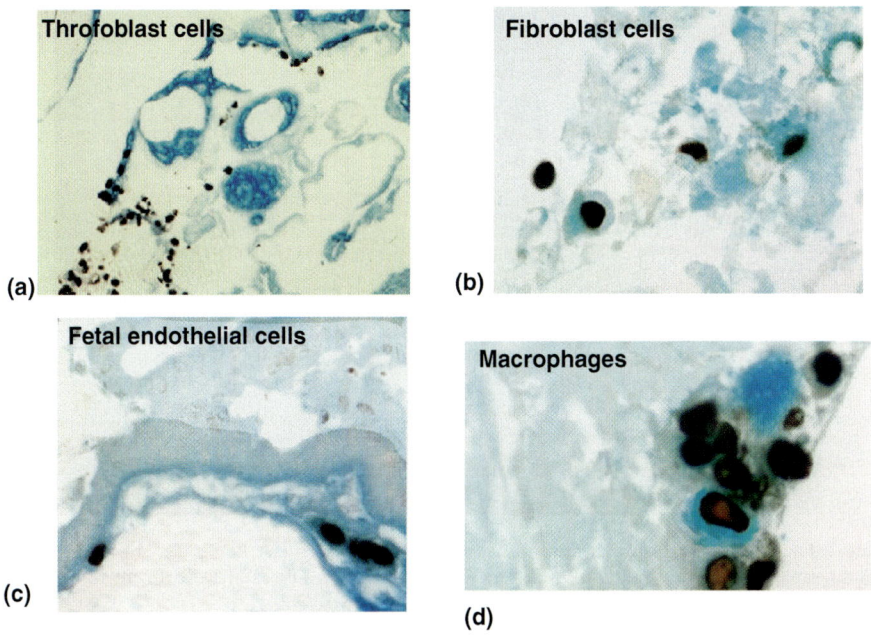

Plate 1 Immunohistochemical double detection of viral and cellular in CMV-infected placenta explants. (A) In blue, the cytokeratin marker showing the trophoblast layer and in brown CMV-early antigen (× 200); (B) In blue, the vimentin-positive cells showing fibroblast cells and in brown CMV-immediate early antigen (× 400); (C) In blue, the endothelial cell marker and in brown CMV-early antigen (× 400); (D) In blue, the CD68 marker showing macrophages and in brown CMV-early antigen (× 500). From Gabrielli et al. (2001) (see also page 6 of this volume).

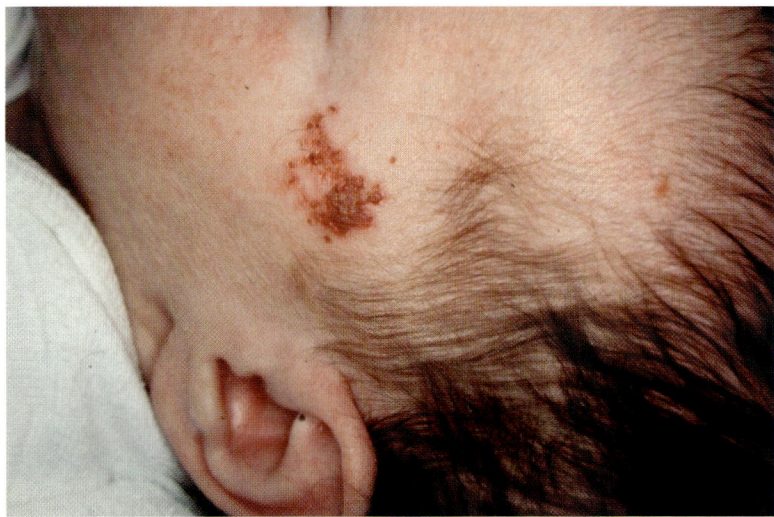

Plate 2 Facial vesicular rash indicative of neonatal HSV infection (see also page 25 of this volume). (Photograph courtesy of Andrew Pavia, Division of Infectious Diseases, Department of Pediatrics, University of Utah School of Medicine.)

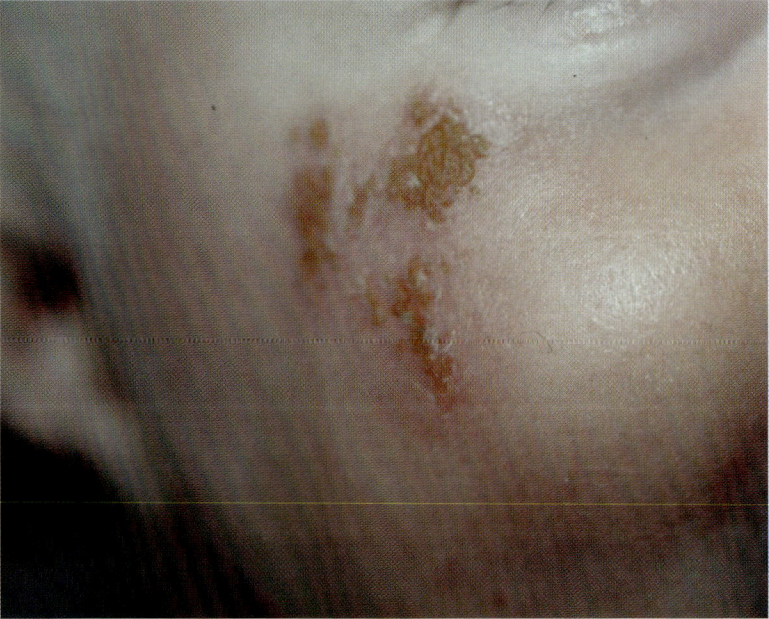

Plate 3 Recurrent HSV rash in a young infant with a history of neonatal HSV infection (see also page 31 of this volume). (Photograph courtesy of Andrew Pavia, Division of Infectious Diseases, Department of Pediatrics, University of Utah School of Medicine.)

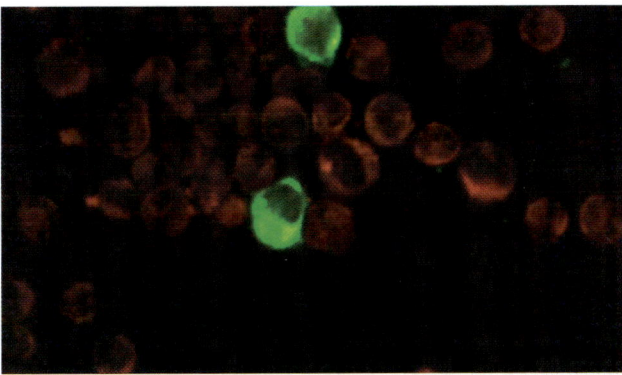

Plate 4 Peripheral blood lymphocytes isolated on Ficoll from a patient with roseola infantum (caused by HHV-6) and stained with monoclonal antibody to gp 60/110. Approximately 2–3% of the cells are positive for HHV-6 antigens. With permission from Dr. Janos Luka, Ph.D, associate professor, Department of Pathology, Eastern Virginia Medical School (1993 to present). http://herpesvirus. tripod.com/gallery/pictures/imfluo/ar202.JPG (see also page 43 of this volume).

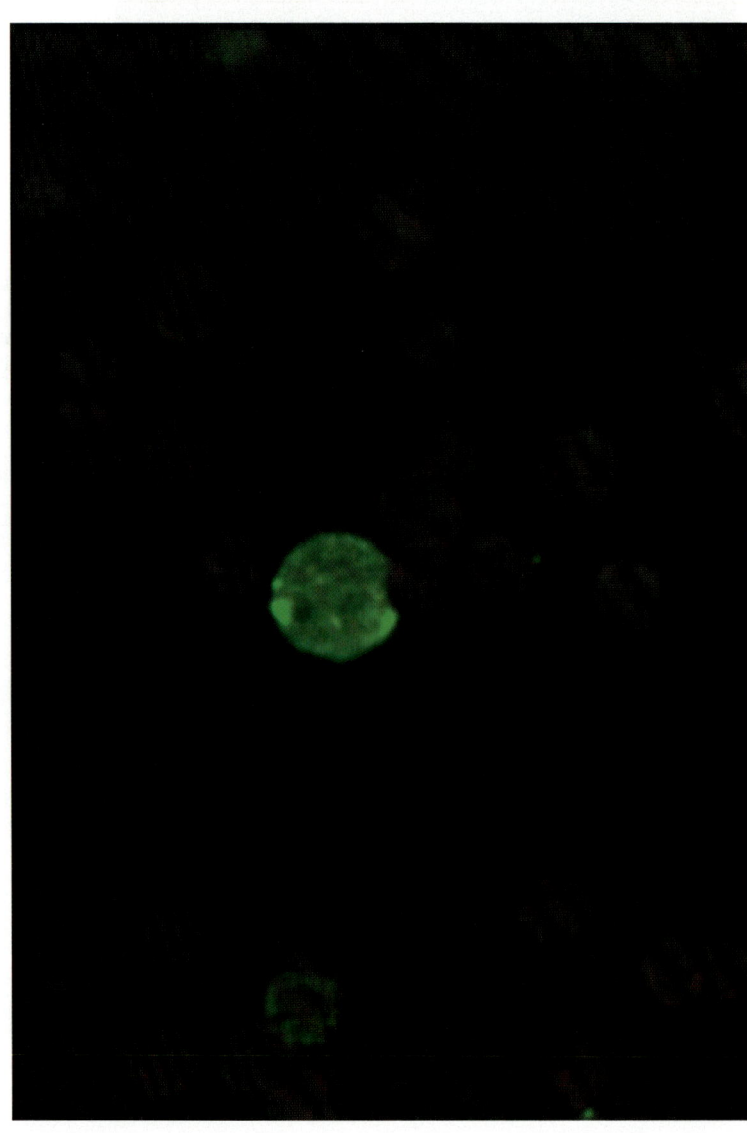

Plate 5 SUP-T1 cell line infected with HHV-7 and stained at day 7 with monoclonal antibodies to gp 110 envelop antigen. With permission from Dr. Janos Luka, Ph.D, associate professor, Department of Pathology, Eastern Virginia Medical School (1993 to present) (see also page 44 of this volume). http://herpesvirus.tripod.com/gallery/pictures/imfluo/7ve701.JPG.

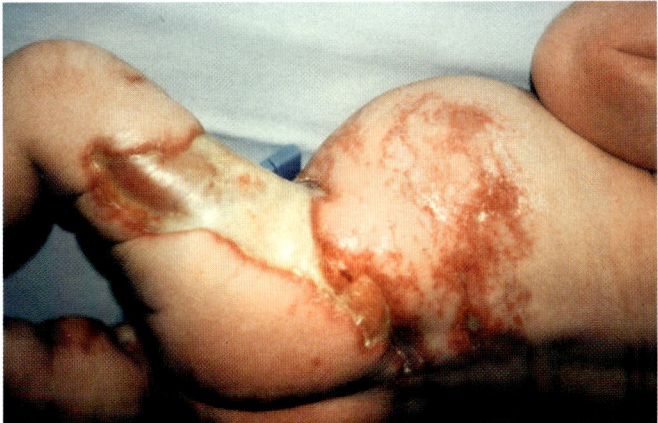

Plate 6 Female stillborn with cicatricial skin lesions involving the left side of chest, axilla, and shoulder as well as hypoplasia of the left upper limb after maternal varicella between the 13th and 15th gestational weeks (see also page 57 of this volume).

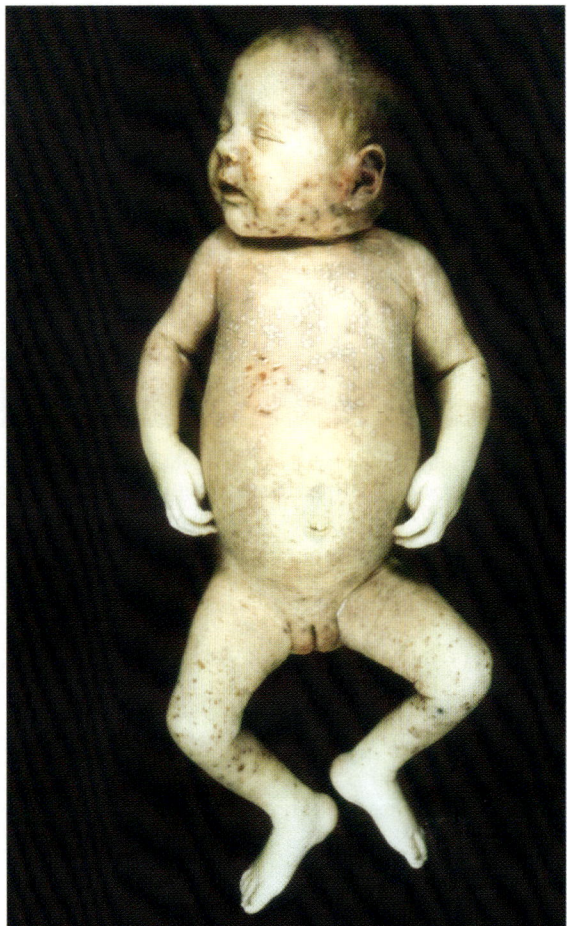

Plate 7 Female neonate with lethal neonatal varicella (see also page 61 of this volume).

Index